MW00837895

Speech Sound Disorders

FOR CLASS AND CLINIC

Fourth Edition

Speech Sound Disorders

FOR CLASS AND CLINIC

Fourth Edition

Ken M. Bleile, PhD

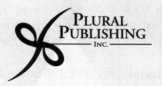

PLURAL
PUBLISHING
INC.

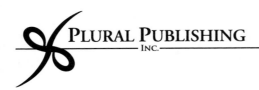

5521 Ruffin Road
San Diego, CA 92123

e-mail: information@pluralpublishing.com
Website: http://www.pluralpublishing.com

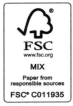

FSC
www.fsc.org
MIX
Paper from
responsible sources
FSC® C011935

Copyright © 2020 by Plural Publishing, Inc.

Typeset in 10.5/13 Times New Roman by Flanagan's Publishing Services, Inc.
Printed in the United States of America by McNaughton & Gunn, Inc.

All rights, including that of translation, reserved. No part of this publication may be reproduced, stored in a retrieval system, or transmitted in any form or by any means, electronic, mechanical, recording, or otherwise, including photocopying, recording, taping, Web distribution, or information storage and retrieval systems without the prior written consent of the publisher.

For permission to use material from this text, contact us by
Telephone: (866) 758-7251
Fax: (888) 758-7255
e-mail: permissions@pluralpublishing.com

Every attempt has been made to contact the copyright holders for material originally printed in another source. If any have been inadvertently overlooked, the publishers will gladly make the necessary arrangements at the first opportunity.

Library of Congress Cataloging-in-Publication Data:

Names: Bleile, Ken Mitchell, author.
Title: Speech sound disorders : for class and clinic / Ken M. Bleile.
Other titles: Manual of speech sound disorders
Description: Fourth edition. | San Diego, CA : Plural Publishing, [2020] |
    Preceded by Manual of speech sound disorders / Ken M. Bleile. Third
    edition. 2015. | Includes bibliographical references and index.
Identifiers: LCCN 2018028733| ISBN 9781635501100 (alk. paper) | ISBN
    1635501105 (alk. paper)
Subjects: | MESH: Speech Sound Disorder--diagnosis | Speech Sound
    Disorder--therapy | Child | Speech Perception--physiology | Phonetics |
    Speech Therapy
Classification: LCC RC424.7 | NLM WL 340.2 | DDC 616.85/5--dc23
LC record available at https://lccn.loc.gov/2018028733

Contents

PART II. SPEECH DEVELOPMENT

PART III. ASSESSMENT

PART IV. TREATMENT

Preface

Welcome to the fourth edition of *Speech Sound Disorders*! I hope you find this to be a useful resource.

Major features of this book include

- Readable and practical discussions of complex clinical topics
- Coverage from infants to adults
- Clear link between speech development and clinical decision making
- Emphasis on underlying principles and procedures
- Student friendly

Content revisions in this new edition include

- About 80% updated and revised
- More treatment chapters
- Every chapter has learning objectives, key words, and review questions
- "Learn by doing" chapters with speech exercises from real children
- Chapters written by invited contributors on AAC, bilingualism, speech production, and speech perception
- More downloadable clinic resources

I wrote this book to support people who help children learn to talk. Whether you are a student who reads the book from beginning to end or a clinician who jumps to the resources and skims through an occasional chapter, if the book ends up marked, dog-eared, and rolled up in your pocket, it will have served its purpose.

Best wishes!
Ken M. Bleile

Companion Website Resources

On the PluralPlus companion website you will find the following additional resources. See the inside front cover of your book for the URL and access code.

For Instructors

- Complete and main idea PowerPoint lecture slides
- Answers to the chapter review questions
- Answers to the "learn by doing" exercises
- Sample undergraduate and graduate course sessions and syllabi

For All Book Users

Assessment Resources

Social Impact
Severity and Intelligibility
Developmental Milestones
  Birth to 3 Years
  Students
Informal Assessments
  Assimilations
  Phonological Processes
  Consonants and Consonant Clusters
  Preschool Consonant Screener
  Phonological Awareness Screener
Published Tests
  Screening Tests
  Complete Tests

Treatment Resources

Talking about Speech
  Descriptions and Demonstrations
  Phonetic Placement and Shaping
Activities
  Birth to 2 Years
  Preschool and Grade School
  School and Daily Life
  Reading and Language

Contributors

Todd A. Bohnenkamp, PhD, CCC-SLP
Associate Professor
Communication Sciences and Disorders
University of Northern Iowa
Cedar Falls, Iowa
Chapter 3. Speech Production

Evette Edmister, PhD, CCC-SLP
Associate Professor
Communication Sciences and Disorders
University of Northern Iowa
Cedar Falls, Iowa
Chapter 20. Supporting Communication

Jaimie L. Gilbert, PhD, CCC-A
Assistant Professor
Communication Sciences and Disorders
University of Northern Iowa
Cedar Falls, Iowa
Chapter 4. Speech Reception and Perception

Lindsey R. Squires, PhD
Assistant Professor
Communication Sciences and Disorders
University of Northern Iowa
Cedar Falls, Iowa
Chapter 12. Assessing a Bilingual Child

Acknowledgments

This book has come full circle—I began the first edition in Iowa and finished the fourth edition in the same state. In between, I worked on book editions in Maryland (Johns Hopkins), Pennsylvania (Children's Hospital of Philadelphia), Hawaii (University of Hawaii), and New Zealand (University of Canterbury). What an odd, wandering journey for a collection of words!

I thank the many people who helped put these words in order through the ideas and experiences they shared with me. I hope you recognize your influence in these pages and that what I wrote pleases you, at least in parts. Thanks especially to faculty, staff, and students at the University of Northern Iowa for your good company all these years. Lastly, I thank my brother and sisters, living and gone (Henry, Cheryl, and Judy), and my wonderful children (Jude and Zoe).

Dedicated to the memory of Sadanand Singh.
A visionary and a great humanist.

PART I

FOUNDATIONS

CHAPTER 1
SPEECH

The world is brimming with fascinating topics, from subatomic particles to supernovas, from Zen to the Zen of baking. Why devote time and energy to study short bursts of sound that pop from a person's mouth, one after another? Of course, one reason may be someone told you to, perhaps saying something like, "Please read Chapter 1." Since you want to pass the course, you read about speech. However, the "why" intended here is of a different sort, something you might paraphrase as, "Why am I learning this stuff when I could be studying ___?" (You fill in the blank.) This chapter addresses three topics:

- Why Study Speech?
- The Nature of Speech
- A Final Thought: Giving Back

Subsequent foundation chapters discuss speech sound disorders, speech production, and speech reception and perception. The section concludes with a "learn by doing" chapter to help brush up—possibly—rusty phonetic skills.

Learning Objectives

I hope on completing the chapter you will

- Appreciate the central role that speech plays in human culture
- Understand that speech has a dual nature
- Know that speech elements in phonology lack meaning
- Understand why phonology is a cornerstone of human communication
- Appreciate the complexity of the channel of communication

Key Words

Key words you will encounter in this chapter

Talk
Thought
Theory of mind
Group identity
Accent
Dialect
Sociolect
Code switching
Cultural transmission
Dual nature of speech
Phonology
Speech perception
Articulation

Why Study Speech?

Speech is a foundation of human culture (Caroll, 2008; Duranti, 2009; Gumperz, 1972; Hymes, 1974). To see this, think of all the things that either you could not accomplish, or you could only accomplish with much greater effort, if speech did not exist to convey language. As summarized in Table 1–1, things that speech facilitates include talking, thinking, being part of a group, and transmitting knowledge from generation to generation.

Talk (Interpersonal Communication)

Talk is how people typically communicate with each other (Carroll, 2008). Stand back and watch a conversation. The mouth of a person opens, emitting a volley of sound. Then the mouth of another person opens and returns a sound volley. As Fillmore (1975) described years ago, the volleys continue—back and forth, back and forth—conveying ideas, memories, and emotions.

Approximately 7,099 different languages exist in the world, a remarkably large number considering they all belong to a single species with the same cognitive system (Ethnologue, 2017). In each of these languages, the primary means of communication is the exchange of sound. Many languages have written systems in addition to spoken ones, allowing the translation of speech into graphic mediums. Modern inventions such as the telephone, computer, film, and television have extended the realm of speech to transmission through electricity.

Of course, speech is not the only form through which humans convey language. Other means include sign language, in which the volleys are gestures rather than sounds (Sacks, 1989; Stokoe, 2005). Although the gestural volleys of sign language are as fascinating to study as those of sound, that intriguing topic lies outside the purview of this book. Nor does this book address fascinating gestural communication systems such as eye gaze and stance, though those forms of communication are rich and increasingly well-researched topics (Burgoon, Guerrero, & Floyd, 2011).

TABLE 1–1. Four Types of Communication Facilitated by Speech

Type of Communication	Definition
Talk	Communication between persons
Thought	Communication with oneself
Groups	Communication within and between groups
Cultural transmission	Communication between generations

Thought (Intrapersonal Communication)

Speech turned inward conveys **thought** (Kozulin, 1990; Smith, 1973). Internal speech and images allow humans to regulate their own behavior, make plans, and reason (Huettig & Harsuiker, 2010). Indeed, sometimes a person does not turn their speech all the way inward and you can hear them muttering—sometimes in whole sentences, though more often in short snatches.

If you introspect, you can mentally overhear speech in your head, perhaps whispering dinner possibilities or planning what you will say to a friend this evening. Or, if you are preparing for an argument you expect with a significant other, the little whisper allows you to play both sides of the projected conflict; a sort of mental script:

Mental Script:

Me: You don't treat me well!

Significant other: I do too!

Me: We never go out to dinner anymore.

Significant other: We do too. We went to dinner on your birthday.

Oops. They're right. Revise the script.

Revised Mental Script:

Me: You don't treat me well!

Significant other: I do too.

Me: We never go out to dinner anymore, except on my birthday.

Significant other: Well, I don't have much money.

Me: That's no excuse.

Good! Much better outcome.

You may notice that inner speech requires some mind reading. In the above example, "me" not only plans their own utterances, but also mind reads what "significant other" likely will reply. The scientific name for this mind reading trick is **theory of mind**, which essentially means that we act on the assumption that other people have minds, thoughts, wishes, motivations, and so forth, just as we do (Firth & Firth, 2005). Theory of mind guides our use of language; difficulties with theory of mind is part of many different communication disorders, including autism spectrum disorder (Schmaafsma, Pfaff, Spunt, & Adolphs, 2015).

Lastly, you may notice that inner speech takes a person out of the moment in which they live and projects them elsewhere—in the example, "me" projects their self into the future. A goal of many meditation practices is to turn off the inner voice so a person may experience more of the now (Lazar, Bush, Gollub, Fricchione, Khalsa, & Benson, 2000). It is not easy! To experience this, try turning off your inner speech and look around the room in which you are reading. The voice disappears for a few moments but soon returns, a little whisper. You can turn it off again, but for most people it soon returns, taking you from the moment to other places.

Groups (Intergroup Communication)

For both good and ill, people use speech to form groups as a means to foster a **group identity** (Gumperz, 1972; Wolfram, 2004). Being a native speaker of a language is a common way people view themselves as belonging to a group. For example, persons born in Spain may group themselves as native Spanish speakers, in contrast to those with foreign **accents** that show they are nonnative Spanish speakers.

Shared speech characteristics of a **dialect** offer another means through which people place themselves in groups. In addition to dialects based on regions, people also may share a dialect based on social relationships: called **sociolects** (Wolfram, 2004). Cockney English is a famous example of a dialect that is both regional and based on social class.

Race, ethnicity, sexual orientation, age, and gender all offer people other ways to build a group identity based on shared speech characteristics. To give just one example, teenagers with similar interests and outlooks may develop a slang (a temporary age- and interest-based dialect) to differentiate themselves from those outside their group. Persons within a dialect group may speak in their dialect with other members of their group and switch dialects when speaking to outsiders: called **code switching** (Wolfram, 2004).

Sharing a common language, dialect, or style of speaking facilitates cohesion within a group, evoking feelings of pride, shared history, and camaraderie (Trudgill, 1995). More negatively, a group may weaponize speech to exclude, mock, debase, or ridicule another group (Labov, 1972). When a group uses speech as a weapon, the attitude may be, "We are ___ (select a favorite adjective: good, superior, intelligent, moral, hip, etc.) because we speak this way, while you are ___ (select a negative stereotype: stupid, inferior, uneducated, ignorant, bad, etc.) because you speak that way."

CLINIC BOX: Do You Speak Bar Bar?

Judging people by their speech is not a recent cultural development. Greeks of antiquity divided the world into two groups: speakers of Greek and those unfortunate souls who spoke other languages. The Greek view was that the latter, because they are unable to speak Greek, were inherently inferior and largely incapable of rational thought. They considered speech of foreigners to be mere noise, a sound like *bar bar bar bar,* giving us the root of the word *barbarian*, or someone who speaks *bar bar* (Kitto, 1951).

Generations (Intergenerational Communication)

Speech and its written forms are primary mechanisms through which a **culture transmits** what it considers needful to know from one generation to the next, allowing a person to learn without direct experience. To illustrate, a parent may tell a child not to touch a hot plate, enabling the child to learn about burns without receiving one. In a broader way, cultures do the same. A few of the multitude of things a culture may consider needful to pass on from one generation to the next include ideas about freedom, morality, and thousands of different technologies. Right this moment you are reading a book as a way of passing on accumulated knowledge of speech sound disorders.

Compared to instinct, speech permits change to occur much more quickly. To illustrate, imagine a terrible drought transforms a forest into desert. To survive in this new environment, an imaginary creature that lived entirely based on its instincts would likely need generations for genes mutations to adapt to the new circumstance. For a species that relies on speech and its written forms to transmit information between generations, all it must do is develop new words to describe what is needful to know in the new environment.

The Nature of Speech

Speech has a **dual nature**, being both an aspect of language and a channel of communication (Hockett, 1960). The dual nature of speech is the basis of the conceptual distinction between phonology and articulation, and, as we shall see in Chapter 2, the basis of the difference between phonological and articulation disorders.

Language

In this book, **phonology** is the knowledge of language rules that underlie speech. Examples of phonological elements include distinctive features, phonemes, syllables, stress, and intonation. The essential characteristic of these and other elements in the phonological system is that they lack meaning. To illustrate, *s*, *t*, and *m* have no meaning in themselves, but other language systems recruit them to create meaning. For example, combined with other consonants and vowels they make words such as *sun*, *see*, *tea*, *toe*, *me*, and *myth*.

Consonants, vowels, syllables, and intonation may seem mundane, relatively insignificant aspects of language, but they are what make the rest of language possible. Because the foundation of our language is meaningless sounds that represent nothing, we can express a nearly infinite number of different meanings, allowing us to express whatever meanings are important in our social and physical environments. To appreciate the role phonology plays in human language, imagine it organized differently. For example, pretend that each consonant and vowel, instead of being meaningless, is associated with a meaning. For example, *s* represents *anger*, *w* represents *sadness*, and *t* represents *touch*. If this were so, *s* could not appear in *sweet* or *sun* or other words, since *s* always represents *anger*.

If phonology had a similar organization, humans could express very few different meanings. In fact, the world of different things to talk about would closely equal the number of sounds we could produce. To illustrate, if our vocal tracts could pronounce

120 different sounds, we could talk about approximately 120 different things, one thing per sound.

In no small measure, human adaptability depends on possessing a language system that allows the expression of an almost infinite number of meanings using a small set of sounds. This allows humans to enter a new environment and create vocabulary to describe the place in which they find themselves. This has allowed humans to spread out across the world and flourish in such diverse places as deserts, mountains, forests, and tundra. Just as easily, phonology would allow us to live on a satellite, the moon, or a distant planet.

Indeed, phonology is so critical to language and so uniquely human that we could define ourselves in the following way:

Humanity is the species whose cornerstone of communication means nothing.

That is, humanity is the species whose language includes phonology.

Channel of Communication

This book follows established practice in dividing the channel of communication into two domains: **articulation** (the motor part of the channel) and **speech perception** (the perceptual part of the channel).

Myths and Otherwise

A myth you sometimes hear about speech is that it is simple. The idea is, "How could speech *not* be simple, since a young child learns to talk and people of all ages chat from morning to night, the sounds and syllables tumbling out, virtually without effort?" Rather than being simple, it is more accurate to say that speech, like many neurological functions, is invisible, occurring automatically or semiautomatically, freeing our attention to focus on the world around us (Fodor, 1993).

In truth, speech is incredibly complex. On average, every second of speech entails producing and perceiving 12 to 14 different sounds (Ostry & Munhall, 1985). Researchers estimate that 140,000 neuromotor commands are required *per one second of speech*, requiring coordination of muscles across half the body, from the diaphragm through the lower half of the face. Chapters 3 and 4 describe this channel. For the present, let's discuss it at a nontechnical level to illustrate this complex and astonishing feat of biology.

The Long Journey of One Short Word

It's easy to think of articulation and perception as being about the mouth and ear, since those are visible structures—the former occupying the lower part of our face and the latter stuck on the side of our head. However, mouths and ears are just the beginning and end of a much more complex, unseen process. To make this process visible, imagine that for some reason you decide to say one little word, *green*.

It Starts in the Brain

The journey of *green* begins when you decide to say *green*. At this point, *green* is not a series of sounds, but rather electricity and brain chemicals. The brain electricity is the same as the electricity that moves through wires in the walls of your home. The brain chemicals are like the light switches on your wall that control the flow of electricity.

At this point, *green* exists only in pieces in various parts of your brain—color in one location and the pronunciation of the word in another. Still, other parts of the brain may contain associations with the word, including perhaps that *green* sometimes means environmentally friendly and other times means a person beginning a new endeavor.

Next, the various parts of *green* assemble in the front part of your brain in preparation for pronunciation. Once assembled, the electrical current that is *green* travels from the front of your brain in several bundles of energy, the biological equivalent of electrical wires. One bundle travels directly to your muscles, and the other circles through the brain to check and correct possible speech errors before they happen. Both bundles meet at your muscles.

Muscle Power

Muscles are cells specialized to contract. The electrical current of *green* causes muscle cell contractions across half your body, from your stomach to your nose. Your diaphragm pushes your lungs, your lungs contract, and your articulators assume shapes for speech.

Air Travel

The muscle contractions push and shape air. *Green* now is air movement flowing from your lungs toward your throat. But the air moves too slowly, so the tube of your throat narrows midway, at your voice box, causing the air to energize—much like how the water in a broad river energizes when the river bed narrows, becoming rapids. The energized air travels through your mouth and nose, where muscle contractions have moved your articulators, so that, like pebbles and boulders in a stream, they shape and configure the energized air.

Green now is a wave of air emitted from your mouth. The air ripples like a stone dropped in a lake causes water to ripple. The rippling air moves away from your mouth and soon encounters a rather strange cauliflower-shaped thing on the side of your head. The cauliflower is the outer part of your ear. It exists there to capture rippling air—not unlike cupping your hand on your ear to create an extra ear when you have difficulty hearing something.

An Earful

The rippling air of *green* pushes on the membranes, ligaments, and muscles of your ear. *Green* is now vibrating flesh. Vibrations rattle your eardrum, travel through the smallest bones of your body, and push against a membrane, which in turn pushes on the water in the inner most part of your ear. *Green* is now rippling, salty, chemical-laden water.

Green ripples along as water, and the water in turn presses down on a membrane lining the inner most part of your ear. Under the membrane are thousands of hair cells. The membrane pushes on the hair cells. *Green* now is a pattern of pressure on thousands upon thousands of hair cells. Attached to the hair cells are nerves of the brain specialized to carry electricity.

Electricity and Chemicals Again

The hair cells press on the nerve fibers and *green* is electricity again. The electricity moves in a bundle from your ear, up the brain, crossing over from one side of the brain to the other. It reaches the upper part of your brain, moves along through several places until it finally reaches a location where your brain reads the electrical current, and translates it into a word: *green*.

And so *green,* slightly less than one half second of speech, is articulated and perceived.

CLINIC BOX: The Speech Chain

Like many students in my generation, *The Speech Chain* (Denes & Pinson, 1993) is the book that first sparked my fascination with the topic that eventually resulted in The Long Journey of One Short Word. I still have a dog-eared copy of *The Speech Chain* on my bookshelves—an early edition, quite old now, but still a fun, readable account of the basic physics of speech.

A Final Thought: Giving Back

Understanding speech disorders begins with the study of speech—it's nature, how it is perceived and produced, and how it is learned.

This chapter explored the role of speech in human society as well as its functions in communication between people, with oneself, between groups, and across generations. We found that speech has a dual nature and discovered that the lack of meaning in speech elements lets our species create a near infinite number of words, allowing us to enter and describe any new environment. We saw how the miracle of speech production and speech perception transforms a word from electricity, to muscle contractions, to rippling air, to vibrating membranes, to rippling water, and back to electricity again. And in the case of *green*, all within half a second.

These ideas, many developed by investigators in other disciplines, are a foundation of speech disorders. To illustrate, speech disorders are important largely because of the central role of speech in human society, and articulation and phonological disorders reflect the dual nature of speech. The following chapters in Part I, "Foundations," deepen our understanding of speech. The discussion of how a child acquires speech is sufficiently large enough to be a section of its own. The concepts and knowledge in Part II, "Speech Development," form the basis for the assessment and treatment of speech disorders.

Importantly, our profession is both a giver and receiver of speech knowledge. Of all the many fields that study speech—linguistics, psychology, anthropology, neuroscience, medicine, and so forth—ours is the one that uses it to achieve a very special purpose: helping a child learn to talk. Researchers in our field "give back" to the study of speech from the unique perspective of attempting to help a child who may struggle with learning it. Questions studied scientifically within our profession are too diverse to catalog, but some general areas include

- Where is speech in the brain?
- How does a child learn to talk?
- Why do some children have difficulty learning speech?

The questions may give the impression—a false one, I believe—that the scientific study of speech is solely the province of university researchers. Clinicians are researchers as much as academicians, are far more numerous than professors, and conduct research far more often. Their research laboratories include the classroom, the preschool, the retirement home, and hospital bedside. Their daily research questions include, "What aspect of communication should I treat?"; "How can I best assess this communication disorder?"; and "What is the research evidence for the best way to treat this speech error?" Their answers are unique "give backs" to the study of speech, offering a perspective on this complex and fascinating topic that others cannot provide. And the best part is if a clinician answers their questions well, a child improves.

CLINIC BOX: Hunting for Treasure

If you'd like a clinical treasure hunt, see if you can uncover the answers to the following questions by the time you finish the book:

- Why don't you want a neonate in your phonetics class if the instructor is grading on a curve?
- How do you do the bilingual dance?
- Why is a speech sound disorder not an illness and speech treatment not a pill?
- What does doing the wave at a football game have to do with hearing?
- Why is augmentative and alternative communication (AAC) like riding a bike?
- Why won't pumping iron help you learn speech?
- Why do students fall down the wabbit hole?

Suggestion: If you are a student, consider asking for extra credit for answering all the questions by the completion of the course.

Conclusions

These are major points in this chapter:

1. Speech plays a central role in human society, facilitating four types of communication: between persons (talking), with oneself (thinking), between groups (group identity), and between generations (cultural transmission).
2. Speech has a dual nature, being both a part of language and a channel of communication, which is the conceptual basis of the distinction between *phonology* and *articulation*.
3. Our profession contributes to speech research both in our universities and as part of clinical work.

Review Questions

1. What roles does speech play in human culture?
2. What is speech turned inward?
3. Explain the idea of intergenerational communication in your own words.
4. What are the two parts of the dual nature of speech?
5. What is the common characteristic of all speech elements in phonology?
6. Explain in your own words what it means that humanity is the species whose cornerstone of communication means nothing.
7. Approximately how many speech sounds does a person say in one second?
8. What are muscle cells specialized to do?
9. Why is it important to narrow the channel of air from your lungs? Where in the throat does this happen?
10. What is the purpose of having a cauliflower shaped thing on the side of your head?

References

Burgoon, J., Guerrero, L., & Floyd, K. (2011). *Nonverbal communication*. Boston, MA: Allyn & Bacon.

Carroll, D. (2008). *The psychology of language* (5th ed.). Belmont, CA: Tomson Delmar.

Denes, P. B., & Pinson, N. (1993). *The speech chain: The physics and biology of spoken language*. Bell Telephone Laboratores. New York, NY: Williams and Wilkins.

Duranti, A. (2009). *Linguistic anthropology: A reader* (2nd ed.). Oxford, UK: Blackwell.

Ethnologue. (2017). Retrieved from http://www.ethnologue.com

Fillmore, C. (1975). *Santa Cruz lectures on deixis: 1971*. Bloomington, IN: Indiana University Linguistics Club.

Firth, C., & Firth, U. (2005). Theory of mind. *Current Biology, 17*, 644–645.

Fodor, J. (1993). *The modularity of mind: An essay on faculty psychology*. Boston, MA: The MIT Press.

Gumperz, J. (1972). *Language and social identity*. New York, NY: Cambridge University Press.

Hockett, C. (1960). The origin of speech. *Scientific American, 203,* 88–111.

Huettig, F., & Harsuiker, R. (2010). Listening to yourself is like listening to others: External, but not internal, verbal self-monitoring is based on speech perception. *Language and Cognitive Processes, 25,* 347–374.

Hymes, D. (1974). *Foundations in sociolinguistics: An ethnographic approach.* Philadelphia, PA: University of Pennsylvania Press.

Kitto, H. D. F. (1951). *The Greeks.* London, UK: Penguin Books.

Kozulin, A. (1990). *Vygotsky's psychology: A biography of ideas.* Cambridge, MA: Harvard University Press.

Labov, W. (1972). *Language in the inner city: Studies in the black English vernacular.* Philadelphia, PA: University of Pennsylvania Press.

Lazar, S., Bush, G., Gollub, R. Fricchione, G., Khalsa, G., & Benson, H. (2000). Functional brain mapping of the relaxation response and meditation. *Neuroreport, 15,* 1581–1585.

Ostry, D., & Munhall, K. (1985). Control of rate and duration of speech movements. *Journal of the Acoustical Society of America, 77*(2), 640–648.

Sacks, O. (1989). *Seeing voices: A journey into the world of the deaf.* Berkeley, CA: University of California Press.

Schmaafsma, S., Pfaff, D., Spunt, R., & Adolphs, R. (2015). Deconstructing and reconstructing theory of mind. *Trends in Cognitive Sciences, 19,* 65–72.

Smith, N. (1973). *The acquisition of phonology.* Boston,, MA: Cambridge University Press.

Stokoe, W. (2005). Sign language structure: An outline of the visual communication systems of the American deaf. *Journal of Deaf Studies and Deaf Education, 10,* 3–37.

Trudgill, P. (1995). *Sociolinguistics: An introduction to language and society* (3rd ed.). New York, NY: Penguin.

Wolfram, W. (2004). Social varieties of American English. In E. Finegan & J. R. Rickford (Eds.), *Language in the USA: Themes for the twenty-first century* (pp 58–73). New York, NY: Cambridge University Press.

CHAPTER 2
SPEECH SOUND DISORDERS

This book is about helping people with speech sound disorders. This chapter addresses foundation topics such as:

■ What Is a Speech Sound Disorder?
■ Why Study Speech Sound Disorders?
■ The Nature of Speech Sound Disorders
■ Will This Help Someone?

Learning Objectives

I hope on completing the chapter you will

■ Know the definition of a speech sound disorder
■ Recognize that speech sound disorders may negatively affect people's lives
■ Recognize health care disparities around the world
■ Appreciate the difference between articulation and phonological disorders
■ Understand the need for additional research to support clinical decisions

Key Words

Key words you will encounter in this chapter

Speech sound disorder
Phonological disorder
Articulation disorder
Evidence-based practice (EBP)

What Is a Speech Sound Disorder?

A **speech sound disorder** is a type of speech difference. Of course, not all speech differences are speech problems, nor is every speech problem a speech sound disorder. A dialect, for example, is a speech difference, but not a speech problem, and a laryngeal anomaly may result in significant speech challenges, but those challenges are not a speech sound disorder.

A speech difference must meet three criteria to be a speech sound disorder:

1. The speech disorder arises during childhood and is not directly attributable to damage to the speech mechanism, sensory systems, peripheral nervous system, or central nervous system.
2. The speech is not the result of dialect or accent.
3. The child or members of the child's community consider it a speech problem.

A Little More Detail

1. *The speech disorder arises during childhood and is not directly attributable to damage to the speech mechanism, sensory systems, peripheral nervous system, or central nervous system.*
   Explanation: Speech sound disorders are different from speech problems arising directly from physical difficulties such as cranial nerve damage, unrepaired cleft palate, laryngeal anomalies, dysarthria, or difficulties in respiratory control. Of course, children with such physical difficulties may also have a speech sound disorder in addition to other speech problems.

2. *The speech is not the result of dialect or accent.*
   Explanation: Speech sound disorders differ from speech variations attributable to dialect and accent. While a speech sound disorder is a learning difficulty, dialect arises from normal language variation and accent represents a learning accomplishment.

3. *The child or members of the child's community consider it a speech problem.*
   Explanation: Individuals, communities, cultures, and ethnic groups may differ both in what they identify as disordered and in what they assign as a priority to remediate. That is, we are not "speech police" who decide for a person or a community what is and is not a speech sound disorder (McCormack, McLeod, McAllister & Harrison, 2010; Taylor & Peters-Johnson, 1986).

Why Study Speech Sound Disorders?

The first chapter discussed the central role of speech in human society. The implication is that speech disorders matter because they interfere with those essential cultural functions. While true, this is not why most of us assess and treat speech sound disorders. What motivates us is that such disorders negatively affect people's lives.

CLINIC BOX: Did You Know?

Within the United States, federal laws provide an overarching legal umbrella to protect children with communication disorders, but access and eligibility for services vary by state and health insurer. As a result, on one side of a state border a child may be diagnosed with a speech sound disorder (and be eligible for treatment), but, if the family drives over the state line or changes health insurance, the child may suddenly be deemed not to have a problem and be ineligible for services.

Children's Lives

No matter where you go in the world, nearly everyone understands that to lead a rich and full life a child needs to communicate. Speech typically is the preferred form of communication, because it allows a person to live most widely in their community. A family in a developing country residing under a tin roof in a dirt-floor shack, cooking from a smoky wood-burning fire, understands this as clearly as a wealthy family in a luxury penthouse in Manhattan, Dubai, or Singapore (Bleile, 2009).

The following five examples of real children provide a "close up" of the many ways a problem in speech may impact a person's life.

Jose

Jose's mother immigrated to the United States from Latin America as a young woman, seeking a better life for herself while sending money home to her family. She found work in restaurants, married, had a son (Jose), divorced, and afterward lived with her son.

Jose grew to be a teenager with a mild to moderate speech disorder affecting [l], [s], and [r]. Because he believed his speech kept girls from going out with him, Jose enrolled in his school's speech treatment program, where he worked hard and had good attendance, except when treatment conflicted with his great passion—playing basketball on the school team.

One summer night when Jose was 15, police raided the restaurant where Jose's mother worked. Jose's mother was in the country illegally and the court began deportation proceedings. Returning to her home country would place them with her family, who lived in a rural area where unemployment was over 90%, electricity was intermittent, and health and education facilities were almost nonexistent. She wondered, *in such a place what will become of my son who sounds so different than his friends?*

Joni

Joni was 5 when she started kindergarten. She was a bright child with a minor speech difficulty that changed "y" into "l" in words such as *yesterday*, which she said as *lesterday*. On the first day of kindergarten, Joni made several new friends. On the second day, as Joni approached her new friends, one said, "Look, it's the *lesterday* girl." Joni felt crushed.

Margaret

Margaret was 5 years old and she had severe cerebral palsy and intellectual impairments. She lived in a developing country with her mother in a dirt floor home. Margaret's mother supported the family by selling trinkets and cigarettes on the street, typically earning less than a dollar a day, often less than twenty dollars monthly.

The most important thing in the world to Margaret's mother was her daughter. For that reason, when she heard that a clinic in the neighborhood provided evaluation services to children with communication disorders, she carried Margaret in her arms to the clinic. Her question to the evaluators was, "Will Margaret ever speak?"

Martin

Martin was 2 years old and spoke four to five different words. The children of his mother's friends spoke several hundred different words at that age, and their pronunciations were much clearer.

At the end of a diagnostic session with a speech-language pathologist, the clinician explained that Martin had something called an expressive language disorder, and that he had a 50% chance of catching up to his peers by the time he was 3 years old (Paul, 1991). However, if he did not catch up, Martin was at risk for speech and language disorders during the preschool years and, possibly, for reading and language difficulties in school (Rice, Taylor, & Zubrick, 2008).

From the parents' perspective, if treatment might reduce the chance of a future speech, language, and reading problems, they were all in for treatment. However, their health insurer denied coverage, explaining, "Why provide speech services when Martin has a 50% chance of recovery without receiving any services at all?"

CLINIC BOX: An Uneven Playing Field

The world is an uneven playing field for a person with a disability, including one in speech (World Report on Disability, 2011). To illustrate, in the world's poorer regions, a family in poverty may only be able to afford to send those children with "the best potential" to school (World Report on Disability, 2011). A child with a communication disorder, even one as mild as pronouncing a few late acquired sounds, is not typically one judged to possess "the best potential." Worldwide, 100 million children remain out of primary school, almost 60% of them girls (World Bank Group, 2005).

Many people around the world believe disability is a stigma created as a punishment from God or from a curse from someone who possesses supernatural powers (Human Rights Watch, 2010). If a culture associates disability with shame or believes it results from God's punishment or a shaman's curse, it is more likely to shut away a child with a communication disorder than to develop laws that mandate clinical services.

Andrea

Andrea's mother consumed narcotics heavily during her pregnancy, and Andrea was born addicted to crack cocaine. Drug withdrawal for Andrea began at birth. The hospital's social worker recommended Andrea immediately begin to receive developmental services, including those for communication.

The Big Picture in Nine Statistics

The children in the previous examples—Jose, Joni, Margaret, Martin, and Andrea—offer a close-up view of speech sound disorders. The following nine statistics provide "the big picture":

1. A speech sound disorder is the world's most common type of communication disorder, affecting approximately 10% to 15% of preschoolers and 6% of students (American Speech-Language-Hearing Association, 2006; Campbell et al., 2003; Law, Boyle, Harris, Harkness, & Nye, 2000; Shriberg & Tomblin, 1999; Slater, 1992).

   What This May Mean: If you choose to work in pediatric settings, expect your caseload to include many children with speech sound disorders.

2. Speech sound disorders are sufficiently severe that nearly four out of five children require treatment (Gierut, 1998).

   What This May Mean: Don't expect most children with speech sound disorders to "get over it" without professional assistance.

3. At least three quarters of preschoolers with speech sound disorders also have language difficulties (Paul & Shriberg, 1982; Ruscello, St. Louis, & Mason, 1991; Shriberg & Kwiatkowski, 1988).

   What This May Mean: Most preschoolers you see for speech sound disorders also need your help in language.

4. A toddler or a preschooler with a speech sound disorder is at increased risk for later academic difficulties during the school years (Anthony et al., 2011; Bird, Bishop, & Freeman, 1995; Felsenfeld, Broen, & McGue, 1994; Shriberg and Kwiatkowski, 1982; Shriberg et al., 2005; Van Dyke & Holte, 2003).

   What This May Mean: Consider a speech sound disorder in a preschooler to be a red flag for possible future academic difficulties.

5. Preschoolers with speech sound disorders have a higher risk for school challenges if they also have language problems, lower nonverbal intelligence, and social disadvantages (Lewis et al., 2015).

   What This May Mean: Your clinical alarm bells for future school challenges should go off loudly if a preschooler with a speech sound disorder also has either language problems, lower nonverbal intelligence, or comes from a deeply impoverished or neglectful environment.

6. Approximately 11% to 15% of 6-year-old students with speech sound disorders also experience specific language impairment (Shriberg & Tomblin, 1999).

   What This May Mean: Evaluate language along with speech, because a first grader referred to you for speech may also have language difficulties.

7. Half or more of students with speech sound disorders struggle academically all the way through high school (Felsenfeld et al., 1994; Gierut, 1998; Lewis, Freebairn, & Taylor, 2000; Pennington & Bishop, 2009; Shriberg & Austin, 1998).

   What This May Mean: Plan that your students with speech sound disorders will probably need academic assistance throughout school to reach their best potential.

8. Even when a student with reduced intelligibility does well in school, one third of grade school teachers perceive them as having less overall academic potential than their classmates (Overby, Carrell, & Bernthal, 2007).

   What This May Mean: The self-image of your student may be "bruised" by the fact that many people falsely believe that their speech difficulties reflect "lack of intelligence."

9. A student with a speech sound disorder is at risk for being bullied, struggling with friendships, and enjoying school less (McCormack, Harrison, McLeod, & McAllister, 2011).

   What This May Mean: Keep your eyes open to the possibility that your student with a speech sound disorder is being ostracized, is socially isolated, or is being bullied.

The Nature of Speech Sound Disorders

Reflecting the nature of speech, speech sound disorders have a dual nature. Persons with **phonological disorders** have knowledge-based difficulties with language rules that underlie speech, while persons with **articulation disorders** have difficulty producing speech. To illustrate, a child with a phonological disorder might not know that [st] is a possible word initial consonant cluster (as in *stop*), whereas a child with an articulation disorder have difficulty shaping the articulators to pronounce [st].

The conceptual distinction between knowing (phonology) and doing (speaking/ articulation) is important because it suggests that seemingly similar difficulties may result from different causes. Possibly, a child with phonological problems may also show difficulties learning other aspects of language, including syntax and reading, while a child whose problem involves more "doing" than "knowing" may have difficulties restricted to pronunciation.

Which Matters Most?

Dodd and McIntosh (2010) assessed the relative contributions of phonology and articulation to speech production. The subjects were 62 two-year-old children who were developing typically. The researchers assessed children in articulation (oral motor skills, speech perception abilities) and phonology (rule abstraction abilities). The researchers then measured the accuracy of their spoken words. The researchers discovered that phonological ability and articulation ability both contributed to speech accuracy, but that the greatest contribution came from a child's phonological abilities.

A Long Discussion

The Dodd & McIntosh study (2010) is part of a long 70-year discussion within the profession regarding the nature of speech disorders.

Articulation Pioneers

The pioneers of our profession largely believed that speech problems arose because a person could not configure the mouth appropriately to produce speech sounds. This idea was reasonable at that time because the primary candidates for treatment were students with good cognition who had pronunciation problems affecting individual late acquired sounds containing notoriously difficult tongue configurations.

The Rise of the Phonologists

Articulation approaches, which dominated the care of speech disorders for two-thirds of the 20th century, began to lose their appeal for many clinicians in the 1970s. The reason was that the primary tenets of articulation treatment (emphasis on individual sounds, phonetic drills, treatment of sounds in isolation and in nonsense syllables, improvements in small increments of change) proved far less successful with newer populations just appearing on the clinical horizon, many of whom were preschoolers with speech problems affecting sound classes. Phonological approaches gained popularity largely because focusing on speech as an aspect of language offered a means to treat newer, more involved populations.

The Present Compromise

Here is a question you may have already asked yourself: what if you do not know if a speech problem arises from a problem with knowledge or doing? Or, what if you suspect that a speech problem arises from difficulties in both phonology *and* articulation? Or, what if you do not really care how a speech problem arises?

In all these situations, you may want a cover term that does not commit you to saying where a problem arises. The name of the cover term you are seeking is speech sound disorder. Though the term seems somewhat dull, it has gained currency in the profession because it is neutral to the disorder's cause (Bowen, 2009; Williams, 2010). In the future, speech sound disorder may develop its own theoretical baggage, but for the present time it seems useful. Some authors, noting that children with speech sound disorders often speak similarly to younger children without speech problems, prefer to use the term delay rather than disorder (Curtiss, Katz, & Tallal, 1992).

CLINIC BOX: Other Terms, Similar Meanings

Disorders of articulation and phonology go by an impressive number of different names, including

- articulation disorder (for both articulation and phonological disorders);
- phonological disorder (for both articulation and phonological disorders);
- developmental ___ (speech, articulation, or phonology) disorder;
- functional speech disorder;
- phonomotor disorder;
- speech disorder;
- functional articulation disorder; and
- idiopathic speech disorder.

Studies: Bauman-Waengler, 2000; Bernhardt & Stemberger, 1998; Bernthal, Bankson, & Flipsen, 2009; Creaghead, Newman, & Secord, 1989; Fey, 1992; Hodson, 1994; Hoffman, Schuckers, & Daniloff, 1989; Locke, 1983; Lowe, 1994; Rvachew & Brosseau-Lapre, 2017; Shelton & McReynolds, 1979; Shriberg & Kwiatkowski, 1982; Smit, 2003; Weiss, Gordon, & Lillywhite, 1987; Williams, 2003; Winitz, 1984.

The Future?

Though articulation and phonology are the dominant perspectives in our profession, they are not necessary ways to consider speech sound disorders. In fact, established ideas have a bad tendency to become blinders, blocking newer perspectives from taking hold. For example, as we learn more about the workings of the brain, perhaps speech treatment will add neurological viewpoints. Or, as we learn more about cognition, perhaps clinicians will say, in effect, "Why describe speech sound disorders in terms of articulation and phonology? Scrap them both. What matters is memory, representation, speech planning, execution, and feedback" (Anthony et al., 2011). Alternately, perhaps a more social perspective will arise and clinicians will say, "No, no: while articulation, phonology, neurology, and cognition matter, what matters most in speech learning is social relations."

My own vote for the future is all the above. One perspective does not preclude insights from other viewpoints. For example, social psychology may offer insights about the social nature of learning, while neurology may help explain how the brain makes speech possible. I suspect the best ideas probably are those we haven't thought of yet. Perhaps the only certain thing about the future study of speech and its disorders is that humans will remain too complex and diverse to fit entirely into the box of any single theoretical framework.

Will This Help Someone?

Most students who study speech sound disorders want to know if learning this will help someone.

CLINIC BOX: Would a Pill Help?

It's tempting to think of a speech sound disorder as an illness and speech treatment as a pill. To illustrate, within the pill perspective you might diagnose a child with an articulation problem and then give an articulation approach pill to correct the condition. The trouble is the analogy becomes stretched very fast. Illnesses tend to be recognized as such regardless of where they occur, while a speech characteristic may be considered a disorder in one community and a normal speech variation in another. As for speech treatment being a pill, a child with an articulation problem may not respond to an articulation approach, but may improve through language activities, or because they want to impress the clinician (or maybe a girl/boy), or they may feel ready to work on speech issues. Perhaps the lesson is that the avenue you follow to helping a child often entails far greater creativity and insight than administering an articulation or phonology pill.

The Short Answer

The short answer: yes. Literally hundreds of studies document the positive effects of speech treatment (Baker & McLeod, 2011). Knowledge of speech sound disorders can help you

- promote vocal development in an infant with medical needs;
- assist a toddler with a developmental disability learn to speak;
- lead a preschooler to unravel the mysteries of speaking in sentences;
- support a student to succeed socially and academically; and
- help persons without communication disorders to learn English as a second language.

A Slightly Less Short Answer

A slightly less short answer: everyone recognizes the need for additional and more rigorous research to support clinical decisions. **Evidence-based practice (EBP)** (the use of research evidence to guide clinical practice) is a major goal of the clinicians in our profession (Apel & Self, 2003).

You may wonder why this area needs more research support. One reason is the subject matter: speaking is astonishingly complex and the people who have speech disorders are far more complex than their speech, and both variables—speech and person—combine in successful treatment. With such complexity, the more we learn about speech and about speech learners, the more our treatments change and the more we need new research to support our work.

Another reason is that the study of speech sound disorders changes in response to evolution of culture, health care, and education. Just a few of the many possible illustrations:

- **Preschoolers:** Forty years ago, the profession debated—sometimes furiously—whether preschoolers should receive treatment for speech sound disorders. The logic was let kids be kids and wait until they reached school to begin treatment. Today, preschoolers regularly receive speech services, and some ask, why not infants and toddlers as well? (Claessen et al., 2016; Williams & Stoel-Gammon, 2016)
- **Diversity:** The world—and our caseloads—are increasingly diverse. To paraphrase a leader in the field: today, if you want to work internationally, just open your front door (Battle, 2012). These welcome cultural changes challenge us to improve our knowledge base and clinical skills.
- **Relooking at students:** Our profession sometimes relooks at familiar populations. Students from kindergarten through high school have been a mainstay of clinicians for so long that you would think there was nothing left to research (American Speech-Language-Hearing Association, 2006, 2010; Shewan, 1988). Then came inclusion of speech as part of a school's curriculum, causing clinicians to rethink basic ways to treat speech sound disorders (Farquharson, 2015; Nathan, Stackhouse, Goulandris, & Snowling, 2004).

In summary, we know a great deal about how to help a child learn to talk, but you can expect the field to change as new theories of speech and human behavior appear and as society changes. Why go through all the effort to learn this topic and to keep updated? Probably everyone who studies speech sound disorders would answer this question differently. My own answer is speech is a fascinating topic and helping a child to communicate is a wonderful use for speech knowledge.

Conclusions

These are the major ideas in this chapter

1. Speech disorders matter because they may negatively affect a person's life.
2. Persons with a speech sound disorder may also have difficulties in school, social relations, and employment.
3. Articulation and phonological disorders reflect the dual nature of speech.
4. Speech sound disorder is a widely accepted cover term for articulation and phonological disorders.
5. Help exists for a person with a speech sound disorder.

Review Questions

1. What are the reasons for the second and third parts of the definition of a speech sound disorder?
2. Do (or did) you know anyone with a speech sound disorder or other type of communication disorder? How does (or did) it affect them?

3. In the example about Andrea, why do you think the social worker recommended developmental services so soon after birth? Why didn't she wait for a developmental problem to arise before making her recommendation?
4. What are the names of the two speech disorders that reflect the dual nature of speech?
5. Why did the pioneers of our profession gravitate toward articulation perspectives?
6. How did treatment of preschoolers lead to the rise of phonological perspectives?
7. What is the name of the cover term for articulation and phonological disorders?

References

American Speech-Language-Hearing Association. (2006). *2006 schools survey report: Caseload characteristics*. Rockville, MD: Author.

American Speech-Language-Hearing Association. (2010). *2010 schools summary report: Number and type of responses, SLPs*. Rockville, MD: Author.

Anthony, J. L., Aghara, R. G., Dunkelberger, M. J, Anthony, T. I., Williams, T. I., & Zhang, Z. (2011). What factors place children with speech sound disorders at risk for reading problems? *American Journal of Speech-Language Pathology, 20*(2), 146–160.

Apel, K., & Self, T. (2003). Evidence-based practice: The marriage of research and clinical services. *ASHA Leader, 8*, 6-7.

Baker, E., & McLeod, S. (2011). Evidence-based practice for children with speech sound disorders: Part 1 narrative review. *Language, Speech, and Hearing Services in Schools, 42*, 102–139.

Battle, D. (2012). *Communication disorders in multicultural and international populations*. St. Louis, MO: Elsevier.

Bauman-Waengler, J. (2000). *Articulatory and phonological impairments: A clinical focus*. Boston, MA: Allyn and Bacon.

Bernhardt, B., & Stemberger, J. (1998). *Handbook of phonological development from the perspective of constraint-based nonlinear phonology*. San Diego, CA: Academic Press.

Bernthal, J., Bankson, N., & Flipsen, P. (Eds.). (2009). *Articulation and phonological disorders: Speech sound disorders in children* (5th ed.). Boston, MA: Allyn & Bacon.

Bird, J., Bishop, D., & Freeman, N. (1995). Phonological awareness and literacy development in children with expressive phonological impairments. *Journal of Speech and Hearing Research, 38*, 446–462.

Bleile, K. (2009). A Nicaraguan experience. In C. Bowen (Ed.), *Children's speech sound disorders*. (pp. 157–160). Oxford, UK: Wiley-Blackwell.

Bowen, C. (2009). *Children's speech sound disorders*. Oxford, UK: Wiley-Blackwell.

Campbell, T., Dollaghan, C., Rockette, H., Paradise, J., Feldman, H., Shriberg, L., . . . Kurs-Lasky, M. (2003). Risk factors for speech delay of unknown origin in 3-year-old children. *Child Development, 74*(2), 346–357.

Claessen, M., Beattie, T., Roberts, R., Leitao, S., Whitworth, A., & Dodd, B. (2017). Is two too early? Assessing toddlers' phonology. *Speech, Language and Hearing, 20*(2), 91–101.

Creaghead, N., Newman, P., & Secord, W. (1989). *Assessment and remediation of articulatory and phonological disorders*. Columbus, OH: Charles E. Merrill.

Curtiss, S., Katz, W., & Tallal, P. (1992). Delay versus deviance in the language acquisition of language-impaired children. *Journal of Speech and Hearing Research, 35*, 373–383.

Dodd, B., & McIntosh, B. (2010). Two-year-old phonology: Impact of input, motor and cognitive abilities on development. *Journal of Child Language, 37*(5), 1027–1046.

Farquharson, K. (2015). After dismissal: Examining the language, literacy, and cognitive skills of children with remediated speech sound disorders. *Perspectives in School Based Issues, 16*(2), 50–59.

Felsenfeld, S., Broen, P., & McGue, M. (1994). A 28-year follow-up of adults with a history of moderate phonological disorder: Educational and functional results. *Journal of Speech and Hearing Research, 37*(6), 1341–1353.

Fey, M. (1992). Articulation and phonology: Inextricable constructs in speech pathology. *Language, Speech, and Hearing Services in Schools, 23*, 225–232.

Gierut, J. A. (1998). Treatment efficacy: Functional phonological disorders in children. *Journal of Speech, Language, and Hearing Research, 41*, S85–S100.

Hodson, B. (1994). Foreword. *Topics in Language Disorders, 14*, vi–viii.

Hoffman, P., Schuckers, G., & Daniloff, R. (1989). *Children's phonetic disorders: Theory and treatment.* Boston, MA: Little, Brown.

Human Rights Watch. (2010). *"As if we weren't human:" Discrimination and violence against women with disabilities in northern Uganda.* New York, NY: Author.

Law, J., Boyle, J., Harris, F., Harkness, A., & Nye, C. (2000). Prevalence and natural history of primary speech and language delay: Findings from a systematic review of the literature. *International Journal of Language and Communication Disorders, 35*(2), 165–188.

Lewis, B., Freebairn, L., Tag, J., Ciesla, A., Iyengar, S., Stein, C., & Taylor, H. (2015). Adolescent outcomes of children with early speech sound disorders with and without language impairment. *American Journal of Speech Language Pathology, 24*, 150–163.

Lewis, B., Freebairn, L., & Taylor, H. (2000). Academic outcomes in children with histories of speech sound disorders. *Journal of Communication Disorders, 33*, 11–30.

Locke, J. (1983). Clinical phonology: The explanation and treatment of speech sound disorders. *Journal of Speech and Hearing Disorders, 48*, 339–341.

Lowe, R. (1994). *Phonology: Assessment and intervention applications.* Baltimore, MD: Williams & Wilkins.

McCormack, J., Harrison, L., McLeod, S., & McAllister, L. (2011). A nationally representative study of the association between communication impairment at 4–5 years and children's life activities at 7–9 years. *Journal of Speech, Language, and Hearing Research, 54*, 1328–1348.

McCormack, J., McLeod, S., McAllister, L., & Harrison, L. J. (2010). My speech problem, your listening problem, and my frustration: The experience of living with childhood speech impairment. *Language, Speech, and Hearing Services in Schools, 41*(4), 379–392.

Nathan, L., Stackhouse, J., Goulandris, N., & Snowling, M. J. (2004). Educational consequences of developmental speech disorder: Key Stage 1 National Curriculum assessment results in English and mathematics. *British Journal of Educational Psychology, 74*, 173-186.

Overby, M., Carrell, T., & Bernthal, J. (2007). Teachers' perceptions of students of students with speech sound disorders: A quantitative and qualitative analysis. *Language, Speech, and Hearing in the Schools, 38*(4), 327–341.

Paul, R. (1991). Profiles of toddlers with slow expressive language. *Topics in Language Disorders, 11*, 1–13.

Paul, R., & Shriberg, L. (1982). Associations between phonology and syntax in speech-delayed children. *Journal of Speech and Hearing Research, 25*, 536–547.

Pennington, B., & Bishop, D. (2009). Relations among speech, language, and reading disorders. *Annual Review of Psychology, 60*, 283–306.

Rice, M. L., Taylor, C. L., & Zubrick, S. R. (2008). Language outcomes of 7-year-old children with or without a history of late language emergence at 24 months. *Journal of Speech, Language and Hearing Research, 51,* 394–407.

Ruscello, D. M., St. Louis, K., & Mason, N. (1991). School-aged children with phonologic disorders: Coexistence with other speech/language disorders. *Journal of Speech and Hearing Research, 34,* 236–242.

Rvachew, S., & Brosseau-Lapre, F. (2017). *Developmental phonological disorders* (2nd ed.). San Diego, CA: Plural.

Shelton, R., & McReynolds, L. (1979). Functional articulation disorders: Preliminaries to treatment. In N. Lass (Ed.), *Introduction to communication disorders* (pp. 263–310). Englewood Cliffs, NJ: Prentice-Hall.

Shewan, C. (1988). 1988 omnibus survey: Adaptation and progress in times of change. *Asha, 30,* 27–30.

Shriberg, L., & Kwiatkowski, J. (1982). Phonological disorders III: A procedure for assessing severity of involvement. *Journal of Speech and Hearing Disorders, 47,* 256–270.

Shriberg, L., & Kwiatkowski, J. (1988). A follow-up study of children with phonologic disorders of unknown origin. *Journal of Speech and Hearing Disorders, 53,* 144–155.

Shriberg, L., & Tomblin, B. (1999). Prevalence of speech delay in 6-year-old children and comorbidity with language impairment. *Journal of Speech, Language, and Hearing Research, 42,* 1461–1481.

Shriberg, L. D., & Austin, D. (1998). Co-morbidity of speech-language disorder: Implications for a phenotype marker of speech delay. In R. Paul (Ed.), *The speech-language connection* (pp. 73–117). Baltimore, MD: Paul H. Brookes.

Shriberg, L. D., Lewis, B. A., Tomblin, J. B., McSweeny, J. L., Karlsson, H. B., & Scheer, A. R. (2005). Toward diagnostic and phenotype markers for genetically transmitted speech delay. *Journal of Speech, Language, and Hearing Research, 48*(4), 834–852.

Slater, S. (1992). Portrait of the professions. *Asha, 34,* 61–65.

Smit, A. (2003). *Articulation and phonology resource guide for school-age children and adults.* New York, NY: Thomson Delmar Learning.

Taylor, O. L., & Peters-Johnson, C. A. (1986). Speech, language, and hearing disorders in Black populations. In O. L. Taylor, *Nature of communication disorders in culturally and linguistically diverse populations.* San Diego, CA: College-Hill Press.

Van Dyke, D. C., & Holte, L. (2003). Communication disorders in children. *Pediatric Annals, 32*(7), 436–437.

Weiss, C., Gordon, M., & Lillywhite, H. (1987). *Clinical management of articulatory and phonologic disorders.* Baltimore, MD: Williams & Wilkins.

Williams, A. (2010). Multiple oppositions intervention. In A. Williams, S. McLeod & R. McCauley (Eds.), *Interventions for speech sound disorders in children* (pp. 73–94). Baltimore, MA: Brookes.

Williams, L. (2003). *Speech disorders resource guide for preschool children.* New York, NY: Thomson Delmar Learning.

Williams, L., & Stoel-Gammon, C. (2016, November). *Identification of speech sound disorders in toddlers.* Seminar session presented at the Annual Convention of the American Speech-Language-Hearing Association, Philadelphia, PA.

Winitz, H. (1984). *Treating articulation disorders.* Baltimore, MD: University Park Press.

World Bank Group. (2005). Retrieved from http://www.worldbank.org

World Report on Disability. (2011). Retrieved from http://www.who.int/disabilities/world_report/en/index

CHAPTER 3

SPEECH PRODUCTION

Todd A. Bohnenkamp

The journey of speech begins in the brain and then arrives in the muscles, which move, channel, and shape air to create sound. This chapter introduces the systems involved in speech production. The nervous system is responsible for high-level functioning as well as the activation and monitoring of the speech production systems. The respiratory system provides the driving force for phonation, which downstream allows articulators to shape sounds for communication. Topics in this chapter include:

- Speech in the Brain
- Speech in the Muscles

Learning Objectives

I hope on completing the chapter you will

- Appreciate the complicated nature of neural control of speech production
- Explain how speakers manipulate the respiratory system to produce speech
- Describe the difference between phonation and speech
- Explain the difference between articulator function for chewing and swallowing and for speech

Key Words

Key words you will encounter in this chapter

Neurons	Glial cells
Action potential	Cell body
Motor neurons	Grey matter
Sensory neurons	Dendrites
Interneurons	White matter

Axons	Phonation
Neurotransmitters	Epiglottis
Synapse	Vestibular (false)
Myelin	vocal folds
Central nervous	True vocal folds
system	Glottis
Peripheral nervous	Adduction
system	Abduction
Corpus callosum	Bernoulli Effect
Cortex	Lamina propria
Lobes	Frequency
Broca's area	Pitch
Primary motor	Speech articulation
cortex	Mandible
Wernicke's area	Tongue
Basal ganglia	Soft palate (velum)
Thalamus	Velopharyngeal
Cerebellum	port
Brain stem	Hypernasal
Lower respiratory	Hyponasal
system	Hard palate
Alveoli	(maxilla)
Pleural linkage	Upper jaw
Larynx	(palatine bone)

Speech in the Brain

Speech begins in the brain as an electrochemical event. Our discussion begins with the neuron before going on to gross anatomy.

Neurons

Your **neurons** are specialized nerve cells that transmit information through an electro-chemical process (**action potential**). Neurons are the basic structure within the neural system. Your brain contains approximately 100 billion neurons (Herculano-Houzel, 2009); there are three basic categories: motor, sensory, and interneurons.

Motor Neurons

Motor neurons bring efferent information out to the body from the brain and spinal cord (central nervous system; CNS) and the spinal cord and cranial nerves (peripheral nervous system; PNS).

Sensory Neurons

Sensory neurons bring sensation from the receptors within the PNS and body into the central nervous system.

Interneurons

Interneurons filter and fine-tune the efferent and afferent information. They greatly outnumber motor and sensory neurons.

Components of Neurons

Although neurons are present in many shapes and sizes, they each have the same core components: cell body, dendrites, axon, and axon terminals (called telodendria). In addition, support cells within the nervous system, or **glial cells**, are responsible for cellular health, maintaining the blood brain barrier, and carrying away metabolic by-products.

Cell Bodies

Each neuron has a **cell body** that is responsible for basic cellular functions. The cell bodies compose the **grey matter** within the nervous system. Large groups of cell bodies are often part of a functionally similar, larger functional system.

Dendrites

These structures are branchlike projections specific to neurons that communicate with the cell body and axons. **Dendrites** are necessary for communication with other neurons through the electrochemical communication of the action potential.

Axons

White matter is a collection of large numbers of **axons**, which are responsible for transmitting impulses throughout the central nervous system. Each neurons has a singular axon that eventually communicates with other neurons via numerous axon terminals (telodendria).

Communication between Neurons

Communication between neurons is dependent upon the release of **neurotransmitters** across the junction between the neurons (**synapse**). Neurotransmitters release from the terminal end buttons and bind on the postsynaptic neuron. The response of the postsynaptic neuron is dependent upon whether the neurotransmitter is excitatory or inhibitory in nature. An excitatory neurotransmitter results in an action potential in the postsynaptic neuron, whereas an inhibitory neurotransmitter will make it less likely to produce an action potential in the postsynaptic neuron. The speed of the electrical current of the action potential accelerates when a **myelin** sheath surrounds the neuronal axon, which also protects and insulates the axon.

Gross Anatomy

Your **central nervous system** (CNS) consists of your brain and spinal cord at its basic level, whereas **the peripheral nervous system** (PNS) consists of the cranial nerves (numbered I–XII) and spinal nerves (31 pairs). Your CNS has a left and right cerebral hemisphere, cerebellum, brain stem, and spinal cord. Meningeal linings surround your two cerebral hemispheres and are there to protect your brain. They are arranged in three levels, from deep (closest to the brain) to superficial (closest to the skin). Cerebrospinal fluid and blood supply run through these layers to nourish and protect the brain and CNS.

Functions of Hemispheres

The functions of your cerebral hemispheres vary considerably. The two hemispheres communicate via commissural fibers called the **corpus callosum**.

Left Hemisphere

Your left hemisphere is responsible for speech, language, sequencing, planning, mathematics, and integration as well as providing cortical control of innervating the spinal nerves to control the right side of the body.

Right Hemisphere

Your right hemisphere is the location for prosody, music, visuospatial recognition (including facial recognition), and creativity as well as controlling the left side of the body.

Cortex

The **cortex** is a 2 to 4 mm thick layer of cells that covers the cerebral hemispheres. Your cortex is the location of the highest-level functions of your brain, including reasoning, executive functioning, voluntary control of structures, memory, vision, hearing, and language and speech production. The cortex of each hemisphere divides into four functional areas called **lobes**.

Frontal Lobe

The largest lobe is the frontal lobe, with a cortical area that composes approximately a third of your entire cortex. It is the location for major cognitive functions, personality, motivation, inhibition, language production, speech production, motor programming, motor sequencing, and executive functioning.

Speech Functions. Speech-related functions in the frontal lobe include planning, sequencing, and motivation prior to the initiation of speech. Cortical locations important for voluntary speech in the frontal lobe include your premotor area, supplementary motor area, and the expressive language center oftentimes referred to as **Broca's area**. Your frontal lobe also contains the **primary motor cortex**, which is responsible for voluntary movement. As you would expect, this is an essential location for speech production.

Parietal, Temporal, and Occipital Lobes

The parietal, temporal, and occipital lobes are instrumental in integrating sensory information for both speech production and perception.

Parietal Lobe. The parietal lobe is the primary cortical area for sensory information, memory, cognition, and perception.

Temporal Lobe. The temporal lobe is an essential component in speech and language production—codifying language, making memories, and integrating with visual input. Language comprehension is located at the juncture of the temporal and parietal lobes at **Wernicke's area**. The lateral surface of the temporal lobe is the location for the primary auditory cortex, responsible for hearing and frequency representation. Connections to your hippocampus, which are essential for converting short-term to long-term memory, are in the temporal lobe.

Occipital Lobe. Your occipital lobe is responsible for visual input and integration of visual material, and contributes to speech and language development.

Subcortical Structures

Your subcortical structures are essential for communication between brain structures and monitoring of background activities. Interaction of the basal ganglia, thalamus, and cerebellum results in fine-tuning of planned voluntary motor movements based on results of previous activity. These structures work together to serve as the quality control system for your CNS.

Basal Ganglia

The **basal ganglia** of your subcortex are responsible for graceful motor movement, essentially functioning as a "filter" that eliminates unwanted voluntary movements and suppresses involuntary movements. A disruption in the basal ganglia can result in disruption to motor control. An example of a motor plan that is "over-filtered," would be Parkinson's disease, whereas Huntington's chorea would be an example of "under-filtering."

Thalamus

The structures of the basal ganglia are part of a larger and complex circuit that includes the cortex and thalamus. Your **thalamus** integrates motor activity with sensory feedback. It receives sensory feedback, particularly the results of previous motor movements, and relays that information to the corresponding portion of the cortex.

Cerebellum

The **cerebellum**, or "little brain," shares information with the thalamus and CNS regarding the location of structures in space (proprioception), the speed or sensation of movement (kinesthesia), and predicting the location of structures as they move (Pellionisz & Llinás, 1979).

Brain Stem

Your **brain stem** is a hub of autonomic involuntary control and integrates with large amounts of efferent and afferent information communicating through the CNS to the PNS. Your brain stem contains large numbers of cell bodies in a structure called the reticular formation, which is responsible for basic life functions such as respiration, digestion, and maintenance of homeostasis.

Cranial Nerves

Your corticobulbar (cranial nerves) and corticospinal (spinal nerves) tracts provide CNS control of the cranial nerves and spinal nerves within the PNS. These tracts decussate, or cross the midline, within the brain stem for contralateral control of the body. Corticobulbar fibers innervate the cell nuclei for 10 of the 12 cranial nerves, whereas corticospinal tract fibers continue to the spinal cord. A short description of each of your cranial nerves and its function in speech production appears in Table 3–1.

Table 3–1. Cranial Nerves

Cranial Nerve	Category	General Function(s)
I Olfactory	Sensory	Smell
II Optic	Sensory	Vision
III Oculomotor	Motor	Medial eye movement
IV Trochlear	Motor	Eye movement
V Trigeminal	Mixed	*M*—Muscles for chewing *S*—Sensory from face, touch from anterior tongue
VI Abducens	Motor	Lateral eye movement
VII Facial	Mixed	*M*—Muscles of the face *S*—Taste from anterior tongue
VIII Vestibulocochlear	Mixed	*M*—Damping of hair cells in cochlea *S*—Hearing and balance
IX Glossopharyngeal	Mixed	*M*—Elevates pharynx *S*—Touch and taste posterior tongue
X Vagus	Mixed	*M*—Larynx and pharynx, velum *S*—Larynx and pharynx, velum
XI Spinal Accessory	Motor	Move head, lift shoulders
XII Hypoglossal	Motor	Tongue movement

Speech in the Muscles

Speech next becomes the movement of muscles. Whereas brain cells are specialized to carry nervous system impulses, muscle cells are specialized to contract. Muscle contractions function to move, channel, and shape air for speech. Speech breathing requires you to make quick inspirations followed by controlled expirations while reducing the number and duration of interruptions to balance gas exchange. This section describes the lower respiratory system, larynx, and speech articulators.

Your **lower respiratory system** within the rib cage includes the lungs, the soft tissues of the trachea, sections of bronchi and smaller airways, and **alveoli**. The alveoli are air sacs within the lung and the location of oxygen and carbon dioxide gas exchange. We use this system to provide the driving pressures for voice and speech via manipulation of the lungs by the inspiratory and expiratory muscles.

Inspiration and expiration are possible because of the interaction of the inherent properties of the rib cage and lungs. Your rib cage, if allowed, would open and move outward if not connected at the sternum, which places the ribs under constant tension. In contrast, your lung tissue would move inward or collapse due to the elasticity of the soft tissues. These forces create a constant negative pressure between the lungs and rib cage resulting in a system that moves in unison. This is called **pleural linkage**.

Inspiration

Inspiration is an active process. The two primary muscles of inspiration are the diaphragm and external intercostals.

Diaphragm

The diaphragm is a large sheet of muscle that separates your thorax from your abdomen. It is mainly active during deep inspirations, pulling the lungs downward as it contracts. The diaphragm is in contact with the 25% of the lung surface. Your diaphragm moves down and forward, resulting in displacement of the incompressible mass of the abdominal viscera to make room for lung movement. You can demonstrate this easily by placing one hand on your rib cage and the other on your stomach. When you take a deep breath, you feel the outward movement of the abdomen. This is the diaphragm forcing the abdominal contents forward. Your diaphragm is active only during inspiratory movements, and any contribution to expiration happens because the passive response of abdominal muscles during speech production force it superiorly.

External Intercostals

Your external intercostals are located between each rib and pull the ribcage up. They work to increase the volume of the lungs, which results in air rushing into the lungs for inspiration. The manipulation of the rib cage by the external intercostals provides volume change due to its contact with 75% of the lung surface area.

Expiration

Expiration can be a passive or forced process. Passive expiration relies on gravity, elasticity of the lungs, and recoil within the rib cage to return the lungs to an equilibrium state following inspiration. However, speech expiration is an active process and requires activity in the many muscles responsible for forced expiration.

Internal Intercostals

The internal intercostal muscles are also located between each rib. In contrast to the externals, this group of muscles is responsible for compressing the rib cage and lungs by pulling the ribs downward. This results in air rushing out of the lungs. These are the muscles responsible for making the subtle airflow and pressure changes necessary for speech.

Abdominal Muscles

The abdominal muscles are not involved in inspiration but are essential muscles for speech production. These four muscles, from deep to superficial, are transversus abdominus, internal oblique abdominus, external oblique abdominus, and rectus abdominus. When contracted, these muscles will force the abdominal contents posteriorly and superiorly. This superior movement will force the diaphragm upward and result in compression of the lungs.

Abdominal activity combines with the activity of the internal intercostal muscles to result in speech expiration. To improve overall speech efficiency, the abdominal muscles are active throughout all speech expirations, but they are not likely to make subtle pressure changes. The rib cage provides the force necessary to indicate stress and emphasis during speech. The abdomen serves a specific role in speech by maintaining activity throughout the expiratory phase, indicating a "speech-specific" posturing of the chest-wall as compared to rest breathing.

CLINIC BOX: The Bucket Handle

Think of movement of air as a "bucket handle." Like a line of bucket handles, each of your ribs is pulled up and out away from the midline to create volume change. As a result, your ribcage is also elevated at the sternum, essentially lifting the entire rib cage out and up in the anterior-posterior plane (Zemlin, 1998). Expiration from this point is passive in nature and a result of the relaxation forces of elasticity in the lungs, recoil in the rib cage, and the effects of gravity.

The Larynx

The biological function of your **larynx** is to protect the airway. It also is the organ for voice production. **Phonation** is a component of speech, but is defined only as the vibration produced by the true vocal folds within the larynx; it is an overlaid function of the larynx. Speech articulators then shape those vibrations into sounds.

Laryngeal Structures

The larynx is located medially within the neck. Your laryngeal structures are primarily cartilaginous. The only bone is the hyoid bone, which forms the upper border of your larynx. It is free-floating and suspended within the body. The hyoid bone connects through membranes, and it articulates with the largest and most pronounced cartilage in the larynx—the thyroid cartilage. The lower border of the larynx is the cricoid cartilage, which articulates with the trachea.

Levels

Three levels, from top to bottom, help protect your airway: **epiglottis**, **vestibular (false) folds**, and **true vocal folds**.

Epiglottis. The function of the epiglottis is to protect the airway during swallow and is not essential for phonation, though it plays a role in the resonance and complexity of the resulting sound.

Vestibular Folds. These thick folds of mucous membrane serve as a layer of airway protection. These are not typically involved in phonation, though they find use in various chanting and singing styles in areas around the world.

True Vocal Folds. Of the three levels, only your true vocal folds are involved in phonation. The space between the true vocal folds is called the **glottis**; closing of the vocal folds is **adduction** and opening is **abduction**. Your true vocal folds perform the many functions essential for phonation.

CLINIC BOX: The Bernoulli Effect

As the velocity of airflow increases through the constriction of your larynx, the pressure perpendicular to that flow will become negative in relation and will result in your vocal folds coming back together. This is the **Bernoulli Effect**. This, in conjunction with the physical properties (e.g., momentum, inertia) of the true vocal folds when forced open, maintains the continued vocal fold vibration needed for phonation.

Pitch

Many muscles in your larynx are involved in glottal configuration, or pitch change. To illustrate, muscles that elevate your larynx during swallow can also activate during phonation to make subtle and discreet changes in the length of the vocal tract to influence resonance. Contraction of the thyroarytenoid muscle decreases your pitch, whereas the cricothyroid muscle elevates pitch. Interaction between the cricothyroid muscle and thyroarytenoid muscle allows pitch changes during phonation, stretching and shortening the covering of connective and mucosal tissue (called the **lamina propria**) that lines each vocal fold.

Voicing

Adduction of the arytenoid cartilages brings your vocal folds together for phonation. The muscles involved include the lateral cricothyroid, the oblique interarytenoid, and transverse interarytenoid. To make an unvoiced sound, the posterior cricoarytenoid muscle opens your vocal folds by rotating the arytenoids open (abduction).

CLINIC BOX: Frequency and Pitch

Frequency and **pitch** are not interchangeable terms. Frequency is the measurement of vibratory cycles per second (Hertz; Hz) and can be objectively measured, whereas pitch is a perceptual correlate to frequency. Frequency is dependent on the amount of the vocal fold mass that is vibrating, which arises from the interaction of the cricothyroid muscle and thyroarytenoid muscle. The greater the mass, the lower the frequency; the lesser the mass, the higher the frequency. This explains why female speakers have a mean speaking fundamental frequency of approximately 210 Hz, whereas males have a mean fundamental frequency nearer 120 Hz (Baken & Orlikoff, 2000). In contrast to frequency, an individual can perceive an increase or decrease in pitch, but it is not quantifiable.

The Speech Articulators

Articulation is the process of joining two structures (Zemlin, 1998). Our topic, **speech articulation,** is the process of shaping of mobile and immobile structures in your vocal tract to produce speech. The overlaid function of speech integrates with the biological functions of airway protection, chewing (mastication), and swallowing (deglutition), requiring the complex coordination of the same structures under entirely different motor programs.

Mobile Structures

Your mobile articulators are the mandible, tongue, velum (soft palate), lips, cheeks, pharynx, and larynx (see previous section).

Larynx. The larynx is the sound source for speech (see previous section).

Mandible. The **mandible** is a mobile articulator that influences the interactions of the teeth, tongue, and lower lip. The function of the mandible varies considerably depending upon the activity. For example, your mandible moves in a rotary direction during mastication to ensure adequate grinding and breakdown of the food or drink (bolus) you manipulate. In contrast, during speech production your mandibular movements are almost exclusively up and down, without the side-to-side movement.

Tongue. Consonant production requires quick and accurate movements of the **tongue.** The tongue lacks a skeletal framework and it completes all shape configurations using its intrinsic muscles. Those intrinsic muscles are responsible for tongue tip elevation (superior longitudinal muscles), tongue tip depression (inferior longitudinal muscles), tongue flattening (vertical muscles), and tongue narrowing (transverse muscles). The variable configurations of these four muscles provide you the ability to produce varied shapes. That ability to reach articulatory targets is in concert with the extrinsic muscles of the tongue, which contribute to protrusion, retraction, and side-to-side movement.

CLINIC BOX: Speech and Swallowing Differences

Speech and swallowing use similar structures in very different ways. Your ability to shape the tongue allows you to produce numerous speech sounds and requires very quick and precise movement of a large structure. Whereas swallowing requires greater amounts of strength, speech requires speed and timing. These differences in strength requirements is one reason why therapy approaches for speech are different from those for swallowing.

To give another illustration of the difference between speech and swallowing, you need much less strength to close the velopharyngeal port during speech than during swallowing. Additionally, during swallowing, the velum elevates and closes during the duration of the oral transit stage of swallowing. This increased closure force ensures you do not have nasal regurgitation during swallow due to the high-pressure buildup in the oral cavity and pharynx. In contrast, speech does not require the same amount of force and its behavior is analogous to a fluttering movement during continuous speech.

Velum (Soft Palate). The **velum (soft palate)** is a slinglike structure that separates the nasal cavity from the oral cavity and pharynx. The velum is one portion of the **velopharyngeal (VP) port** that functions to close the nasal cavity for either speech or swallowing. You do not achieve VP closure by velar movement alone, but rather through a combination of velar elevation with posterior and lateral pharyngeal wall closure. Speech requires rapid and timed movements for you to be able to elevate the velum to close the VP port for oral sounds and to depress it for nasal sounds.

CLINIC BOX: Disorders of Speech

Disorders of speech related to the velum most often occur in craniofacial disorders, but can be present in neurological disorders, motor speech disorders, and oral/head and neck cancer. Craniofacial disorders may or may not result in a cleft of the velum. Typically, if the velum is affected, people perceive affected individuals as **hypernasal** (too much nasal resonance) due to difficulty building up oral pressure for oral sounds. Less often, people perceive affected individuals as **hyponasal** (too little nasal resonance).

Lips and Face. Speech articulation and communication would not be complete without discussion of the muscles of the face. Your lips depend on a surprisingly large number of muscles. The orbicularis is the major muscle of lip rounding; it maintains lip seal during swallowing and when you build up intraoral air pressure during speech. The buccinators and risorius muscles help you retract the corners of your mouth. The speech function of the buccinator is to pull the corners of your lips posteriorly (e.g., producing "eeee"); its biological function is to push your food and drink back into the oral cavity to maintain a cohesive bolus. Your smile comes from the muscles levator anguli oris and zygomatic major, pulling up your lip corners.

Immobile Structures

Your immobile structures are the **maxilla (hard palate)** and **palatine bone (upper jaw)** and teeth.

Maxilla (upper jaw; hard palate). The maxilla is an immobile articulatory structure. Your hard palate and upper jaw separate the oral cavity from the nasal cavity. They are important during mastication and deglutition as your tongue pushes against the maxilla to create a cohesive bolus and then propel the bolus toward the pharynx for swallowing. The horizontal plates of the upper jaw (palatine bone) lie behind your maxilla and compose the posterior third of your hard palate. A disruption of this fusion of hard palate and upper jaw may result in a cleft, which may vary in severity anywhere from the lips to the velum.

Teeth. The biological functions of your teeth are to cut, shear, and grind food for chewing and swallowing (Zemlin, 1998). The teeth also play an essential role in the production of certain speech sounds (e.g., [f] and [v]) and contribute to the articulation of many other sounds. The loss of, or missing, teeth can have direct effects on speech.

Conclusions

These are major ideas in this chapter:

1. The foundation for speech is 100 billion neurons in the nervous system.
2. Nervous system control of speech is reliant on high-level cortical function in addition to other structures of the CNS and PNS.
3. Your respiratory system is the driving force for speech.
4. The biological function of your larynx is airway protection; it also serves as the organ responsible for phonation.
5. Although they use the same structures, movement and control of the speech articulators is markedly different from that for chewing and swallowing.

Review Questions

1. What are the main components of a neuron?
2. What is the importance of the action potential?
3. What is the importance of the synapse?
4. What are the functions of myelin?
5. How do the functions of the left and right cerebral hemispheres differ?
6. Where does gas exchange in the lungs occur?
7. Is speech categorized as forced or passive expiration?
8. What is the biological function of the larynx?
9. How does phonation differ from speech?
10. What structures within the larynx are the sound source?

11. Contraction of which muscle raises pitch? Which muscle decreases pitch?
12. How does mandibular movement differ between speech production and chewing?
13. What separates the nasal and oral cavities?
14. What structure is responsible for determining whether a sound is oral or nasal?
15. What structures are needed to close the velopharyngeal port?

References

Baken, R. J., & Orlikoff, R. F. (2000). *Clinical measurement of speech and voice.* San Diego, CA: Singular.

Bhatnager, S. C. (2012). *Neuroscience for the study of communicative disorders* (4th ed.). Philadelphia, PA: Lippincott Williams & Wilkins.

Draper, M. H., Ladefoged, P., & Whitteridge, D. (1959). Respiratory muscles in speech. *Journal of Speech and Hearing Research, 2,* 16–27.

Herculano-Houzel, S. (2009). The human brain in numbers: A linearly scaled-up primate brain. *Frontiers in Human Neuroscience, 3*(31). https://doi.org/10.3389/neuro.09.031.2009

Hixon, T. J., Goldman, M. D., & Mead, J. (1973). Kinematics of the chest wall during speech production: Volume displacements of the rib cage, abdomen, and lung. *Journal of Speech and Hearing Research, 16,* 78–115.

Hixon, T. J., Mead, J., & Goldman, M. D. (1976). Dynamics of the chest wall during speech production: Function of the thorax, rib cage, diaphragm, and abdomen. *Journal of Speech and Hearing Research, 19,* 297–356.

Hoit, J. D., & Lohmeier, H. L. (2000). Influence of continuous speaking on ventilation. *Journal of Speech, Language, and Hearing Research, 43*(5), 1240–1251.

Kahane, J. C. (1982). Growth of the human prepubertal and pubertal larynx. *Journal of Speech and Hearing Research, 25,* 446–455.

Kent, R. D. (1997). *The speech sciences.* San Diego, CA: Singular.

Lubker, J. F. (1968). An electromyographic-cinefluorographic investigation of velar function during normal speech production. *Cleft Palate Journal, 5,* 1–18.

Ochs, M., Nyengaard, J. R., Jung, A., Knudsen, L., Voigt, M., Wahlers, T., & Gundersen, H. J. (2004). The number of alveoli in the human lung. *American Journal of Respiratory and Critical Care Medicine, 169*(1), 120–124. https://doi.org/10.1164/rccm.200308-1107OC

Pellionisz, A., & Llinás, R. (1979). Brain modeling by tensor network theory and computer simulation. The cerebellum: Distributed processor for predictive coordination. *Neuroscience, 4*(3), 323–348.

West, J. B. (2000). *Respiratory physiology: The essentials* (6th ed.). Philadelphia, PA: Lippincott, Williams & Wilkins.

Winkworth, A. L., Davis, P. J., Adams, R. D., & Ellis, E. (1995). Breathing patterns during spontaneous speech. *Journal or Speech and Hearing Research, 38*(1), 124–144.

Zemlin, W. (1998). *Speech and hearing science: Anatomy and physiology* (4th ed.). Boston, MA: Allyn & Bacon.

CHAPTER 4

SPEECH RECEPTION AND PERCEPTION

Jaimie L. Gilbert

Speech entails passing a volley of sound from a speaker to a listener. This chapter follows sound on its journey from a speaker's mouth, through the air, into and through the ears, and to a listener's brain, where it is processed and interpreted. Major topics in this chapter include:

- Introduction
- Sound in the Air
- Sound in the Ear
- Sound in the Brain

Learning Objectives

I hope on completing the chapter you will

- Know basic properties of sound waves
- Recognize important elements of ear anatomy and physiology
- Understand how sound goes from a wave in the air to neural impulses which listeners can assign meaning

Key Words

Key words you will encounter in this chapter

Speech reception	Ossicular chain
Speech perception	Malleus
Rarefaction	Incus
Compression	Stapes
Longitudinal wave	Oval window
Time	Cochlea
Frequency	Organ of Corti
Wavelength	Hair cells
Period	Auditory nerve
Intensity	Brain stem
Inverse square law	Medulla
Impedance	Pons
Pinna	Midbrain
Tympanic	SPLICE
membrane	Percept

Introduction

This chapter explores how sound travels through the air, through the ear, and to the brain. For verbal communication, a listener must both *receive* and *perceive* speech sounds. Here's what I mean by these two terms, **speech reception** and **speech perception**.

Speech Reception

This is the process of converting a physical sound wave to different types of energy. This energy is encoded in the ear and conducted along the auditory pathway to the brain.

Speech Perception

This is the comprehension of a spoken communicative message using a combination of sensory input, linguistic context, indexical cues, a perceiver's cognitive skills, and environmental cues.

Sound in the Air

Speech reception begins as a sound wave in the air.

Sound Generation

Sound, as we typically experience it, is a vibration that travels as a wave through the air particles around us. Three requirements for sound are a source of energy, a source of vibration (a.k.a., sound source), and an elastic medium (Emanuel & Letowski, 2009). An energy source causes a sound source to move (vibrate). Sound source motion causes a change in pressure in the elastic medium (air) adjacent to the sound source. The pressure change pushes the air particles right next to the sound source closer to air particles on their other side (farther away from the sound source).

Dominos

This pushing of some air particles together forms an area of compression. It works this way: one air particle bumps the one next to it, like a chain of dominos, transferring energy to the next particle in line. Because air is an elastic medium, the first air particle that moved recoils and tries to go back to its original position. The second air particle in line, after transferring energy to the third air particle in line, also recoils, moving back closer to its original position, and so on and so forth.

Now you have air particles moving back to their original spot and some air particles moving away from their original spot, creating areas with fewer air particles in it (with air particles spaced farther apart)—this is a **rarefaction**. Because there are also some particles moving closer to the next particle in line, there are also areas where air particles are spaced closer together—this is **compression**. The alternating areas of compression and rarefaction (alternating pressures) form a **longitudinal wave**. The longitudinal wave (areas of compression and rarefaction) travels (or propagates) through the medium (the air).

Properties of Particle Motion

Think of sound this way: there are two elements "moving" in a sound wave—the particles and the wave itself. Each particle moves a certain distance, at a certain speed, and in a certain direction. The direction particles move in comparison to the direction the wave moves determines which type of wave it is. Particle motion can be parallel or perpendicular to wave motion. In a longitudinal wave, the air particles are moving parallel in the same direction the wave is travelling, and there are areas of compression and rarefaction. Also, in a longitudinal wave, a cycle consists of one compression and one rarefaction.

CLINIC BOX: Do the (Transverse) Wave

Sound is a longitudinal wave. There is another type of wave, a transverse wave, where particles move perpendicular (at a 90° angle) to the direction in which the wave is travelling. When people in a sports stadium "do the wave," they are demonstrating a transverse wave. If you consider the people's arms to be the particles, these move up and down. The wave itself, however, moves from one side to another side, making particle motion perpendicular to wave motion.

Sound Waves in 3-D

Sound has three important characteristics: *time, frequency,* and *intensity.* I call these the three dimensions, or 3-D, of sound.

Time

The first 3-D of sound is time. **Time**, as a dimension of sound, refers to the speed of sound. Speed of sound is how far the wave travels in a certain amount of *time.* Speed of sound is a property of the elastic medium through which the sound wave is travelling and not a property of the sound wave itself. For example, speech typically travels through air. Sound waves may differ in other properties, but if the medium is the same, all waves will travel at the same speed. This means that in the same medium—in air, for example—all sounds will travel the same amount of distance in a specific amount of time.

Frequency

The second 3-D of sound is frequency. **Frequency** is a measure of how many completed cycles of the waveform occur *per second*. Frequency correlates with the human perception of pitch. Higher frequency is associated with higher pitch (e.g., treble), and lower frequency with lower pitch (e.g., bass). A Hertz is one cycle of compression and rarefaction per second. To illustrate, a sound at 20 Hz has 20 cycles of compression and rarefaction. Researchers estimate the human ear can hear a frequency range of approximately 20 Hertz (Hz) up to 20,000 Hz. The actual frequency range important for speech reception and perception is narrower—only about 250 to 8000 Hz.

Frequency, Waves, and Distance. In addition to frequency (wave cycles per second), you can also measure sound by its distance, or how far the wave travels. **Wavelength** is the distance in space traveled by one cycle of the wave. **Period** is the amount of time it takes to complete one cycle. That is, wavelength is a measure of distance and period is a measure of time. Frequency, period, and wavelength, are related: frequency is the number of cycles completed per second, period is how many seconds it takes to complete one cycle, and wavelength is the distance traveled in one cycle.

Intensity

The third 3-D of sound is intensity. **Intensity** correlates with the human perception of loudness. Another way to describe intensity is the strength of a sound, or how much "oomph" the sound wave has. More technically, intensity is proportional to pressure. Intensity factors in time and distance: the farther a sound wave travels, the more area it needs to cover. As the distance travelled increases, the intensity of the sound decreases. This is the inverse square law.

Inverse Square Law. The **inverse square law** relates intensity and distance. I can guarantee that you already know and understand this law, you just might not have known there was a specific name for it. For example, if you really want to hear someone speak, what do you do? You move closer to the person so you can hear them better and louder. The farther away you are (increased distance) from the talker (sound source), the less intense his/her voice is when it reaches you. Therefore, as distance increases, intensity decreases. As one goes up, the other goes down—this is the definition of an inverse relationship. The actual amount intensity decreases involves squaring (calculating an exponential value to the second power). Thus, you have the inverse (one goes up as the other goes down) square (by an amount related to the square of the measure of distance) law.

Measuring Intensity. Intensity is measured in decibels (dB). Decibels are a relative measurement, meaning that they can only be interpreted by knowing what you are comparing the sound to, that is, a reference. To illustrate the need for a reference, if you start a new pizza restaurant, you could advertise that your pizza tastes two times better!

However, this is meaningless to potential customers unless you state what you are using as a reference—to what are you comparing your pizza? You could be comparing your pizza to the most popular pizza restaurant in your area, or you could be comparing your pizza to the taste of the cardboard box containing a delivery pizza. Without knowing the reference, giving a value of "two times better" is not informative.

In the study of communicative sciences and disorders, three different references exist to interpret the intensity of a sound. The three decibel reference scales are

- Sound pressure level (SPL): A physical pressure measurement, for example, a standard atmospheric pressure.
- Hearing level (HL): Average, normal, human hearing sensitivity.
- Sensation level (SL): An individual's hearing sensitivity.

Using the HL scale, the range of intensity that humans (with normal hearing) can hear is about 10 dB HL to 120 dB HL.

Summary: Time, Frequency, and Intensity

Frequency and intensity both inherently involve time. Frequency is a measure of how many cycles of compression and rarefaction are completed in one second. The unit of measurement is Hertz (Hz). The frequency range important for human speech is 250 Hz to 8000 Hz. Intensity is a measure of the strength of the wave and is measured in decibels (dB) referenced to a specific sound pressure (dB SPL), average human hearing (dB HL), or a specific individual's hearing sensitivity (dB SL).

Sound in the Ear

Sound does not travel unopposed. Physical forces try to stop the sound wave from moving, which is why a sound wave can "die out" and not last forever. Opposition to sound wave movement is called impedance. Sound can also encounter obstacles that affect how it travels and redirects it. One of the obstacles a sound wave encounters is the ear.

Ears

In this stage, speech reception continues as vibration of bones, membranes, and fluids. Ears on both sides of the head collect sound waves from the air. When a sound wave encounters the obstacle of the head, some sound waves travel into the ear canal on one side of the head. Some sound waves also "bend" around the head and travel into the ear canal on the other side of the head. Sounds with lower frequencies are more likely to reach the other side of the head. The brain stem analyzes differences between the waves that reach the two ears to determine spatial orientation—in other words, where are we in space compared to other objects around us.

The Outer Ear

Pinna

The ear is a transducer—meaning it changes the sound as it moves sound on its way. The first change is the direction of the sound wave. The **pinna**, the name for the part of the ear visible on the side of the head, has many folds facing in different directions. When the pinna catches sound (that is, when the sound wave encounters the obstacle of the pinna), some of the sound wave reflects and then travels in a different direction. If the sound wave encounters another fold, it is redirected again. By the process of reflection, the sound wave eventually is funneled into the external auditory canal.

External Auditory Canal

The entrance to external auditory canal is in the bowl of the pinna. The external auditory canal is a "tube" through which sound travels. The tube's shape emphasizes specific frequencies of sound. At the end of the tube is the ear drum, which is technically called the **tympanic membrane** (TM).

The Middle Ear

Up until this point in the auditory pathway, sound travels through air. In the next change, or transition, sound travels through tissue and bone, causing those structures to vibrate.

Tympanic Membrane

The first tissue encountered by the sound wave in the auditory pathway is the tympanic membrane, which separates the outer and middle ear. As sound energy reaches the air particle next to the TM, the last air particle in the "dominos chain" strikes the TM, just like a drumstick hits a drum, causing the TM to vibrate. The middle ear side of the tympanic membrane is connected to a chain of bones, causing them to vibrate.

Ossicular Chain

Three bones stretch across the middle ear space. The name of the entire set of three bones is the **ossicular chain.** The vibration set in motion by the TM travels from one bone, to the next, to the next. The first bone in the chain is the **malleus**, which transfers the vibration to the **incus**, which sends the vibration on to the **stapes**. At the end of the ossicular chain, the stapes attaches to a membrane that is part of the inner ear called the oval window. You may have heard these bones referred to more colloquially as the hammer, anvil, and stirrup.

Getting More "Oomph"

The middle ear performs a vital role in transmitting sound to the inner ear. Its job is to transduce sound from a medium of air (outer ear) to a medium of fluid (inner ear). Fluid has a greater impedance than air (there is more opposition trying to prevent the medium of fluid from moving/vibrating). A main function of the middle ear is to increase the pressure of the sound wave so that it will be able to travel through fluid and not just fizzle out when it reaches a medium with greater impedance. The middle ear achieves this impedance matching through two means: an ossicular lever and difference in window size.

Ossicular Lever. The ossicular chain acts like a lever. If you have ever shoveled snow, you know that if you press down at the top of the shovel handle, you can pick up more snow than if you press down on the handle closer to the shovel. With the increased length and a pivot point, you can move more snow at the end of the shovel. The ossicular chain functions similarly, causing pressure to increase at the end of the chain, which causes more fluid in the inner ear to move.

Window Size. Relatively speaking, the TM is HUGE compared to the oval window. When the sound wave "hits" the tympanic membrane, the ossicular chain funnels this sound wave to the oval window at the end of the chain, distributing a lot of energy across a small surface area, resulting in an increase of pressure at the oval window.

CLINIC BOX: Hearing Loss

There are three types of hearing loss: conductive hearing loss, sensorineural hearing loss, and mixed hearing loss. The job of the outer and middle ear is to conduct sound; together they form the conductive mechanism. The job of the inner ear and nerve are to sense sound and transmit it to the brain; together they form the sensorineural mechanism. Conductive hearing loss arises in the outer or middle ear, sensorineural hearing loss arises in the inner ear or nerve, and mixed hearing loss arises in both the conductive and sensorineural mechanisms.

If there is a difficulty in the conductive mechanism, it may be possible to treat this problem so that the mechanism functions relatively normally. For example, a surgeon could remove an overgrowth of bone that affects the mass and stiffness of the ossicular chain. Alternately, a surgeon may replace the ossicular chain with a prosthetic.

Given the more complicated encoding that takes place in the sensorineural mechanism, if there is a problem in this mechanism, current knowledge is limited in the ability to return it to normal function. Treatments for cochlear lesions generally involve either attempting to increase likelihood of neural firing (e.g., amplifying sound with hearing aids) or bypassing the outer, middle, and inner ear to directly stimulate the auditory nerve (i.e., cochlear implants).

The Inner Ear

As indicated in the preceding section, the **oval window** is a membrane that separates the middle and inner ear. The last bone in the ossicular chain, the stapes, covers the oval window, causing it to vibrate along with the ossicular chain. On the inner ear side of the oval window is the cochlea. The **cochlea** is a sensory organ shaped like a snail circling around on itself. The outside of the cochlea consists of bone and is part of the temporal bone of the skull.

The cochlea has three layers inside it, each filled with fluid, with membranes separating one layer from the next. When the bones of the middle ear shake the oval window, fluid in the cochlea starts to "slosh" around, creating a wave or motion. Sound that previously traveled through air, tissue, and bone now is traveling through fluid. The membranes inside the cochlea are affected by this wave in the fluid and start to move back and forth (vibrate).

Organ of Corti

The **Organ of Corti** is a structure in the middle layer of the cochlea. The Organ of Corti contains many different types of cells, including **hair cells**, which have an electrical charge due to their chemical composition. When the membrane is pressed on by fluid, the electrical discharge is picked up by nerve endings from the auditory nerve in the center core of the cochlea.

CLINIC BOX: Hearing by the Numbers

Here is a quick summary of what we have discussed so far about sound in the air and the ear—a sort of hearing by the numbers:

- 3-D of sound: Time, frequency, and intensity
- Three requirements for sound: Energy source, sound source, and elastic medium
- Three decibel scales: Sound pressure level (SPL), hearing level (HL), and sensation level (SL)
- Three parts of the ear: Outer, middle, and inner
- Two mechanisms of hearing: Conductive and sensorineural
- Two methods of middle ear impedance matching: Ossicular lever and window size

CLINIC BOX: Ion Channels and Positivity: How the Magic Happens

Motion in the cochlea turns into electrical impulses in the auditory nerve. The hair cells and fluids in the cochlea have unique and different chemical compositions. As the fluid sloshes back and forth in the cochlea, parts of the hair cells flip and flop back and forth. When the hair cell is "flipped" a door on its side opens. When the hair cell is "flopped" the door on its side closes. The name of that door is an ion channel. When the ion channel is open, the chemical compositions of the hair cell and the fluid it is in mix together. The biggest change that happens is that positively charged particles (a type of ion) move from the fluid into the hair cell. When the ion channel is closed, the hair cell resets to go back to its original chemical composition. For that to happen, it has to get rid of those extra positive ions. It sends those positive ions out, and that discarding of charged particles is picked up by the auditory nerve. That is, when the hair cells discharge, they send an electrical signal to the auditory nerve. This is how motion in the inner ear becomes an electrical signal traveling up the auditory nerve to the brain.

Sound in the Brain

In this final stage, speech reception concludes and speech perception begins.

The Auditory Nerve

The **auditory nerve** is a branch of the vestibulocochlear nerve, or cranial nerve VIII. The cochlea is wrapped around a branch of this nerve so that the nerve is in the center of the cochlea. The electrical impulse in the auditory nerve leaves the center of the cochlea and travels until it connects to the brain stem.

Central Auditory Pathway

The **brain stem** is the connector or junction between the spinal cord and the brain—so it is a part of the human central nervous system. There are three structures within the brain stem: the **medulla**, the **pons**, and the **midbrain**, the latter of which is the part of the brain stem closest to the brain.

The electrical signal travels up the brain stem. The pons is the first location to receive input from both the right and the left ears, allowing the process of comparing differences between sounds received at both ears to begin, leading to spatial orientation. From there, the electrical signal travels to the midbrain and then to the thalamus. From the thalamus, the electrical signal goes to Heschl's Gyrus, which is the primary auditory cortex in the temporal lobe of the brain. Information then travels to other cortical areas, including auditory association areas.

The End is the Beginning

Speech reception entails sound traveling via air, bone and tissue, fluid, and electricity. Where speech reception ends, speech perception begins, turning these electrical impulses into meaningful speech and communication.

Splice It

An end goal of speech sound production is to communicate a message or intent. That is, listeners not only need to *receive* speech, but also *perceive* speech. So how do humans make sense of the received coded auditory information? My suggestion is that we **SPLICE** it, using Sensory cues, Perceptual decisions, Linguistic cues, Indexical cues, Cognitive skills, and Environmental cues.

S: Sensory Cues

The auditory pathway and the encoding of sound obviously play a critical role in speech reception and speech perception. However, remember that other senses are simultaneously providing sensory input and information that can influence speech reception and speech perception. To illustrate, while a listener hears speech, they may also *see* the speaker, may *feel* the ground beneath their feet, or *smell* a cup of coffee in their hand, all of which may influence their speech perception.

P: Perceptual Decisions

A **percept** is the meaning assigned to the sensory input. The decision of what meaning to assign to sensory input is influenced by past knowledge and experiences. Given this, we interpret sensory input and make decisions about what our senses are telling us, which may or may not be the same as the intended message.

L: Linguistic Cues

Language and linguistics impose a sort of structure on which to map the received sound and determine which possible meaning (allowed according to linguistic rules) it best matches. That is, when making perceptual decisions regarding speech, listeners apply their knowledge of language(s). Specifically, knowing which sounds are present in a language and how they can be connected (phonology) limits the possibilities of what a speaker said. Similarly, knowledge of how a language sequences sound may alter its acoustic characteristics and can affect the ability to correctly interpret and perceive speech. At the syllabic or morphemic level, knowing what prefixes or endings words can take (morphology), meanings they represent (semantics), how morphemes are sequenced (syntax), and how language is shaped by context (discourse-pragmatics), all influence perceptual decisions.

I: Indexical Cues

Different talkers have differently shaped vocal tracts, leading to variations in the acoustic characteristics of their voices. *Who* produced the speech sound can influence a listener's perception of the speech in different ways (Kreiman & Sidtis, 2011). For example

- A speaker may have specific quirks in how they speak.
- A listener may be very familiar with the speaker, or perhaps doesn't know the speaker at all (see, for example, Nygaard, Sommers, & Pisoni, 1994).
- A speaker may have an either familiar or unfamiliar accent or a dialect (see, for example, Bradlow & Bent, 2008).

C: Cognitive Skills

Connected speech entails rapid processing, even when the speech is slow, requiring our speech reception and perception systems to keep pace with masses of incoming information. Memory and attention, among many other cognitive skills, helps us process speech and make use of linguistic knowledge.

Memory. Some information needs to be stored in memory as we make the best match or the best guess as to what a speaker said (see, for example, Pisoni, 1973, 1993). Receiving and perceiving speech memory systems require

- Short-term memory (what was said just prior, what were the characteristics of the prior speech)
- Working memory (ability to manipulate short-term memory to, for example, weigh different possibilities of the intended message based on speech characteristics)
- Long-term memory (knowledge of semantics and syntax)

Attention. Attention skills influence our ability to focus on incoming auditory information, especially when the message competes for a listener's attention. For example, speech perception occurs while a listener might also be checking notifications on their phone, texting, or wondering what they will have for lunch.

E: Environmental Cues

Do you remember that sound wave we discussed at the beginning of this chapter? That travels through air to reach the ear and start the journey up the auditory pathway? Now imagine that sound wave mixing with one, two, three, or a dozen different sound waves occurring in the environment at the same time. Perhaps you can picture a family gathering where many people are all talking at once, or a restaurant with sounds from the kitchen, utensils clattering on dishes, and multiple conversations. These examples illustrate that the speech you want to hear does not often occur in an isolated environment. It competes with other sounds.

Another environmental feature (although it could also be considered another branch of linguistics) is the pragmatic environment. What is the purpose of the communication? Is it personal or professional? What is the social context? For example, are you interviewing for a job, trying to impress someone, talking with your mom on the phone, or goofing off with your best friend? All these varied contexts may influence speech perception.

Conclusions

Major topics addressed in this chapter include

1. The three important dimensions of sound waves are time, frequency, and intensity.
2. The main parts of the ear are the outer, middle, and inner ear.
3. Many factors affect how listeners perceive speech sounds, including sensory input as well as lexical, indexical, cognitive, and environmental features and knowledge.

Review Questions

1. What are some examples of the different mediums a sound wave travels through after it is produced by a talker and before it is fully perceived by a listener?
2. What are examples of different properties of a sound wave, and how would you define them?
3. What is the difference between a longitudinal wave and a transverse wave? Which type of wave is sound?
4. What does the inverse square law mean?
5. Other than how sound travels through the auditory pathway, what are some examples of other features that might influence how a listener perceives speech?
6. What are the names of the bones in the ossicular chain, and in which part of the ear are they located?
7. What are the two ways that the middle ear makes sure the sound wave has enough "oomph" to travel through the fluid in the inner ear (that has a higher impedance)?
8. What does it mean to receive and to perceive speech?

Recommended Readings

If you want to read further about topics in speech reception and perception, here is a list of books and articles that may interest you.

Denes, P. B., & Pinson E. N. (2007). *The speech chain: The physics and biology of spoken language* (2nd ed.). New York, NY: W. H. Freeman.

Hamill, T. A., & Price, L. L. (2014). *The hearing sciences* (2nd ed.). San Diego, CA: Plural.

Hughes, G. B., & Pensak, M. L. (2007). *Clinical otology* (3rd ed.). New York, NY: Thieme.

Katz, J., Chasin, M., English, K., Hood, L. J., & Tillery, K. L. (2015). *Handbook of clinical audiology* (7th ed.). Philadelphia, PA: Wolters Kluwer.

Martin, F. N., & Clark, J. G. (2015). *Introduction to audiology* (12th ed.). Boston, MA: Pearson.

Mattys, S. L., & Wiget, L. (2011). Effects of cognitive load on speech recognition. *Journal of Memory and Language, 65,* 145–160.

McGurk, H., & MacDonald, J. (1976). Hearing lips and seeing voices. *Nature, 264,* 746–748.

Nolte, J. (2002). *The human brain: An introduction to its functional anatomy* (5th ed.). St. Louis, MO: Mosby.

Pisoni, D. B., & Remez, R. E. (Eds.). (2005). *The handbook of speech perception.* Malden, MA: Blackwell.

Tye-Murray, N. (2015). *Foundations of aural rehabilitation: Children, adults, and their family members* (4th ed.). Stanford, CT: Cengage Learning.

References

Bradlow, A. R., & Bent, T. (2008). Perceptual adaptation to non-native speech. *Cognition, 106,* 707–729.

Emanuel, D. C., & Letowski, T. (2009). *Hearing science.* Philadelphia, PA: Wolters Kluwer, Lippincott Williams & Wilkins.

Kreiman, J., & Sidtis, D. (2011). *Foundations of voice studies: An interdisciplinary approach to voice production and perception.* Malden, MA: Wiley-Blackwell.

Nygaard, L. C., Sommers, M. S., & Pisoni, D. B. (1994). Speech perception as a talker-contingent process. *Psychological Science, 5*(1), 42–46.

Pisoni, D. B. (1973). Auditory and phonetic memory codes in the discrimination of consonants and vowels. *Perception & Psychophysics, 13*(2), 253–260.

Pisoni, D. B. (1993). Long-term memory in speech perception: Some new findings on talker variability, speaking rate and perceptual learning. *Speech Communication, 13*(1–2), 109–125.

CHAPTER 5

PHONETICS WARM-UP

This is the first "learn by doing" chapter. Its topic is phonetics, an essential tool in assessment and treatment of children with speech sound disorders. Topics include:

- Transcription
- International Phonetic Alphabet
- Notations
- Exercises

Learning Objectives

I hope on completing the chapter you will

- Appreciate the need for phonetic transcription
- Know where to find consonant and vowel charts
- Understand basic phonetic notations
- Complete speech exercises on phonetics

Key Words

Key words you will encounter in this chapter

International Phonetic Alphabet
Brackets
Slashes
Phonemes
x becomes y
Broad transcription
Narrow transcription
Trochaic stress

Transcription

If you ever wondered why we transcribe speech, consider four short words

Knee

Key

King

Peak

In these words, four different letters and letter combinations represent a single vowel: the "e" sound in *knee* (*ee*), *key* (*ey*), *king* (*i*), and *peak* (*ea*). Further, in *knee* the *k* is silent and in *king* the *n* and *g* coalesce to form a single sound. Similar inconsistencies between pronunciation and spelling occur throughout English. If this weren't confusing enough, remember that the same letter can also represent different sounds, as in *peck* and *Pete*.

Blame the confusion on the printing press, which five centuries ago helped cement the English spelling system (Baugh & Cable, 2002). Since then, spelling of words has changed much more slowly than changes in pronunciation. If you suffered mastering (or not mastering) the oddities of English spelling in grade school, you may envy speakers of Hawaiian, a language which was set in writing far more recently than English and shows a much closer approximation between its spoken and written forms. In Hawaiian and other languages with relatively new written traditions, spelling typically is a reasonable approximation of pronunciation (Elbert & Pukui, 2001).

International Phonetic Alphabet

The **International Phonetic Alphabet** (IPA) of the International Phonetic Association (2005) offers the most widely used system of phonetic transcription. Tables 5–1 through 5–3 list the most frequently encountered IPA symbols for English consonants, vowels, and diphthongs. You will notice there are two vowel charts. That is because there are two widely used ways to describe vowels. Other systems of transcription also exist. If your training is a system other than IPA, you will have a small extra step translating between that system and the one this book uses.

CLINIC BOX: A Caution

Have some caution with articulatory definitions on consonant and vowel charts. For example, IPA lists [i] as made with the tongue tip raised, though a quick survey of friends and a little introspection shows most make [i] with the tongue tip down. Many sounds show similar articulatory variability, including [s] (tongue tip raised or lowered). Consonant and vowel charts typically do not show such variations.

TABLE 5–1. Consonants

Manner	Place							
	Bilabial	**Labiodental**	**Interdental**	**Alveolar**	**Postalveolar**	**Palatal**	**Velar**	**Glottal**
Oral stop	p b			t d			k g	
Fricative		f v	θ ð	s z	ʃ			
Affricate					tʃ dʒ			
Nasal stop	m			n			ŋ	
Liquid								
Central				rᵃ				
Lateral				l				
Glide	w					j		hᵇ

ᵃFor convenience, the book transcribes the central liquid as [**r**].

ᵇ[**h**] is categorized as a glide because in many ways it behaves as a glide in English. For example, [**h**], [**w**], and [**j**] can begin syllables but not close them. If you define [**h**] as a fricative, you will only need to make a few slight alterations in the analyses in this book.

TABLE 5–2. Vowels and Diphthongs

	Tongue Position				
	Front	**←**	**Central**	**→**	**Back**
Close	i				u
	ɪ				ʊ
Close mid	eɪ		ə	ɚ	oʊ
Open mid		ɛ	ʌ		ɔ
		æ			
Open			a		ɑ
Tongue Position	**Spread**	**←**	**Lips**	**→**	**Rounded**

Notes.

1. For convenience, the vowels [i] and [u] (which are often pronounced as diphthongs) are transcribed as [i] and [u], respectively.

2. *Open* replaced *low* and *close* replaced *high* in the revised International Phonetic Alphabet (International Phonetics Association, 2005).

3. Diphthongs:

    [ɔɪ] = tongue begins as for [ɔ] and moves toward [ɪ]
    [aɪ] = tongue begins as for [a] and moves toward [ɪ]
    [aʊ] = tongue begins as for [a] and moves toward [ʊ]
    [ɚ] = tongue shape has both [ə]-like and [r]-like qualities

TABLE 5–3. Vowels and Diphthongs

	Tongue Position				
	Front	**←**	**Central**	**→**	**Back**
High	i				u
	ɪ				ʊ
High mid	eɪ		ə	ɚ	oʊ
Low mid		ɛ	ʌ		ɔ
		æ			
Low			a		ɑ
Tongue Position	**Spread**	**←**	**Lips**	**→**	**Rounded**

Note. Instead of close and open, some vowel diagrams use high and low.

Notations

Extensive use of notations is rare in clinic practice and I generally avoid their use in this book. Still, some notations are necessary; and others, although not necessary, prove extremely convenient.

[ ] or / /?

Brackets (sometimes also called square brackets) indicate a phonetic transcription, and **slashes** indicate a phonemic transcription. Within our profession, the convention is you can place single sounds, groups of sounds, and entire words or phrases within brackets or slashes. The following examples demonstrate the use of this notation:

1. **Example:** The consonant *b* as in *bet*.
   Notation: [b] or /b/
2. **Example:** Voiceless stops.
   Notation: [p t k] or /p t k/
3. **Example:** The word *deep*.
   Notation: [dip] or /dip/

I typically transcribe a child's speech within square brackets (e.g., *bee* as [bi]), because they imply nothing about the phonological status of the transcribed sounds. Slashes (e.g., *bee* as /bi/) indicate that the transcribed sounds are **phonemes**; that is, the sounds can distinguish between words in the child's speech, just as *p* and *b* do in adult English *pea* and *bee*.

Determining which sounds are phonemes in a child's speech is a controversial procedure and clinicians seldom perform it in most clinic settings. For this reason, except when a clinician undertakes a phonemic analysis, I enclose a transcription in square brackets rather than slashes. Ball, Müller, and Rutter (2009) offer a similar perspective. Additionally, they recommend the addition of straight vertical lines when a clinician believes sounds are constrastive in a child's phonological system.

x → y or y/x?

The literal meaning of the first notation is "**x becomes y**"; the literal meaning of the second notation is "**y for x.**" Both notations provide simple ways to describe speech changes. The arrow appears in linguistically oriented approaches, and the slash in more traditional approaches. The book favors "x becomes y" because I find it more intuitive. The following examples demonstrate these notations:

1. **Example:** The child says [w] for [r].
   Notation: r → w or w/r

2. **Example:** The child says fricatives as stops.
   Notation: fricatives → stops or stops/fricatives

3. **Example:** The child deletes both members of consonant clusters.
   Notation: CC → ø or ø/CC

x → y/z

This algebraic-looking notation literally means, "x becomes y in the environment of z." The notation describes how a phonetic or word environment affects production of speech. The *x* and *y* can be any articulation and phonological unit—features, consonants, vowels, individual sounds, syllables, or stress. The *z* typically is a distinctive feature, consonant, vowel, a syllable boundary (symbolized as *S*), or a word boundary (symbolized as "#"). The following examples demonstrate the use of this notation:

1. **Example:** The child says liquids as glides in the beginning of words.
   Notation: liquids → glides/# ____

2. **Example:** The child says [s] as [z] between vowels.
   Notation: s → z/V____V

3. **Example:** The child says [g] as [k] at the end of syllables.
   Notation: g → k/____S

4. **Example:** The child deletes the first member of a consonant cluster in the beginning of words.
   Notation: CC → øC/#____

Exercises

Exercise 1

This and Exercise 2 provide practice using distinctive features to classify speech sounds. The first exercise asks you to identify speech sounds within a sound class, and the next exercise asks you to identify sound classes based on the sounds they contain. (***Hint:*** If you don't remember—or don't know—a phonetic term, Appendix B contains a long list of speech terms.)

Problem

1. Which sound classes are obstruents? *This is an example.*
2. Which consonant places of production are labial?
3. Which vowels are front?
4. Which consonant is a voiceless alveolar fricative?
5. Which feature distinguishes [f] from [v]?
6. Which features distinguish [p] from [d]?
7. Which sound is voiced, interdental, and fricative?
8. Which sound is palatal?
9. Which sound is liquid and central?
10. Which sounds are voiceless stops?
11. Which sounds are approximants?
12. Which sound is lateral?

Answer Sheet

1. Obstruents: *oral stops, fricatives, affricates*
2. Labial:
3. Front:
4. Voiceless alveolar fricative:
5. [f] from [v]:
6. [p] from [d]:
7. Voiced, interdental, fricative:
8. Palatal:
9. Liquid and central:
10. Voiceless stops:
11. Approximants:
12. Lateral:

Exercise 2

Understanding a child's speech abilities often requires identifying the sound class to which groups of sounds belong. This exercise provides practice in this important aspect of clinical care. Unless specifically asked, it isn't necessary to list all of a sound's distinctive features. To illustrate, the complete list of distinctive features for [l] is voiced, alveolar, liquid, and lateral. However, as [l] is the only lateral in English, the distinctive feature lateral is sufficient to distinguish [l] from all other sounds.

Problem

Use distinctive features to define the sounds and groups of sounds listed on the answer sheet. *The first word is an example.*

Answer Sheet

1. f v: *labiodental*
2. l:
3. p t k:
4. s:
5. l r:
6. j:
7. i (Table 2):
8. i (Table 3):
9. t d n s z l r:
10. k g ŋ:

Exercise 3

Special notations are a convenient type of shorthand. This exercise provides practice in their use.

Problem

1. Make a phonemic transcription of *k* in *key*. *This is an example.*
2. Make a phonetic transcription of *k* in *key*.
3. Make a phonetic transcription of bilabial oral stops.
4. Make a phonetic transcription of *duke*.
5. Indicate that a child says [t] as [d], using both linguistically based and traditional notations.
6. Indicate that a child says liquids as glides, using both linguistically based and traditional notations.
7. Indicate that a child deletes the second consonant in clusters containing two consonants, using both linguistically based and traditional notations.
8. Indicate that a child says [g] as [k] at the ends of words.
9. Indicate that a child says voiceless fricatives as voiced fricatives between vowels.
10. Indicate that a child says *two* as [tu] or [du].

Answer Sheet

1. phonemic: /k/
2. phonetic:
3. bilabial oral stops:
4. duke:
5. [t] as [d]:
6. liquids as glides:
7. deletion:
8. [g] as [k]:
9. between vowels:
10. [tu] or [du]:

Exercise 4

Speech sounds (consonants, vowels, and diphthongs) are often the major focus of evaluation and treatment. A transcription that includes only the sounds in the consonant and vowel charts is a **broad transcription**. A more detailed transcription of speech is a **narrow transcription**. Appendix A at the end of this book contains diacritics and special symbols for narrow transcription. This and Exercise 5 provide practice in broad transcription.

Problem

Transcribe each word on the answer sheet as you would say them carefully in isolation; or, better yet, have someone say each word carefully and slowly and transcribe that person's speech. *The first word is an example.*

Answer Sheet

1. Cat: *kæt*
2. Thin:
3. Unite:
4. Brew:
5. Giving:
6. Fingernail polish:
7. Century:
8. Please:
9. Winter:
10. Between:

Exercise 5

For additional practice, use a broad transcription to transcribe the following words, giving special attention to any sounds you may have mistranscribed in Exercise 4.

Problem

As in the previous exercise, transcribe each word as you would say it carefully in isolation; or, better yet, have someone say each word carefully and slowly and transcribe that person's speech.

Answer Sheet

1. Dog:
2. Money:
3. Sat:
4. Judge:
5. Mastering:
6. Phonetic symbols:
7. Sheep:
8. Loud:
9. Ketchup:
10. Yes:

Exercise 6

Syllables play an important role in the assessment and treatment of speech sound disorders. Many children in earlier developmental stages, for example, have difficulty pronouncing voiceless sounds in the beginning of syllables and words, leading them to say words such as *pen* and *toe* as *bee* and *doe*, respectively. Many children also experience difficulties pronouncing voiced sounds at the end of syllables, leading them to pronounce words such as *pig* and *bib* as *pick* and *bip*, respectively. Other influences of syllables on speech also occur in more advanced developmental stages. This exercise deals with syllable structure and the Exercise 7 focuses on syllable sequences.

Problem

Transcribe the words and phrases on the answer sheet and then place *S* (for syllable) above your phonetic transcription, drawing lines between *S* and each speech sound in the syllable. Say the words slowly and carefully. *The first word is an example.* Next, transcribe the phrases "it is" and "this time," again, saying the phrases once slowly and carefully and then quickly and casually. Describe in the discussion question how their syllable structure changes in more rapid and casual speech. (***Hint:*** Listen carefully to the last consonant in "it" and "this.")

Answer Sheet

1. Diaper: daɪ pɚ

2. Pretend:

3. Banana:

4. Branches:

5. Abalone:

6. Winter:

7. It is:

8. This time:

9. For discussion:

Exercise 7

Not all sequences of sounds in syllables are equally difficult. For example, all other things being equal, a child is likely to experience less difficulty with a CV sequence (as in *two*) than a CCCVC sequence (as in *strap*). This exercise provides opportunities to identify sequences of syllables in words.

Problem

Describe the words on the answer sheet in terms of sequence of consonants and vowels within the syllable. Indicate syllable boundaries with a period (.). *The first word is an example.* (***Hint:*** Indicate syllable boundaries as you would say the words and phrases slowly and carefully.)

Answer Sheet

1. Below: *CV.CV*
2. Sunday:
3. Infatuate:
4. Eye:
5. Winter:
6. Egg:
7. Etch:
8. Powerful emotions:
9. Spread:
10. Knight:

Exercise 8

Stress is yet another dimension of speech that can influence a child's ability to pronounce words and phrases. For example, because English favors words with stress on the first syllable (called a **trochaic stress** pattern), a child in an earlier stage in development may delete the first unstressed syllable in words such as *banana* and *beginning*, while a more developmentally advanced child may continue to have difficulty with unstressed syllables in longer words such as *refrigerator* and *astronomy*. This exercise provides opportunities to identify primary stress in multisyllabic words.

Problem

Identify which syllable in each word receives primary stress. Although it is not necessary to do so, you may also wish to capitalize all the letters in the syllable that receives primary stress. *The first word is an example.* (**Hint:** If you experience problems identifying the syllable that receives primary stress, say each word several times, changing the syllable that receives primary stress. For example, pronounce balloon with exaggerated primary stress as BA lloon and ba LLOON. The pronunciation that sounds most natural is likely the one with primary stress on the correct syllable.)

Answer Sheet

1. Begin: *be GIN*
2. Bishop:
3. Happiness:
4. Astronomy:
5. Telescope:
6. Meadow:
7. Failure:
8. Apologize:
9. Believer:
10. Astrophysics:

Exercise 9

This exercise focuses on analyzing assimilations in words, a frequent occurrence in the speech of younger children. The first two questions ask you to define the difference between progressive and regressive types of assimilation. The remaining seven questions ask you both to identify the type of assimilation—progressive, regressive, or both progressive and regressive—and, much more importantly, provide a reasonable phonetic explanation for why the assimilation occurs.

Problem

1. What is progressive assimilation? *This is an example.*
2. What is regressive assimilation?
3. Why is [n] usually a dental consonant in the word *tenth*? (*Hint:* For this and the following questions, provide a reasonable phonetic explanation for why the assimilation occurs along with identifying whether the assimilation is progressive, regressive, or both.)
4. Why is [r] usually voiceless in *pride*?
5. Explain in your own words why some speakers say *sandwich* as *samwich*.
6. Explain in your own words why people often pronounce *something* with a [p] between the [m] and [θ]. (*Hint:* The same explanation illustrates why most speakers place a [p] between [m] and [s] in *Chomsky*, leading that well-known linguist's name to be pronounced *Chompsky*.)
7. Explain in your own words why a child might pronounce the final [d] in *bead* as [b].
8. Explain in your own words why a child might pronounce *peak* as [kik].
9. *For discussion:* Explain in your own words why a child might correctly pronounce [t] as [t] when the sound occurs before front vowels (for example, in words such as *tea*), but might pronounce [t] as [k] when the sound occurs before back vowels (for example, in words such as *two*).

Answer Sheet

1. Progressive assimilation: *influence of an earlier sound on a later sound*
2. Regressive assimilation:
3. Tenth:
4. Pride:
5. Sandwich:
6. Something:
7. Bead:
8. Peak:
9. *For discussion:*

Conclusions

Topics addressed in this chapter, the first of four "learn by doing" chapters, include

1. Phonetic transcription provides an unambiguous record of speech.
2. The International Phonetic Alphabet (IPA) provides a well-established catalogue of phonetic symbols.
3. Special notations sometimes are convenient in transcribing and analyzing speech.
4. Practice exercises prepare you for the analysis of speech sound disorders.

Review Questions

1. What is the definition of IPA?
2. What do some phonetic transcription systems use instead of close and open?
3. What do square brackets imply about the phonological status of the transcribed sounds?
4. What are phonemes?
5. Give an example to show you understand the use of the notation "x → y."
6. What is the difference between a broad transcription and a narrow transcription?
7. What does the symbol *S* mean?
8. What does CV mean?

References

Ball, M. J., Müller, N., & Rutter, B. (2009). *Phonology for communication disorders*. Hove, UK: Psychology Press.

Baugh, A., & Cable, T. (2002). *A history of the English language* (5th ed.). London, UK: Routledge.

Elbert, S., & Pukui, M. (2001). *Hawaiian grammar.* Honolulu, HI: University of Hawaii Press.

International Phonetic Association. (2005). *International phonetic alphabet*. Retrieved from http://www.langsci.ucl.ac.uk/ipa/index

PART II
SPEECH DEVELOPMENT

CHAPTER 6
INFANTS

Because an infant cannot know beforehand which language they will learn, a child is born able to learn any language. This means, for example, that an infant who grows up learning English also can learn approximately 7,099 other languages (Ethnologue, 2017). Understanding *what* a child learns about speech, *when* (at which ages) they learn it, and *how* they learn it, gives us tools to help a child with speech challenges. This chapter focuses on the youngest learners. Topics include:

- Speech Perception
- Vocal Production
- Sound Communication

The three major topics—speech perception, vocal production, and sound communication—in the chapter interact with one another. Think of speech perception and vocal production as the building blocks that create the foundation on which sound communication stands. Subsequent chapters in this section discuss the same topics in toddlers (1 to 2 years), preschoolers, (2 to 5 years), and students (5 years and older). The section concludes with a "learn by doing" chapter focusing on classic studies in speech development.

Learning Objectives

I hope on completing the chapter you will

- Understand why an infant begins life capable of learning any language.
- Describe how intonation helps an infant communicate when the meaning of words is unclear.
- List three contributions of babbling to future speech development.
- Describe how an infant learns to speak.

Key Words

Key words you will encounter in this chapter

Categorical perception
Primary auditory cortex
Reflexive vocalizations (vegetative sounds)
Cooing
Vocal play
Canonical babbling (babbling)
Reduplicated babbling
Nonreduplicated babbling
Variegated babbling (jargon)
Bonding
Speech input
Motherese
Familiar social routines

Speech Perception

You don't want a newborn in your phonetics class if it is graded on a curve. The world's languages contain approximately 600 different consonants and 200 different vowels (Ladefoged, 2001; Ladefoged & Johnson, 2010), and an infant is born potentially able to hear all of them. Development of speech perception in infants largely consists of fine-tuning a child's abilities to fit the sounds in the language of the community (Kuhl, 2004, 2007; Mehler, Bertoncini, & Barriere, 1978; Vihman, 1996; Werker & Hensch, 2015; Zhao & Kuhl 2016). Major perceptual developments occur in intonation and speech sounds.

Intonation

An infant's education in speech begins before birth while floating in the womb and hearing mother's voice as she speaks. Do you remember that swimming pool game in which children speak to each other under water? That may be like what an unborn child hears when their mother speaks: mostly intonation, very little information about consonants and vowels.

I Know That Voice

Researchers know that an unborn infant hears mother's voice because a newborn will turn toward a recording of her voice when it plays from a speaker on one side while another's voice plays on the other side (Mehler et al., 1978). Such recognition may foster bonding between infant and parent early in life when a child is maximally dependent on others to survive. Infants continue to pay attention to intonation as they grow.

Development

At 3 months, an infant may imitate the intonation contour of a caregiver (Gratier & Devoucher, 2011). Throughout infancy, intonation helps a child communicate even when the meaning of words is unclear. To illustrate, near six months, a child may stop an activity when a parent says *no* in a commanding voice (Hedrick, Prather, & Tobin, 1984). Parents often assume this shows a child understands *no* and, by ceasing the action, is demonstrating compliance. However, compliance is based on intonation, rather than knowing what *no* means. It's too perverse to recommend, but if parents wished, they could say *yes* instead of *no* (or *dog* or *bus*, for that matter) with a commanding voice and a 6-month-old child would likely respond as if *no* were spoken.

Speech Sounds

To acquire a language, an infant must discover individual sounds buried in the rapid flow of speech—not an easy task, since people seldom speak sounds in isolation. Sounds change in pronunciation depending on syllable position and presence of adjoining sounds, and people speak at rates of nine or more sounds per second. Finding speech sounds would probably be impossible were it not for an infant's mammalian heritage, which includes possessing a cochlea and hearing mechanism capable of **categorical perception**—that is, able to divide the speech stream into individual sounds (Eimas, Siqueland, Jusczyk, & Vigorito, 1971; Jusczyk, 1992).

Categorical Perception

Categorical perception divides the flow of speech. It exists at birth. When tested in the weeks following delivery, an infant's perception of speech sounds in the ambient language is the same as their perception of speech sounds in other languages. During infancy, experience shapes a child's speech perception abilities, and by the first birthday, a child has superior perception for sounds in the language spoken in the community compared to those in other languages (Kuhl, 2010; Zhang & Merzenich, 2001). According to Kuhl, during infancy, a child moves from "a citizen of the world" to a citizen of a specific language. The presumed neurological basis of this change in speech perception is maturation of the **primary auditory cortex**, which is a sensory area adjacent to Wernicke's area in the temporal lobe (Pascallis, de Hann, & Nelson, 2002).

Vocal Production

Infant vocalizations provide "practice" for later speech development (Bleile, 1998; Bleile, Stark, & Silverman McGowan, 1993; Jusczyk, 1992; Locke, 1983; Locke & Pearson, 1992; Vihman & Miller, 1988). Infant vocalizations establish a connection between their speech perception and vocal production systems, a link between ear and mouth. An infant who vocalizes *mmm,* for example, learns that closing the mouth, vibrating the larynx, and emitting air through the nose creates the perception of *m* (Goldstein & Schwade, 2008).

As Table 6–1 indicates, vocal production in infants proceeds in five stages (Goldstein & Schwade, 2008; Gratier & Devouche, 2011; Stark, 1980). Of the five stages, give special attention to canonical babbling (the fourth stage), because, arguably, it is the one most relevant to future speech development. Infancy ends with the child vocally in control of a small repertoire of sounds and syllables that serve as material for future word building.

TABLE 6–1. Vocal Development in Infants

Age	Vocalizations
0–2 months	Reflexive vocalization
2–4 months	Cooing
4–6 months	Vocal play
6–10 months	Canonical babbling
10–12 months	Variegated babbling

Sources: Stark (1980) and Oller (1992).

Reflexive Vocalizations

Mammalian oral tracts are noisy, as anyone who has spent time around cows and pigs will agree. During the first few months, an infant's sound making consists of **reflexive vocalizations** (also called **vegetative sounds**), which occur as a by-product of breathing in and out while moving the tongue and jaw. When the mouth is relatively wide open, a sound may emerge that seems vowellike, and when the articulators are relatively close together, a sound may emerge that seems consonantlike.

Something like an [e]

To illustrate, suppose an infant is sitting up with the tongue lying flat in their mouth, and they breathe out. The result will likely be a sound something like an [e]. However, the sound is not a true vowel because it lacks the fine motor coordination and timing of an adult vowel. Another way to say it: [e] is just a sound that occurs when the tongue lies flat in the mouth and the other articulators are far apart. Similarly, if an infant's articulators are closer together when they exhale (or inhale, for that matter), they will make a consonantlike sound. The origin of vowels and consonants lies in those first few months as an infant makes reflexive sounds while opening and closing the mouth.

CLINIC BOX: Wow! Quite a Difference

One reason an infant doesn't sound like an adult is that their vocal tract is startling different than ours (Kent & Murray, 1982). An infant's vocal tract is approximately 7 to 8 cm at birth (our adult vocal tracts are 15 to 18 cm) and an infant's larynx lies high in the throat, providing protection against choking, while ours lies midway in our throats (Vorperian et al., 2009). The larynx gradually descends during infancy, though it does not reach its mature throat position until the middle of the second year. Additionally, an infant's tongue lies more forward in the mouth than ours, and their vocal tract is a gradual slope and ours is right bending. Their velopharynx and epiglottis also lie closer together compared to ours (Bosma, 1986).

Cooing

Near two to four months, sounds made toward the back of the mouth (**cooing**) become more prevalent among an infant's vocalizations. You may hear sounds that are [**k**]-like, [**g**]-like, and [**x**]-like, and other sounds that you can only classify as "velar or pharyngeal fricative maybe kinda voiced sorta things." Here are three alternative explanations for why an infant's vocalizations change from reflexive to cooing:

1. Around three months, myelination (myelin is a white fatty substance that covers axons), which proceeds rapidly during the first year, reaches the area of an infant's motor homunculus (an electrical depiction of the nerve endings of the body) that

controls movements to the back of the mouth, somehow favoring production of those sounds (Evans & Hutchins, 2002).

2. Another possible explanation is that the larynx, which descends the throat during the first and second year, allows an infant to produce a wider variety of sounds.

3. Other possible explanations for this intriguing developmental change could involve the oral structure, which changes considerably during infancy.

Vocal Play

Near four to six months, sounds near the front of the mouth (**vocal play**) become prominent among an infant's vocalizations. Sometimes investigators call this stage *sound play*. During this stage, you may hear raspberries, trills, and [**b**]-like and [**d**]-like sounds.

Canonical Babbling

Canonical babbling (or simply **babbling**, if you prefer) is defined as sound making in which 20% or higher of the vocalizations contain a consonant and vowel within the same syllable. These vocalizations occur among an infant's sound making between six to ten months.

Chickens and Eggs

Canonical babble consists either of repetitions of a same consonant in a syllable, such as [**ba ba ba**] (called **reduplicated babble**), or repetitions of different consonants in the same syllable, such as [**ba da da**] (called **nonreduplicated babble**). Which comes first, reduplicated or nonreduplicated babbling? Researchers once believed that reduplicate babbling preceded nonreduplicated babble, but research now indicates that the two typically co-occur in infant vocalizations and that one type need not precede the other.

Why It Matters

Canonical babbling matters because it advances speech development in at least three ways: syllables, speech sounds, and individual differences.

- **Syllables:** Syllables are a foundation of language. Think of them as train cars that carry consonants and vowels. Canonical babbling represents an infant's growing ability to pack consonants and vowels into syllables, controlling time transitions between sounds lasting less than one-third of a second.
- **Speech Sounds:** Amazingly, under five months, infant vocalizations around the world sound similar (Boysson-Bardies, & Vihman, 1991). To illustrate, a 4-month-old in France vocalizes the same sounds as one in the United States, Indonesia, or Tibet. By 7 months, something has changed: French babies babble more French sounds, American babies babble more English sounds, and so forth. Canonical babbling reflects the effect of an infants' increasing exposure to and

experiences with the ambient language (Vihman, 1996). These babbled sounds provide building blocks for a child's spoken words.

■ **Individual Differences:** Infants vary in the sounds they babble. For example, you may hear one infant babble [**ba ba ba**], another [**da da da**], and yet another [**ba da ga**]. Years ago, Menn (1976) proposed that this variation results from an interaction between three factors: size and shape of the oral tract, the articulators, and chance. To illustrate the general idea, an infant who is breathing out and happens to close and open the lips at the same time may babble [**ba**], while another infant who happens to raise and lower the tongue tip to the alveolar ridge while breathing out may babble [**da**], or if the velum is lowered, [**n**].

Why do infants tend to babble certain sounds but not others? That is, why can you observe many infants babble [**ba ba ba**] or [**da ma ba**], but you will have great difficulty finding one babbling [**ra ra ra**]? Within Menn's perspective, the reason lies in the size and shape of an infant's oral tract and articulators, which make it more likely to stumble vocally on certain sounds than on others. To illustrate, an infant is more likely to vocally stumble on [**b**], [**d**], and [**m**] than [**l**] or [**r**]. This does not preclude the possibility of you someday discovering an infant who babbles [**la la la**], [**ra ra ra**], or even [**la ra la**]. However, given the size and shape of the oral tract and articulators, you will probably have to wait a long time to find an infant who vocally stumbles on those sounds.

Variegated Babbling

Variegated babbling (also called **jargon**) is canonical babbling under an adult-sounding intonation contour. It appears in the sound making of some—though not all—infants near ten to twelve months. Variegated babbling may reflect an infant's awareness of intonation combined with a growing ability to control canonical syllables. The result: to a listener, it sounds like an infant is babbling in sentences.

CLINIC BOX: A Comfort Zone

An infant vocalizes more when they are in their comfort zone, a state of well-being that can occur any time of day or night, with or without someone being present. Waking and drifting off to sleep are often preferred times for an infant to vocalize. To discover if an infant vocalizes when no one is present, consider asking a family member to purchase a baby monitor. If a baby monitor is not an option, listening behind an open doorway will do. Chapter 16, "Developmental Goals," discusses this topic from a clinical perspective.

Summary: In a Word

In a word—more accurately, in several sentences—in the first year, an infant makes great progress in speech perception and vocal development, the two building blocks of sound communication:

- Infants pay close attention to intonation.
- Categorical perception helps an infant discover individual sounds within the stream of speech.
- The earliest vocalizations arise while breathing and moving the mouth.
- Vocalizations progress to sounds in the back and then front of the mouth.
- Babbling establishes an infant's ability to make sounds in syllables.
- The first year of life closes with infant babbling occurring under an adult-sounding intonation contour.

Sound Communication

Through a combination of brain growth, stimulation from the environment, fine-tuning of perceptual abilities, and vocal practice, an infant lays down the foundations for future developments in communication. The major topics in sound communication in infants are

- What an Infant Learns
- How an Infant Learns
- Pulling It Together

What an Infant Learns

A child does not begin life knowing that sound plays a special role in communication. Learning such basic things as sound can mean and the "my turn–your turn" pattern of conversation are major accomplishments in infancy (Bruner, 1983; Wittmer & Petersen, 2017).

Sound Can Mean

An infant's world is a rich stew of sights, touches, smells, and noises, including machines rumbling, animals barking and mewing, air moving, and fabric rustling—not to mention people laughing, grunting, crying, and speaking. Categorical perception leads to an early realization that sounds people make may carry meaning (Chang & Thompson, 2011; Jusczyk, 1992). Thus, even as young as 4 to 6 months, an infant may turn on hearing their name, and a few months later, may look when someone names a family member (for example, "Where is mommy?").

My Turn–Your Turn

Conversations are like a game of catch in which people toss sound back and forth (Fillmore, 1975). As discussed in Chapter 1, "Speech," during a conversation, one person tosses a ball of sound and the other person catches it, tosses it back, and so the conversation goes: back and forth, back and forth. During the first year, a child acquires rudiments of "serve and return" conversational turn taking. By as early as 3 to 4 months, an infant may vocalize when spoken to, and by 5 to 6 months, may play sound and gesture games such as "peek-a-boo," though the parent may need to "take both sides of the conversation," moving their own and the infant's hands (Hedrick, Prather, & Tobin, 1984). By 9 to 10 months, an infant may initiate such games.

CLINIC BOX: Nature or Nurture?

Today almost all researchers agree that speech acquisition requires both a brain capable of learning and an environment dedicated to teaching. Thirty years ago, this reasonable sounding perspective would have been scientific heresy. At that time, much of the academic world interested in child development divided itself into two camps. A strong nativist view, which dominated much of linguistics, held that language learning resulted from the unfolding of a genetically determined program (Chomsky, 2002, 2006). An equally uncompromising version of behaviorism, which dominated much of psychology, held that learning in children resulted solely from environmental factors (Skinner, 2014, 2011). Thirty years of research suggests that strong versions of both nativism and behaviorism are incorrect: speech learning in children is not "all genes" or "all environment," but results from an interaction between the two.

How an Infant Learns

How does an infant discover that one lump of sound means *mommy* and that another lump means *daddy* or *cat* or something else entirely? How does an infant learn that in conversations sound volleys back and forth? Answering *how* questions are critical to helping an infant at risk for future speech difficulties (see Chapter 16, "Developmental Goals"). Probably every clinician offers a different explanation for *how*. I suggest that bonding, speech input, and familiar social routines are critical to placing an infant on the road to language.

Bonding

Bonding provides the emotional connection a parent needs to devote the enormous time and effort required to raise an infant. In the absence of bonding, would a caregiver go without all but a few hours of sleep during the first months of an infant's life? Care for a sick infant? Change 3,000 diapers (the average number of changes in a child's life)? Probably not.

Promoting Bonding. Successful interactions between a caregiver and an infant help to promote bonding. An early success for a mother may occur when a newborn hears her voice and looks toward her. Guiding an infant to sleep through the night can be another form of success, as can providing the care that helps a sick infant become well. Even diaper changing, not typically a caregiver's favorite occupation, provides opportunities for successful interactions and a feeling of taking care of a basic need of your child.

Speech Input

Adult speech has the power to transform the noise in a child's world into a ladder for learning (see Chapter 18, "Talking with Children"). **Speech input** that facilitates learning holds a child's interest, changes in response to a child's shifts in attention, and contains modifications that accommodate a child's experiences and developmental level (Goldstein & Schwade, 2008; Kuhl, 2004, 2007; Ramírez-Esparza, García-Sierra, & Kuhl, 2014, 2017). **Motherese**, Fatherese, and, more recently, Parentese are names of speech modifications made by adults when talking with infants.

Capturing an Infant's Attention. Motherese characteristics are vocal "ploys" to capture and hold an infant's wayward attention. They include

- Higher than usual pitch
- Talking about shared perceptions
- Exaggerated intonation
- Use of repetitions
- Calling attention to objects

Speech characteristics of Fatherese are somewhat different than Motherese (Shute & Wheldall, 1999), especially when fathers play with boys. Father's speech to infant girls has characteristics like those in Motherese (Lewis & Gregory, 1987).

Familiar Social Routines

The third critical factor for speech learning is **familiar social routines** (a reoccurring event or situation involving at least two people) (Bruner, 1983; Conboy & Kuhl, 2011; Metzoff, Kuhl, Movelian, & Sejnowski, 2009; Snow & Goldfield, 1983). The following analogy (hopefully) gives some insights into why familiar social routines matter so much in speech learning.

The Strange Case of Deeb. Picture yourself on a busy street in a far country (I don't know where, just someplace far away). People are hurrying by, talking and gesturing, cars and buses beeping, lights flashing, displays in gaudy store windows beckoning. People utter streams of sound at one another, gesturing. Maybe someone stops, looks at her companion, waves her arms, and among her stream of noise you hear something that sounds like *deeb*. You wonder: What does *deeb* mean? Is it a noun? A verb? Or is it even a word? Or is it part of a word, or several small words?

If learning the meaning of *deeb* seems hard in such a situation, imagine how much more challenging it would be for an infant. After all, at least you know that language underlies the human noise, and that the rushing air contains such things as sentences, words, and speech sounds. Also, you and the other people on the street share a common knowledge about communication, so, though you may not know what their words mean, you know that sound carries meaning and you have some sense of things that people likely talk about. Not so for an infant, who has a far less well-developed brain and does not share an adult's communication knowledge. And remember, talk is fast—9 to

13 speech sounds reach an infant's ear every second—and understanding speech requires interpreting events lasting one-third of a second.

Finding Deeb. Now imagine a different situation: you are in a grocery store in the same far country, purchasing food. You place your food on the conveyer belt, the clerk rings up the costs, stretches out his hand, and says, *deeb*. You put money in the clerk's hand, he takes your money, and returns your change. You then pick up your bags and walk out the door having successfully purchased your groceries because you figured out that *deeb* means something like *Please, pay me*.

How did you do it? That is, how did you figure out what *deeb* means? The answer is that you know the social routines of grocery stores: the customer collects food, brings it to a checkout counter, the clerk rings it up, and then asks for payment. In this way, your knowledge of a familiar social store routine, acquired over many repetitions of the experience, allows you to narrow down the possible meanings of *deeb* and buy your groceries.

Insight into Infants. If that analogy makes sense to you, then you have an insight into the value of familiar social routines in speech learning. Rather than a grocery store, an infant's routines include mealtime, diaper changing, bedtime, and playtime—all interactions with caregivers that occur over and over, in which an infant hears the same words every day referring to objects and activities that they can see and touch. If bonding *motivates* a caregiver to raise a child, and if speech input *simplifies* language for a child, then familiar social routines *provide the location* where learning speech for communication typically occurs.

Pulling It Together

These are major ideas in sound communication in infants

- An infant learns that sound can mean and that conversations involve taking turns with sound.
- A child needs both a brain able to learn and an environment dedicated to teaching speech.
- Bonding provides the emotional connection a parent needs to raise an infant.
- Speech input in the form of Motherese transforms the noise in a child's world into a ladder for learning.
- Familiar social routines provide an important location for learning.

Conclusions

This chapter discussed the following topics:

1. During infancy, a child lays down foundations for future speech development.
2. An infant begins with a speech perception mechanism capable of potentially hearing all sounds in the world's languages, but they end the first year with a perceptual system largely restricted to the sounds in the child's language community.

3. Whereas perception abilities begin widely and then narrow, vocal production begins narrowly and then broadens, growing during infancy from vegetative sounds to a small stock of consonants, vowels, and syllables.
4. An infant learns such fundamental communication building blocks as the "my turn–your turn" structure of conversation and a small stock of word meanings.

Review Questions

1. Why does an infant begin life with a speech perception mechanism able of learning any language?
2. Describe how intonation helps an infant communicate when the meaning of words is unclear.
3. What is categorical perception?
4. List three contributions of canonical babbling to future speech development.
5. Explain in your own words why commonalities and individual differences arise in canonical babbling.
6. At what age does an infant begin to demonstrate that they understand that sound can mean?
7. At what age does an infant begin to demonstrate that they understand "my turn–your turn" in conversations?
8. Explain in your own words why bonding is important to speech learning.
9. What is Motherese? Why is it important and what are its characteristics?
10. Why are familiar social routines important to speech learning?

References

Bleile, K. (1998). Speech development in the absence of babbling. In R. Paul (Ed.), *Speech/language connection* (Vol. 6). Baltimore, MD: Paul H. Brookes.

Bleile, K., Stark R., & Silverman McGowan, J. (1993). Evidence for the relationship between babbling and later speech development. *Clinical Linguistics and Phonetics, 7*, 319–337.

Bosma, J. F. (1986). *Anatomy of the infant head (Johns Hopkins series in contemporary medicine and public health)*. Baltimore, MD: Johns Hopkins University Press.

Boysson-Bardies, B., & Vihman, M. (1991). Adaptation to language: Evidence from babbling and first words in four languages. *Language, 67*, 297–319.

Bruner, J. (1983). *Child talk: Learning to use language*. Oxford, UK: Oxford University Press.

Chang, R., & Thompson, N. (2011). Whines, cries, and motherese: Their relative power to distract. *Journal of Social, Evolutionary, and Cultural Psychology, 5*, 131–141.

Chomksy, N. (2002) *Syntactic structures*. New York, NY: Mouton de Groyer.

Chomsky, N. (2006). *Language and mind*. New York, NY: Cambridge University Press.

Conboy, B., & Kuhl, P. (2011). Impact of second-language experience in infancy: Brain measures of first- and second-language speech perception. *Developmental Science, 14*(2), 242–248.

Eimas, P. D., Siqueland, E., Jusczk, P., & Vigorito, J. (1971). Speech perception in infants. *Science 22*, 303–306.

Ethnologue. (2017). Retrieved from http://www.ethnologue.com

Evans, O. B., & Hutchins, J. B. (2002). Development of the nervous system. In D. E. Haines (Ed.), *Fundamental neuroscience* (pp. 71–89). New York, NY: Churchhill Livingstone.

Fillmore, C. (1975). *Santa Cruz lectures on deixis: 1971.* Bloomington, IN: Indiana University Linguistics Club.

Goldstein, M., & Schwade, J. (2008). Social feedback to infants' babbling facilitates rapid phonological learning. *Psychological Science, 19*(5), 515–523.

Gratier, M., & Devouche, E. (2011). Imitation and repetition of prosodic contour in vocal interaction at 3 months. *Developmental Psychology, 47*(1), 67–76.

Hedrick, D., Prather, E., & Tobin, A. (1984). *Sequenced Inventory of Communication Development-R.* Seattle, WA: University of Washington Press.

Jusczyk, P. (1992). Developing phonological categories from the speech signal. In C. Ferguson, L. Menn, & C. Stoel-Gammon (Eds.), *Phonological development: Models, research, implications* (pp. 17–64). Timonium, MD: York Press.

Kent, R., & Murray, A. (1982). Acoustic features of infant vocalic utterances at 3, 6, and 9 months. *Journal of the Acoustical Society of America, 72*, 353–365.

Kuhl, P. (2004). Early language acquisition: Cracking the speech code. *Nature Reviews: Neuroscience, 5*, 831–843.

Kuhl, P. (2007). Is speech learning "gated" by the social brain? *Developmental Science, 10*, 110–120.

Kuhl, P. (2010). Brain mechanisms in early language acquisition. *Neuron, 67*, 713–727.

Ladefoged, P. (2001). *Vowels and consonants.* Cambridge, MA: Blackwell.

Ladefoged, P., & Johnson, K. (2010). *A course in phonetics* (6th ed.). New York, NY: Cengage.

Lewis, C., & Gregory, S. (1987). Parents' talk to their infants: The importance of context. *First Language, 7*, 201–216.

Locke, J. (1983). Phonological acquisition and change. New York: Academic Press.

Locke, J., & Pearson, D. (1992). Vocal learning and the emergence of phonological capacity: A neurobiological approach. In C. Ferguson, L. Menn, & C. Stoel-Gammon (Eds.), *Phonological development: Models, research, implications* (pp. 91–130). Timonium, MD: York Press.

Mayo Clinic. (2011). *Multiple sclerosis.* Retrieved from http://www.mayoclinic.com/health/multiple-sclerosis

Mehler, J., Bertoncini, J., & Barriere, M. (1978). Infant recognition of mother's voice. *Perception, 7*(5), 491–497.

Menn, L. (1976). *Pattern, control and contrast in beginning speech: A case study in the development of word form and word function* (Unpublished doctoral dissertation). University of Illinois, Champagne-Urbana, IL.

Metzoff, A., Kuhl, P., Movelian, J., & Sejnowski, (2009). Foundations for a new science of learning. *Science, 17*, 284–288.

Oller, K. (1992). Description of infant vocalizations and young child speech: Theoretical and practical tools. *Seminars in Speech and Language, 13*, 178–192.

Pascallis, O., de Haan, M., & Nelson, C. (2002). Is face processing species specific during the first year of life? *Science, 296*, 1321–1323.

Ramírez-Esparza, N., García-Sierra, A., & Kuhl, P. K. (2014). Look who's talking: Speech style and social context in language input to infants are linked to concurrent and future speech development. *Developmental Science, 17*(6), 880–891.

Ramírez-Esparza, N., García-Sierra, A., & Kuhl, P. K. (2017). Look who's talking NOW! Parentese speech, social context, and language development across time. *Frontiers in Psychology, 20.* https://doi.org/10.3389/fpsyg.2017.01008

Shute, B., & Wheldall, K. (1999). Fundamental frequency and temporal modifications in the speech of British fathers to their children. *Educational Psychology, 19*, 221–233.

Skinner, B. F. (2011). *About behaviorism.* New York, NY: Vintage Books.

Skinner, B. F. (2014). *Verbal behavior.* Cambridge, MA: J. F. Skinner Foundation Reprint Series.

Snow, C., & Goldfield, B. (1983). Turn the page please: Situation-specific language acquisition. *Journal of Child Language, 10,* 551–569.

Stark, R. (1980). Stages of speech development in the first year of life. In G. Yeni-Komshian, J. Kavanagh, & C. Ferguson (Eds.), *Child phonology: Production* (pp. 73–92). New York, NY: Academic Press.

Vihman, M. (1996). *Phonological development: The origins of language in the child.* Cambridge, MA: Blackwell.

Vihman, M. & Miller, R. (1988). Words and babble at the threshold of lexical acquisition. In. M. D. Smith & J. L. Locke (Eds), *The emergent lexicon: The child's development of a linguistic vocabulary.* New York, NY: Academic Press.

Vorperian, H., Wang, S., Chung, M., Schimek, E., Durtschi, R., Kent, R., . . . Gentry, L. (2009). Anatomic development of the oral and pharyngeal portions of the vocal tract: An imaging study. *Journal of the Acoustic Society of America, 125*(3), 1666–1678.

Werker, J., & Hensch, T. (2015). Critical periods in speech perception: New directions. *Annual Review of Psychology, 66,* 173–196.

Wittmer, D., & Petersen, S. (2017). *Infant and toddler development and responsive program planning* (4th ed.). New York, NY: Pearson.

Zhang, L., & Merzenich, M. (2001). Persistent and specific influences of early acoustic environments on primary auditory cortex. *Nature Neuroscience, 4,* 1123–1130.

Zhao, T., & Kuhl, P. (2016). Effects of enriched auditory experience on infants' speech perception during the first year of life. *Prospects, 46,* 235–247.

CHAPTER 7

TODDLERS

Between their first and second birthday, a toddler goes from communicating through pointing, eye gaze, noises, and pulling by the arm, to expressing themselves primarily with words. This impressive developmental advance is the subject of this chapter. Topics include:

- Speech Perception
- Speech Production
- Sound Communication

Learning Objectives

I hope on completing the chapter you will

- Explain why toddlers with good speech perception make perceptual errors.
- Understand why endpoint sounds are earlier acquisitions than midpoint sounds.
- Describe the difference between independent and relational analyses.
- Explain how a growing brain may influence play behaviors.
- Understand a toddler's challenge to communicate.

Key Words

Key words you will encounter in this chapter

Expressive vocabulary
Phonetic inventories
Independent analysis
Relational analysis
Endpoints
Midpoints
Facilitative talk
Strategic errors
Modeling
Bombardment
Requests for confirmation or clarification
Parallel talk
Expansions
Communication strategies
Lexical selection (selectivity)
Word-based learning
Favorite sounds and word recipes
Gestalt learning (mature jargon)

Speech Perception

During the first year, the environment shaped an infant's speech perception mechanism to fit the language of the child's community. This development provided the infant a reliable modality through which to obtain information about the world. As the second year of life begins, a child increasingly turns these advanced speech perception abilities to the task of learning word meanings. A toddler perceives, for example, that one sound sequence means *dog* and another means *cat*.

Development

Thanks to an early maturing primary auditory cortex, a toddler comes to the challenge of speaking with the aid of advanced speech perception abilities (Maurer, 2005; Pascallis, de Hann, & Nelson, 2002). However, speech perception errors still occur; in fact, they occur so often and sometimes are so funny you find them sprinkled in comics and jokes. To illustrate, a toddler may call a *picnic table* a *pick me table* or a New Zealand toddler may call *email* an *emu*. Such errors are less a problem of a misfiring perceptual system and more to do with inattention, distraction, and lack of world and cultural knowledge (Brungart, 2001; Liebold, 2017).

Speech Production

During the first year, early sound making was a by-product of breathing in and out while opening and closing the mouth; later, sound making included babbling a small stock of sounds, syllables, and stress patterns. In the second year, a child increasingly expands this small phonetic stock to build their first **expressive vocabulary** (words that a child produces). As a toddler says these first words, they vocally "stumble on" other sounds, which further increases the stock of speech elements available for word building.

During the second year, clinically relevant developments in speech production occur in

- Consonants
- Vowels
- Syllables
- Stress

Two notes before beginning

1. This chapter does not discuss phonological processes (errors affecting sound classes) because they overlap in toddlers and early preschoolers; and so, to avoid redundancy, the topic appears only in the preschooler chapter.
2. The chapter focuses on general patterns in development. The "learn by doing" chapter contains exercises that focus on individual differences in development.

Consonants

Probably more information exists about consonant development than for any other aspect of speech. Easily, the most complete information is for English, though—increasingly—information about other languages exists as well (McLeod, 2007). Clinically, you typically analyze consonant development in toddlers in one of two ways:

- Consonant inventories
- Consonants correct

Consonant Inventories

Phonetic inventories list the speech elements a child can produce. Most often, the speech element is a consonant, though you can make an inventory of any aspect of speech (vowels, stress, syllable shapes, etc.). The important thing to remember about consonant inventories (or an inventory of any speech element) is that it doesn't tell you if a child says it correctly—they only tell that a child produces it. Because you do not specify correctness relative to the adult language, investigators call a phonetic inventory an **independent analysis** (Stoel-Gammon & Dunn, 1985).

Why Would I Want to Do This?. A phonetic inventory describes a child's universe of speech-making abilities. Another way to say it: a phonetic inventory analysis tells you what a child *can* do, rather than what they *cannot* do. To illustrate, an inventory analysis may show a toddler makes an [**m**], even though the sound occurs—incorrectly from an adult perspective—beginning the word *bee*.

Inventory analyses find their greatest use with toddlers, when many pronunciations are inaccurate relative to the adult language. Table 7–1 shows the progression in consonant development in toddlers based on consonant inventory (Stoel-Gammon,

TABLE 7–1. Consonant Inventories			
Age	**Position**	**Number of Consonants**	**Typical Consonants**
15 months	Initial	3	b d h
	Final	none	—
18 months	Initial	6	b d m n h w
	Final	1	t
24 months	Initial	11	b d g t k m n h w f s
	Final	6	p t k n r s

Source: Stoel-Gammon (1985).

1985). Robb and Bleile (1994) report similar, though not identical, inventories. The progression is

- **15 months:** A typical inventory might include three different consonant word initially and none or one consonant word finally.
- **18 months:** A typical inventory might include six word-initial consonants and one word-final consonant. The word-initial consonant inventory may contain voiced oral and nasal stops and one or two glides, while the word-final consonant inventory may consist of a voiceless stop, perhaps [t].
- **24 months:** A typical consonant inventory may contain 9 to 11 consonant word initially and five to six consonant word finally. Word initial consonant inventories may contain both voiced and voiceless stops, nasal consonants, and several glides and voiceless fricatives. A word final consonant inventory may contain voiceless oral stops, a nasal stop, and a fricative.

Correct Consonants

You can also look at speech development in toddlers by analyzing the consonants they pronounce correctly. Because correctness is determined relative to the adult language, investigators call this a **relational analysis** (Stoel-Gammon & Dunn, 1985). Relational analyses of consonant development in toddlers have found

1. Under 2 years, a toddler typically pronounces [**m n h w p b**] correctly in at least two positions (word positions are initial, medial, final) (Sander, 1972).
2. By 24 months, a toddler's list of correct consonants expands and the child may also pronounce [**m n h w p b ŋ t k d g**].
3. Also near 24 months, a toddler pronounces approximately 70% of consonants correctly (Stoel-Gammon, 1987; Watson & Scukanec, 1997).

General Pattern. Both phonetic inventory and relational analyses suggest that early in life, a child's consonants tend to be stops and glides, along with a few fricatives. Data shown in McLeod (2007) and the review by McLeod (2011) of consonant acquisition in 17 languages show a similar pattern, with the earliest occurring consonants across languages produced correctly by 75% of children being [**m n h w j p b d to k g ŋ f**]. The review of studies in Mandarin Chinese by Li and Carol (2017) show similar patterns.

Why? There is a reason stops and glides tend to be early acquisitions. Tables 7–2 (consonant inventories) and 7–3 (correct consonants) make this easier to see. The tables show consonant classes organized by degree of constriction between articulators, organized from most closure (articulators touching) to most distance (articulators farthest apart).

Endpoints and Midpoints. The general pattern is that toddlers' first consonants tend to be endpoints, primarily stops and glides. Think of those sound classes as **endpoints** in a continuum of distance between articulators. Stops (nasals and oral stops) lie at one endpoint with complete closure between articulators. Glides lie at the other end of the

TABLE 7–2. Consonant Inventories: Relationship between Development and Articulator Distance

	15 months	18 months	24 months
Stops	b d	b d	b d g t k m n ŋ
Affricates			
Fricatives			f s
Liquids			
Glides	h	h	h w

TABLE 7–3. Consonants Correct: Relationship between Development and Articulator Distance

	Under 24 months	24 months
Stops	b p m n	b d g p t k ŋ
Affricates		
Fricatives		
Liquids		
Glides	h w	h w

continuum with there being so much distance between articulators to almost be vowels. Affricates, fricatives, and liquids are **midpoint** sound classes.

Vowels

Toddlers are more advanced in vowel development than in consonant development (Selby, Robb, & Gilbert, 2000). Early acquisitions typically include "corners" of the vowel quadrangle [i u a ɑ]. Mid vowels tend to come in somewhat later than open and closed pure vowels (Bleile, 1988). Between 1;6 to 1;11, a toddler correctly produces approximately 80% of their non-rhotic vowels (Pollack & Berni, 2003).

Syllables

Open syllables (syllables ending in a vowel) predominate, especially early in the second year. Toward the year's end, a toddler often shows improved ability to close syllables with a consonant, typically a nasal or voiceless stop.

Stress

Words containing a single syllable predominate, though some two and even three syllable words may also occur (Kehoe, 1997). Multisyllabic words most often consist of two syllables and have primary stress on the first syllable. Pronunciation of *banana* as [nana] and *umbrella* as **[bɛlə]** illustrate this pattern.

Summary: Puzzle Pieces

Putting the pieces of the toddler speech perception and production puzzle together:

- Speech perception confusions result largely from lack of world knowledge and inattention.
- A toddler's first consonants tend to be endpoints (stops and glides).
- Vowel development is in advance of consonant development.
- Open syllables predominate.
- Words with two syllables tend to follow a stress–unstressed pattern.

Sound Communication

Through a combination of brain growth and environmental stimulation, during the second year a child gradually discovers the power of speech for communication. During this period, a family may frequently remind a toddler to "use your words." Topics in sound communication in toddlers include

- What a Toddler Learns
- How a Toddler Learns
- Pulling It Together

What a Toddler Learns

Major advances during the second year occur in speech for communication and expressive vocabulary.

Speech for Communication

A child's discovery of speech for communication is not like a light bulb, dark one moment and bright the next, but more like a new plant that grows roots, establishes itself, and then spreads. By 12 to 13 months, a toddler may possess a few spoken words, though they primarily communicate through voice and gestures (Hedrick, Prather, & Tobin, 1984). A few months later, words take their place alongside gestures and vocalizations, and by 16 to 18 months, become the primary form of communication. During this period, a toddler may also begin combining words together, further expanding the range of things about which they can communicate. By 24 months, a child's communication may include the regular use of two and three-word sentences (Brown, 1973).

Expressive Vocabulary

The size of a child's expressive vocabulary grows in conjunction with increased use of words to communicate, perhaps spurred by a growing neocortex in conjunction with a rapidly maturing hippocampus, creating more things to talk about and a memory system that retains more of what it learns (Dekaban & Sadowsky, 1978; Liston & Kagan, 2002). As shown in Table 7–4, at 12 or 13 months, a toddler's expressive vocabulary may include two or three different words (Capute, Palmer, Shapiro, Wachtel, Schmidt, & Ross, 1986). A few more words appear by 14 to 15 months. The pace of acquisition quickens from 7 to 20 words between 16 to 17 months, and expands even more rapidly after that, so that at 20 to 21 months, a child's expressive vocabulary may include 50 different words, approximately a 25-fold increase in expressive vocabulary in 6 months. By 24 months, a child's expressive vocabulary typically consists of more than 200 different words.

How a Toddler Learns

As with infants, toddlers depend on bonding, speech input, and familiar routines to acquire speech for communication. Bonding moves a caregiver to devote the enormous time and energy required to support the development of a child. Speech input translates the complexities of language into a form that a toddler can learn. Familiar social routines evolve, adapting to a child's developmental changes. Important developmental changes in communication during a child's second year include

- Changes in Motherese
- Meeting a Challenge

TABLE 7–4. Growth in Size of Expressive Vocabulary in Toddlers

Age	Number of Words
12 to 13 months	2 to 3 words
14 to 15 months	4 to 6 words
16 to 17 months	7 to 20 words
20 to 21 months	50 words

Source: Capute, Palmer, Shapiro, Wachtel, Schmidt, & Ross (1986).

Changes in Motherese

Motherese changes along with a child. To understand the need for this change, perform a thought experiment: imagine yourself speaking in Motherese to an infant of 3 months and then speaking that exact way to a toddler of 23 months. The high-pitched voice, exaggerated intonation, and other speech changes you need to grab and hold an infant's attention would seem grossly out of place with a toddler. Stated differently, infants and toddlers both require modified speech input to learn, but the form of the input adjusts to fit a child's level of development.

Facilitative Talk. This book calls toddler Motherese **facilitative talk** to differentiate it from Motherese with infants. If you prefer, you can call it advanced Motherese, toddler Motherese, or simply Motherese. Whatever we call it, it is a primary means of instruction for caregivers and clinicians alike (see Chapter 18, Talking with Children, for discussion and illustrations). These are the major forms of facilitative talk:

- **Strategic Errors:** A **strategic error** is an adult-made error that focuses a child on communication. To give a speech example, if a child pronounces word-initial [t] as [d] during play, the caregiver or clinician might point to a doll's toe and say, *doe*. The hoped-for response is that the child looks confused or laughs and, perhaps, attempts to say the word with an initial [t].
- **Modeling:** Modeling, as the name suggests, provides a child an example (a model) of the behavior a caregiver wants a child to learn.
- **Bombardment:** Bombardment increases the relative frequency of a speech element. The logic behind bombardment is that a child tends to learn earlier what they hear more often.
- **Requests for Confirmation or Clarification:** Requests for confirmation or clarification focus a child's attention on the purpose of speech, which is to communicate. The technique's value lies in focusing a child on speech to communicate a message from one person to another.
- **Parallel talk:** Parallel talk provides a child words and sentences to describe either their activities or aspects of the environment to which the child is attending. Parallel talk supports the well-known truth that a child is more likely to acquire aspects of language that refer to things and actions they find interesting.
- **Expansions:** Expansions "fill in the missing parts" in a child's utterances.

Meeting a Challenge

A toddler faces a challenge familiar to every adult second language learner: hearing a speech sound is not the same as knowing how to produce it. Arguably, a toddler faces a greater challenge, because, thanks to their early-maturing primary auditory cortex, their speech perception abilities are far in advance of their speech production skills, which will not reach maturity until grade school (Maas & Mailend, 2017).

Do you see the communication challenge a toddler faces? They have a growing brain, which gives them many things they say, and they have an advanced speech perception system, which lets them hear differences between many sounds. Their difficulty is that hearing a sound does not tell them how to say it. Compounding the challenge, their speech production system develops much more slowly than their perception system. To meet this challenge, a toddler develops **communication strategies** that "get around" their speech limitations by simplifying the speaking task.

Lexical Selection. *Say words with sounds you already make.* Many toddlers follow a **lexical selection** strategy (also called selectivity), "picking and choosing" words to say based on their ability to pronounce them. This strategy allows a toddler to ignore the multitude of sounds they cannot pronounce and communicate instead with words that contain those sounds lying within their narrow range of speech abilities. First described by Ferguson and Farwell (1975) and studied experimentally by Schwartz and Leonard (1982), lexical selection appears to be a widespread speaking strategy among both typically developing toddlers and those with speech sound disorders (Leonard, 1985).

Word-Based Learning. *Say words just well enough for someone to understand you.* **Word-based learning** is another frequently encountered communication strategy. A word-based learner says words just well enough for someone to (hopefully) understand them, giving little attention to the accuracy of the pronunciation. A word-based learner is somewhat analogous to a person in a foreign country who learns a few words of the language and pronounces them just well enough for someone to understand them. As a result, a word-based learner may pronounce words that contain a word initial [**m**] in the adult language as [**m**] in some words, [**p**] in others, and [**b**] in others.

Favorite Sounds and Word Recipes. *Say many different words in a few simple ways.* While some children "pick and choose" (lexical selection) and others pronounce haphazardly (word-based learning), still others simplify the challenge of speaking through **favorite sounds and word recipes** that allow them to render a wide variety of sounds through a few simple means. To illustrate, a favorite consonant could be [**s**], which the child uses to begin nearly all words that he says (Ferguson & Macken, 1983).

Word recipes are like favorite sounds, though word recipes involve the entire word rather than a single sound. To illustrate, a toddler's word recipe might be all words they say are CVC and the first consonant is [**b**], the vowel is lax, and the second consonant is [**m**] or [**n**]. The term *word recipe* conveys that a toddler, like some inexperienced cooks, repeatedly uses the same very few recipes (Menn, 1976; Waterson, 1971). For a novice cook, all meals may end up tasting like spaghetti. For a child with a word recipe strategy, all words may end up sounding like [**di**].

Gestalt Learning. *Say the sentence intonation and let speech sounds be placeholders.* **Gestalt learning** (sometimes called **mature jargon** to differentiate it from infant jargon) simplifies speech by bypassing words in favor of phrase and sentence melody. The speech of a toddler following this strategy may contain phrases with good intonation and relatively poor pronunciation of individual sounds. In a colorful and insightful phrase, Ann Peters has said that such children "learn the tune before the word" (Peters, 1977, 1983).

Pulling It Together

These are the major ideas in sound communication in toddlers:

- A toddler grows their expressive vocabulary and increasingly communicates with words.
- Facilitative talk shapes language into a lesson a toddler can learn.
- A toddler perceives more speech than they can produce.
- A toddler develops strategies that help them communicate despite their speech challenges.
- Strategies toddlers use to communicate include
  - *Say words with sounds you already make* (lexical selection)
  - *Say words just well enough for someone to understand you* (word-based learning)
  - *Say many different words in a few simple ways* (favorite sounds and word recipes)
  - *Say the sentence intonation and let speech sounds be placeholders* (gestalt learning)

CLINIC BOX: A Simple Experiment

Try a simple experiment to discover for yourself that a toddler's development of speech perception is in advance of speech production. For the experiment, present a toddler several different objects that they pronounce similarly, and then ask them to pick up each object that you name. For example, if a child pronounces *dog* and *cat* as [ga], present the child with a toy cat and a toy dog. If you do this, you will find that even when you are extremely careful not to use eye gaze or other means to assist in object identification, a child experiences little difficulty pointing to or picking up the appropriate objects.

Here's what the experiment shows: if a child's perceptual knowledge (sometimes called a representation) was the same as the way they pronounce the word, selecting the right object should be impossible, since the child pronounces each similarly. The fact that most children experience little difficulty picking out the right object suggests that they know more (that is, have more advanced perceptual knowledge) than shown by their speech production. Interestingly, in all species of mammals studied to date, perception systems develop earlier than production systems (Hauser, 1996).

Conclusions

Major ideas in this chapter include

1. A toddler increasingly uses words to communicate.
2. Perceptual errors occur through lack of knowledge and inattention.

3. A toddler's first words contain sounds, syllables, and stress patterns learned during the first year, and they "stumble on" new speech elements as they increasingly use words to communicate.

4. Communication strategies allow a toddler to communicate when he perceives more distinctions than he can produce.

Review Questions

1. Explain in your own words why misperceptions occur in toddlers even though their speech perception system is mature.
2. What is a consonant inventory? Is it an independent analysis or a relational analysis?
3. What does the term endpoint mean?
4. What consonant classes are endpoints?
5. What consonant classes are midpoints?
6. Is a correct consonant analysis an independent analysis or a relational analysis?
7. At approximately what age does a toddler's expressive vocabulary contain 50 different words?
8. List three forms (techniques) for facilitative talk (or advanced Motherese, if you prefer) with toddlers, explaining for each form the type of instruction it provides.
9. In your own words, explain a toddler's challenge to communicate.
10. Explain in your own words why lexical selection might help a toddler to communicate through words.

References

Bleile, K. (1988). A note on vowel patterns in two normally developing children. *Clinical Linguistics and Phonetics, 3,* 203–212.

Brown, R. (1973). *A first language: The early stages.* Cambridge, MA: Harvard University Press.

Brungart, D. S. (2001). Informational and energetic masking effects in the perception of two simultaneous talkers. *The Journal of the Acoustical Society of America, 109,* 1101–1109.

Capute, A., Palmer, F., Shapiro, B., Wachtel, R., Schmidt, S., & Ross A. (1986). Clinical Linguistic and Auditory Milestone Scale: Prediction of cognition in infancy. *Developmental Medicine and Child Neurology, 28,* 762–771.

Dekaban, A. S., & Sadowsky, D. (1978). Changes in brain weights during the span of human life: Relation of brain weights to body heights and body weights. *Annals of Neurology, 4,* 345–356.

Ferguson, C., & Farwell, C. (1975). Words and sounds in early language acquisition: English initial consonants in the first fifty words. *Language, 51,* 419–439.

Ferguson, C., & Macken, M. (1983). The role of play in phonological development. In K. Nelson (Ed.), *Child language IV* (pp. 256–282). Hillsdale, NJ: Lawrence Erlbaum.

Hauser, M. (1996). *The Evolution of communication.* Boston, MA: The MIT Press.

Hedrick, D., Prather, E., & Tobin, A. (1984). *Sequenced Inventory of Communication Development-R.* Seattle, WA: University of Washington Press.

Kehoe, M. (1997). Stress error patterns in English-speaking children's word productions. *Clinical Linguistics and Phonetics, 11,* 389–409.

Leonard, L. (1985). Unusual and subtle behavior in the speech of phonologically disordered children. *Journal of Speech and Hearing Disorders, 50,* 4–13.

Li, X. X., & To, C. K(2017). A review of phonological development of Mandarin-speaking children. *American Journal of Speech Language Pathology, 26,* 1–17.

Liebold, L. (2017). Speech perception in complex acoustic environments: Developmental effects. *Journal of Speech, Language, and Hearing Research, 60,* 3001–3008.

Liston, C., & Kagan, J. (2002). Memory enhancement in early childhood. *Nature, 419,* 896.

Maas, E., & Mailend, M. (2017). Fricative contrast and coarticulation in children with and without speech sound disorders. *American Journal of Speech Language Pathology, 26,* 649–663.

Maurer, D. (Ed.). (2005). Special issue: Critical periods re-examined: Evidence from human sensory development. *Developmental Psychobiology, 46*(3), 155–292.

McLeod, S. (Ed.). (2007). *The international guide to speech acquisition.* Clifton Park, NY: Thomson Delmar Learning.

McLeod, S. (2011). Laying the foundations for multilingual acquisition: An international overview of speech acquisition. *Journal of Linguistics and Language Teaching, 2,* 53–71.

Menn, L. (1976). *Pattern, control and contrast in beginning speech: A case study in the development of word form and word function* (Unpublished doctoral dissertation). University of Illinois, Champagne-Urbana, IL.

Pascallis, O., de Haan, M., & Nelson, C. (2002). Is face processing species specific during the first year of life? *Science, 296,* 1321–1323.

Peters, A. (1977). Language learning strategies: Does the whole equal the sum of the parts? *Language, 53,* 560–573.

Peters, A. (1983). *The units of language acquisition.* New York, NY: Cambridge University Press.

Pollock, K. E., & Berni, M. C. (2003). Incidence of non-rhotic vowel errors in children: Data from the Memphis Vowel Project. *Clinical Linguistics and Phonetics, 17,* 393–401.

Robb, M., & Bleile, K. (1994). Consonant inventories of young children from 8 to 25 months. *Clinical Linguistics and Phonetics, 8,* 295–320.

Sander, E. (1972). When are speech sounds learned? *Journal of Speech and Hearing Disorders, 37,* 55–63.

Schwartz, R., & Leonard, L. (1982). Do children pick and choose: An examination of phonological selection and avoidance in early lexical acquisition. *Journal of Child Language, 9,* 319–336.

Selby, J. C., Robb, M. P., & Gilbert, H. R. (2000). Normal vowel articulations between 15 and 36 months of age. *Clinical Linguistics & Phonetics, 14*(4), 255–265.

Stoel-Gammon, C. (1985). Phonetic inventories, 15–24 months: A longitudinal study. *Journal of Speech and Hearing Research, 28,* 505–512.

Stoel-Gammon, C. (1987). Phonological skills of 2-year-olds. *Language, Speech, and Hearing Services in Schools, 18,* 323–329.

Stoel-Gammon, C., & Dunn, C. (1985). *Normal and disordered phonology in children.* Baltimore, MD: University Park Press.

Waterson, N. (1971). Child phonology: A prosodic view. *Journal of Linguistics, 7,* 179–221.

Watson, M., & Scukanec, G. (1997). Profiling the phonological abilities of 2-year-olds: A longitudinal investigation. *Child Language Teaching and Therapy, 13,* 3–14.

CHAPTER 8
PRESCHOOLERS

Speech is faster and more motorically complex than hitting a home run, playing a piano, or dancing a ballet. Yet, while baseball, a musical instrument, and dance require years to master, children acquire major aspects of speech before beginning school. It is as if they mastered calculus before learning addition, subtraction, multiplication, and division. The remarkable ability of preschoolers as speech learners is the subject of this chapter. Topics include:

- Speech Perception
- Speech Production
- Sound Communication

Learning Objectives

I hope on completing the chapter you will

- Understand the nature of perceptual errors in preschoolers.
- Identify sound classes mastered during the preschool years.
- Know how social development influences speech development.

Key Words

Key words you will encounter in this chapter

Distinctive features
Phonological processes
Childhood apraxia of speech (CAS)
Onset
Rime (also called Rhyme)
Primary stress
Excessive stress or equal stress (EES)

Speech Perception

As with toddlers, most often a preschooler's perceptual confusions result from inattention, limited knowledge, and the presence of competing sounds that impact higher cognitive processing, rather than from a child having a "broken" speech perception system (Brungart, 2001; Liebold, 2017). My personal Champion Misperceiver was a preschooler who I met many years ago (Bleile, 1987). During a 10-week period, this clever child's misperceptions included

> *Dandelion* is *dandy flower*
>
> *Picnic table* is *pick me table*
>
> *Clothes pin* is *pin clothes*
>
> *Lawnmower* is *lawnmotor*
>
> *Elbow* is *el-bone*
>
> *Fire siren/noon whistle* is *fire whistle*
>
> *Butterfly* is *buzzerfly*
>
> *Tater tot* is *little rock*

Like many preschooler misperceptions, his has a kind of wonderful logic: What is a plant more likely to be, a dandy lion or a dandy flower? And what else is a Tater tot other than a crunchy little rock?

Speech Production

Preschoolers are better speech learners than adults, who cannot match the perfection of their mastery of speech and accent (Johnson & Newport, 1989). Major developments in speech production from 2 to 5 years occur in

- Consonants
- Vowels
- Syllables
- Stress

For each area, the discussion focuses on correct productions first and speech errors second. Although both **distinctive features** and **phonological processes** provide useful terminology to describe errors affecting sound classes, this chapter tends toward the terminology of phonological processes because I like its transparency.

Consonants

During a brief 3-year period, a child too young for school masters all but the most challenging consonants of their language.

Correct Productions

Table 8–1 summarizes acquisition for consonants and [ɚ]; Table 8–2 does the same for consonant clusters. The rhotic vowel [ɚ] is included because a clinician often treats it along with [r].

What's in Those Tables?. If you spend some time looking at Tables 8–1 and 8–2, you'll find the following patterns:

- The preschool years are when a child largely masters midpoint consonant classes (affricates, fricatives, liquid; see Chapter 7, "Toddlers," for discussion of midpoints and endpoints).
- 50% of children have acquired the consonants in all sound classes by 4 years, 6 months.
- Although acquisition of consonant clusters is delayed relative to individual consonants, 50% of children acquire all consonant clusters by their 5th birthday.

TABLE 8–1. Age of Acquisition (50% Correct) of Consonants and [ɚ]

Consonant	50%	Consonant	50%
m	<3;0	f	<3;0
n	<3;0	v	3;6
ŋ	<3;0	θ	4;6
h	<3;0	ð	4;6
w	<3;0	s	3;6
j	<3;0	z	4;0
p	<3;0	ʃ	3;6
t	<3;0	tʃ	3;6
k	<3;0	dʒ	3;6
b	<3;0	r	3;6
d	<3;0	l	3;6
g	<3;0	ɚ	4;6

Note. Tables 8–1 and 8–2 are a reanalysis of Smit, Hand, Frelinger, Bernthal, & Byrd (1990). The tables depict the ages at which 50% of children produced the consonant or consonant cluster correctly; whereas Smit et al., because their interest was treatment eligibility, focused on when 90% of children produced it correctly. The listed sounds were acquired by both genders at the given ages and never by less than 50% by children at a later age. Acquisition ages for consonants in Table 8–1 are averaged across word positions. Acquisition ages for consonant clusters in Table 8–2 are for word initial position.
Source: Smit, Hand, Frelinger, Bernthal, & Byrd (1990).

TABLE 8–2. Age of Acquisition (50% Correct) of Consonant Clusters in Word Initial Positions

Cluster	50%	Cluster	50%
tw	3;0	pr	4;0
kw	3;0	br	3;6
sp	3;6	tr	5;0
st	3;6	dr	4;0
sk	3;6	kr	4;0
sm	3;6	gr	4;6
sn	3;6	fr	3;6
sw	3;6	θr	5;0
sl	4;6	skw	3;6
pl	3;6	spl	5;0
bl	3;6	spr	5;0
kl	4;0	str	5;0
gl	3;6	skr	5;0
fl	3;6		

Note. The Smit et al. data does not contain information for [ʃr] consonant cluster.
Source: Smit, Hand, Frelinger, Bernthal, & Byrd (1990).

Other Studies, Similar Findings. McLeod's (2002) meta-analysis and McLeod, van Doorn, and Reed (2001a, 2001b) reveal similar, though not identical, patterns in acquisition of Australian English. McLeod (2002) and McLeod et al. (2001a, 2001b) show the following patterns in the development of consonant clusters in Australian English:

- Consonant clusters are pronounced correctly approximately one-third of the time in connected speech by 3 years.
- Word-final consonant clusters are more likely to be correct than consonant clusters in word-final position.
- Consonant cluster acquisition is nearly complete by the time a child is 5.
- Of 27 different word-initial consonant clusters, all but six are acquired by 50% of children before 5 years. Of the remaining six, two are clusters in which the second consonant is [r] and four are clusters with three consonants.

Speech Errors

A preschooler's speech production system, while developing rapidly, still lags behind that of their speech perception system (Huttenlocher, 1994; Pascallis, de Haan, & Nelson, 2002; Schade & van Groenigen, 1961; Scheibel, 1993; Simonds & Scheibel, 1989). To communicate with those around them, a preschooler discovers regular ways to say words that contain sounds and sound combinations they struggle to pronounce. These ways may include

- Delete the part of a word they cannot say
- Replace a midpoint consonant with an endpoint consonant
- Make sounds in a word more similar
- Give equal stress to all syllables in a word

Phonological Processes. Phonological processes provide a convenient way to describe how a preschooler communicates "around" their speech limitations. Here are three guideposts for the following discussion:

1. Speech errors of toddlers and preschoolers overlap; many phonological processes occur in the speech of children of both ages.
2. The phonological processes in this section focus primarily on consonants; those primarily affecting vowels, syllables, and stress appear in their respective sections.
3. Typical errors found in production of consonants and consonant clusters are bolded. are examined; the names of less common errors appear in italics.

Place Changes

- **Fronting:** Substitution of an alveolar stop for a postalveolar or velar consonant.
- **Velar assimilation:** Consonants assimilate to the place of production of a velar consonant.
- **Labial assimilation:** Consonants assimilate to the place of production of a labial consonant.
- *Backing:* Alveolar (and sometimes postalveolar) consonants are pronounced as velar stops.
- *Glottal replacement:* Replacement of a consonant with a glottal stop.

Manner Changes

- **Stopping:** Substitution of a stop for a fricative or affricate.
- **Gliding:** Substitution of a glide for a liquid.
- **Lateralization:** Sounds typically produced with central air emission (most commonly [s] and [z], but sometimes [ʃ], [ʒ], [ʧ], and [ʤ]) are pronounced with lateral air emission.

- *Affrication:* Stops or fricatives (both usually alveolars) are pronounced as affricates.
- *Nasalization:* Nasal stop replace nonnasal consonants (usually oral stops).
- *Denasalization:* Oral consonants (usually oral stops) replace nasal consonants.

Sound Reversals

- **Metathesis (meTAthesis):** The reversal of two sounds in a word; for example, saying *pet* as [tɛp].

Consonant Cluster Changes

- **Cluster reduction:** Deletion of a consonant in a consonant cluster.
- **Epenthesis (ePENthesis):** Insertion of a vowel between consonants in a consonant cluster.

Vowels

Correct Productions

- Children typically acquire vowels earlier than consonants.
- Vowel development is largely complete by 3 years (Pollack & Berni, 2003; Selby, Robb, & Gilbert, 2000). Late acquisitions include r-colored vowels and unstressed vowels in multisyllabic words.

Speech Errors

- The speech of approximately 24% to 65% of children less than 3 years contains a high incidence of vowel errors (Pollack & Berni, 2003).
- Extensive or inconsistent vowel errors may occur in preschoolers diagnosed with moderate to severe speech sound disorders and are a hallmark of **Childhood apraxia of speech (CAS)**, a neurological childhood speech sound disorder in which the precision and consistency of movements underlying speech are impaired in the absence of neuromuscular deficits (American Speech-Language-Hearing Association, 2007; Gibbon, 2009; Pollack & Berni, 2003).

Phonological Processes

Two major substitution phonological processes affect vowels:

- **Vowel neutralization:** A neutral vowel (schwa, [ʊ], or [ɪ]) replaces another vowel.
- **Vocalization:** A neutral vowel (schwa, [ʊ], or [ɪ]) replaces a syllabic consonant.

Syllables

Correct Productions

- Syllables develop rapidly during the preschool years.
- At the beginning of the preschool period, a child's speech may contain syllables that are V, VC, CV, CVC, CVCV, and CVCVC.
- Reflecting the adult language, CV is likely to be the most frequently occurring syllable.
- As the preschool years proceed, syllable beginnings and endings (called **onsets** and **rhymes**) increasingly contain diverse consonants and consonant clusters.

Speech Errors

The following phonological processes may affect syllables.

Entire Syllable

- **Reduplication:** Repetition of a syllable.
- **Syllable deletion:** Deletion of an unstressed syllable.

Beginning of Syllables

- **Prevocalic voicing:** Consonants before a vowel are voiced.
- *Initial consonant deletion:* The initial consonant in the word is deleted.

End of Syllables.

- **Final consonant devoicing:** Obstruents are voiceless at the ends of words.
- **Final consonant deletion:** Deletion of a consonant at the end of a syllable or word.

Stress

Correct Productions

- In common with other speech areas, acquisition of stress patterns shows major development during the preschool years.
- Whereas a toddler's speech showed a preference for the major stress (**primary stress**) on the first syllable, early preschoolers show sufficient mastery of the speech mechanism to allow words beginning with unstressed syllables, as in *banana* and *umbrella* (Kehoe, 1997).
- As a child develops during the preschool years, three-syllable words with primary stress on the first, second, or third syllable become more common.

Speech Errors

- A child who finds stress patterns challenging may either delete syllables or resort to excessive stress or equal stress on syllables, called EES (**excessive stress or equal stress**) (Bowen, 2011).
- Difficulties with stress in words may be a central challenge for a preschooler or a student with childhood apraxia of speech (Ballard, Robin, McCabe, & McDonald, 2010).

Summary: A Challenge That Stretches

Speech development progresses rapidly during the preschool years, both challenging and stretching a child's speech production abilities. During this brief 3-year period

- Perceptual errors arise as a preschooler's world expands.
- A preschooler typically masters midpoint consonants.
- Fifty percent of preschoolers complete acquisition of consonant clusters before beginning school.
- Vowel errors become less common after 3 years.
- More syllable and stress patterns emerge.
- To communicate around their speech production limitations, a preschooler
  - ◆ May delete the part of a word they cannot say (final consonant deletion, syllable deletion)
  - ◆ May replace a midpoint consonant with an endpoint consonant (gliding, stopping)
  - ◆ May make sounds in a word more similar (velar assimilation, prevocalic voicing)
  - ◆ May give equal stress to all syllables in a word (excessive stress or equal stress)

Sound Communication

Speech for communication makes major strides during the preschool years. The major topics in sound communication in preschoolers are

- What a Preschooler Learns
- How a Preschooler Learns
- Pulling It Together

What a Preschooler Learns

Important advances in the preschool years occur in expressive vocabulary and in syntax and morphology.

Expressive Vocabulary

You may remember that the toddler period ended with words well established as a means of communication. Look back at the arc of a child's progress: it took an infant nearly one year to *begin* to use words to communicate and to learn to speak two or three different words, and it took a toddler nearly six months to establish words as a primary means of communication and to learn to say 50 different words. Compare that to a preschooler who speaks thousands of words.

Syntax and Morphology

Not only does a preschooler say an enormous number of different words, they also put them in sentences. Table 8–3 shows the growth of average sentence length at yearly intervals between 2 years (24 months) and 5 years (60 months) (Brown, 1973).

Additionally, a preschooler learns to modify word and sentence meaning (morphology). Listen to a preschooler and you discover that they alter words to indicate that an activity is ongoing (*He is running.*), that they use speech signify that there is more than one thing (*dogs and cats*), and that they can tell you something occurred in the past (*He left.*).

How a Preschooler Learns

Previous sections in this chapter focused on speech development as a matter of *what* and *when* (what age) a preschooler learns about speech. Our final topic is, *how does a child learn?* Combining *what*, *when*, and *how* together for children developing typically provides a foundation to help a child with speech challenges (see Chapter 16, "Developmental Goals").

Perspectives

Of course, you can answer *how* a child learns in many different ways. Certainly, bonding between child and parents, speech input to simplify "the speech and language lesson,"

TABLE 8–3. Growth MLU in the Preschool Years

Age	Mean Length of Utterance
2 years	1.92
3 years	3.16
4 years	4.40
5 years	5.63

and familiar social routines all continue to support preschooler learning as they did with infants and toddlers. Brain development offers a different answer to *how*. The brain grows to 85% of its adult size during the preschool years, the hippocampus is mature, and Broca's area is developing. All those developments help with speech learning as the environment continues to shape the child's brain at the cellular level, pruning unused brain cell connections, and elaborating connections between the remaining cells.

A Social How

This chapter offers a "social answer" to how a preschooler learns speech.

A Small World. To see how a preschooler's social world may spur speech development, first imagine a young child, a toddler, walking up to their mother or father and saying, *ball*. The child's parent thinks a moment, lies down, reaches under the couch, pulls out the ball, and says, "Here you go." A parent successfully performs this mind reading trick based on a single word, *ball,* because they know their child's routines extremely well—knows, perhaps, that the child likes to smack the ball, often causing it to roll under the couch.

A World Grows Larger. Now imagine the same child as a preschooler in preschool class or daycare center. They walk up to a teacher and say, *ball*. For a preschooler interacting with less familiar conversational partners, the one-word utterance would likely prove insufficient to obtain what they want. Not knowing the child as well, the teacher may wonder, "Do you want a ball? Did someone take your ball? Do you want a ball from home?" That is, the teacher fails this particular mind reading test because one-word speech often proves insufficient in a world of less familiar persons.

Effect of an Expanding World

Interacting with more and less familiar people in an expanding social network, helps spur a preschooler to put words together into longer strings to express the expanding range of things permitted by their growing brain. This both challenges and expands a child's speech making abilities. The challenge means a child must learns to pronounce an increased and varying number of sounds in combination with each other under flowing intonation contours (Velleman, 2002). At the same time, this challenge expands a child's speech making abilities because it encourages them to improve speech to communicate more successfully.

Pulling It Together

These are the major ideas in sound communication in preschoolers:

- A preschooler's ability to learn words and make sentences expands rapidly.
- Foundations of speech learning includes support from social relationships and rapid brain development.

- A preschooler's social world typically expands to include less familiar people.
- Vocabulary growth, maturing syntactic skills, and an expanding social world combine to both challenge and stretch a preschooler's speech abilities.

Conclusions

Ideas in this chapter include

1. A child possesses relatively advanced speech perception abilities, though they may still make knowledge-based perceptual errors.
2. Early on, a child's speech contains a limited variety of sounds and syllables, but by 5 years old, has grown to contain most major sound classes.
3. Rapid developments in vocabulary and syntax provide a greater means of expression.
4. During the preschool years, a child increasingly communicates with persons outside the immediate family.
5. An expanding social world both challenges and stretches a child's speech abilities.

Review Questions

1. Why do speech perception errors abound in preschoolers despite them having mature speech perception systems?
2. Explain in your own words why a preschooler could misperceive *dandelion* as *dandy flower*.
3. Give an example of substituting an endpoint consonant for a midpoint consonant.
4. List two typical place errors and two manner errors.
5. What does *metathesis* mean?
6. What are the names of the two most common vowel errors?
7. What is the name of the most common syllable error affecting consonants at the beginning of syllables?
8. How may social development influence a child's speech development?

References

American Speech-Language-Hearing Association. (2007). *Childhood apraxia of speech* [Position statement]. Retrieved from http://www.asha.org/policy

Ballard, K. J., Robin, D. A., McCabe, P., & McDonald, J. (2010). Treating dysprosody in childhood apraxia of speech. *Journal of Speech, Language, and Hearing Research, 53*(5), 1227–1245.

Bleile, K. (1987). *Regressions in the phonological development of two children.* Iowa City, IA: University of Iowa.

Bowen, C. (2011). *Prosody work in a child 4;2.* Sydney, Australia: Phono Groups.

Brown, R. (1973). *A first language: The early stages.* Cambridge, MA: Harvard University Press.

Brungart, D. S. (2001). Informational and energetic masking effects in the perception of two simultaneous talkers. *The Journal of the Acoustical Society of America, 109*, 1101–1109.

Gibbon, F. E. (2009). Vowel errors in children with speech disorders. In C. Bowen (Ed.), *Children's speech sound disorders*. Oxford, UK: Wiley-Blackwell.

Huttenlocher, R. (1994). Synaptogenesis, synapse elimination, and neural plasticity in human cerebral cortex. In C. Nelson (Ed.), *Threats to optimal development: The Minnesota Symposia on Child Psychology* (Vol. 27, pp. 35–54). Hillsdale, NJ: L. Erlbaum.

Johnson, J., & Newport, E. (1989). Critical period effects in second language learning: The influence of maturational state on the acquisition of English as a second language. *Cognitive Psychology, 21*, 60–99.

Kehoe, M. (1997). Stress error patterns in English-speaking children's word productions. *Clinical Linguistics and Phonetics, 11*, 389–409.

Liebold, L. (2017). Speech perception in complex acoustic environments: Developmental effects. *Journal of Speech, Language, and Hearing Research, 60*, 3001–3008.

McLeod, S. (2002). Part I: The plethora of available data on children's speech development. *ACQuiring Knowledge in Speech, Language, and Hearing, 4*, 141–147.

McLeod, S., van Doorn, J., & Reed, V. A. (2001a). Normal acquisition of consonant clusters. *American Journal of Speech-Language Pathology, 10*, 99–110.

McLeod, S., van Doorn, J., & Reed, V. A. (2001b). Consonant cluster development in two-year-olds: General trends and individual difference. *Journal of Speech, Language, Hearing Research, 44*, 1144–1171.

Pascallis, O., de Haan, M., & Nelson, C. (2002). Is face processing species specific during the first year of life? *Science, 296*, 1321–1323.

Pollock, K. E., & Berni, M. C. (2003). Incidence of non-rhotic vowel errors in children: Data from the Memphis Vowel Project. *Clinical Linguistics and Phonetics, 17*, 393–401.

Schade, J. P., & van Groenigen, W. B. (1961). Structural organization of the human cerebral cortex. I. Maturation of the middle frontal gyrus. *Acta Anatomica, 47*, 72–111.

Scheibel, A. B. (1993). Dendritic structure and language development. In B. de Boysson-Bardies (Ed.), *Developmental neurocognition: Speech and face processing in the first year of life*. Dordrecht, the Netherlands: Kluwer.

Selby, J. C., Robb, M. P., & Gilbert, H. R. (2000). Normal vowel articulations between 15 and 36 months of age. *Clinical Linguistics & Phonetics, 14*(4), 255–265.

Simonds, R. J., & Scheibel, A. B. (1989). The postnatal development of the motor speech area: A preliminary study. *Brain and Language, 37*, 42–58.

Smit, A., Hand, L., Frelinger, J., Bernthal, J., & Byrd, A. (1990). The Iowa articulation norms project and its Nebraska replication. *Journal of Speech and Hearing Disorders, 55*, 779–798.

Velleman, S. L. (2002). Phonotactic therapy. *Seminars in Speech and Language, 23*(1), 43–56.

CHAPTER 9
STUDENTS

The speech accomplishments of preschoolers become the foundations of speech development in students, who then go on to master the most challenging sounds in their language, learn to decode written language, and acquire increasingly complex intonation and stress patterns in discourse and literature. Major topics in this chapter include:

- Speech Perception
- Speech Production
- Sound Communication

Learning Objectives

I hope on completing the chapter you will

- Recognize that speech development is lifelong.
- Understand the difference between discrimination and awareness.
- Explain why the late 8 are late.
- Know why the curriculum matters in speech learning.

Key Words

Key words you will encounter in this chapter

English language learners (ELL)
The late 8
Phonological awareness
Syllable segmentation
Rhyme awareness
Alliteration awareness
Phoneme isolation
Phoneme segmentation

Speech Perception

Misperceptions continue during the school years and into adulthood. For example, a student may misconstrue sarcasm as compliment, mistake insult for praise. To illustrate, a student may misinterpret pitch and intonation markers of sarcasm in sentences such as, "Now THAT is really nice," understanding it to mean, "Now that is REALLY nice." Like adults, a student may also parse a sentence incorrectly; for example, mishearing *peace* as *peas* in a John Lennon lyric, "All I am saying is give peas a chance."

It is common that some students with speech sound disorders are well-known for having difficulty hearing their own misperceptions, failing to recognize that they pronounce a word differently than they intend to say it. To illustrate, when a clinician points out that they say *rabbit* as *wabbit,* they may reply, "No I don't. I say *wabbit* as *wabbit*." Perspectives to treat speech perception difficulties are in Chapter 17, "Treatment Sounds," and in Chapter 22, "Sound Decisions."

Speech Production

Incredibly, by the beginning of the school years, many students have mastered major areas of speech production (see Chapter 8, "Preschoolers"). For some students, further speech development occurs in the following areas:

- Consonants and [r] colored vowels
- Consonant clusters
- Difficult words (vowels, syllables, and stress)

As in previous chapters, the order of topics in each section is acquisition, correct productions, and speech errors. Due to the nature of the speech difficulty, vowels, syllables, and stress appear together in the section on Difficult Words. The section concludes with a capsule summary of perceptual and production development in students.

Consonants + [r] Colored Vowels

Most clinicians spend large amounts of their time treating consonants and [r] colored vowels. Importantly, treatments for those sounds may also assist people without speech challenges who are acquiring English as a nonnative language (**English language learners**), children and adults alike (McLeod, 2011).

Table 9–1 lists consonants acquired by less than 75% of children before they begin school. Collectively, these consonants have a name: **the late 8** (Table 9–2). The tables also show [r] colored vowels, which are included because a school clinician often treats that vowel alongside consonants. Technically, then, Tables 9–1 and 9–2 show the late 8 + 1.

TABLE 9–1. Age of Acquisition (75% Correct) of Late-Acquired Consonants Averaged Across Both Word Initial and Word Final Positions

Consonant	75%
s	5;0
ʃ	5;0
θ	6;0
ð	5;6
z	6;0
ʧ	6;0
r	6;0
l	6;0
ɚ	5;6

Note. Tables 9–1 and 9–3 are a reanalysis of Smit, Hand, Frelinger, Bernthal, & Byrd (1990). The tables depict the ages at which 75% of children produced the consonant or consonant cluster correctly; whereas Smit et al., because their interest was treatment eligibility, focused on when 90% of children produced it correctly. The listed sounds were acquired by both genders at the given ages and never by less than 50% by children at a later age. Acquisition ages for consonants in Table 9–1 are averaged across word positions. Acquisition ages for consonant clusters in Table 9–3 are for word initial position.

Source: Smit, Hand, Frelinger, Bernthal, & Byrd (1990).

Table 9–2. The Late 8 + 1

Consonant
s
ʃ
θ
ð
z
ʧ
r and ɚ
l

A Collection of Challenges

If a student with speech difficulties looks at Table 9–2, they might see a collection of challenges:

- **Stick out your tongue and hiss:** [θ] and [ð] places the tongue tip between the teeth.
- **Hiss behind your teeth:** [s] and [z] places your tongue tip close enough behind either your top or bottom front teeth to make a hiss.
- **Raise your tongue blade:** [ʃ] raises your tongue blade close enough to the roof of your mouth to produce a hiss.
- **Stop and start:** The affricate [tʃ] coalesces a stop and fricative into one consonant.
- **Over the sides:** [l] is the only English sound where air flows over the sides of the tongue.
- **Multiple tongue gymnastics:** [r] entails some truly challenging tongue movements, requiring you to either bunching up the tongue body or curl back your tongue tip.
- **Retract your what? Your tongue root?:** [r] colored vowels entail saying a vowel while retracting the tongue root.

Correct Productions

Approximately 75% of students acquire the late 8 + 1 "in a bunch" between their 5th and 6th birthdays. Specifically,

$$5;0 = s \ ʃ$$
$$5;6 = ð \ ɚ$$
$$6;0 = θ \ z \ tʃ \ l \ r$$

Speech Errors

Students with challenges affecting late sounds often make the same speech errors as preschoolers. For example, a student's closest approximation of [s] could be [t] (stopping), or their closest approximation for [r] could be [w] (gliding).

Additionally, students make speech errors you might paraphrase as "almost there," "not quite," or "just a little off." Formerly, researchers called these distortions. Speech errors you are most likely to encounter when treating students with late 8 challenges include

- **Lisp:** A student may pronounce alveolar consonants (especially fricatives) either on or between the teeth. They may also occur with air flowing over the sides of the tongue, creating a lateral lisp.
- **Lateralize:** A student may pronounce [s] and [z] (sometimes [ʃ] and [tʃ]) with lateral air emission, like [l], though the air may flow over one side of the tongue rather than both sides.

■ **Bladed:** A student may pronounce [s] and [z] (and sometimes [l]) by raising the tongue blade rather than raising or lowering the tongue tip.

■ **Derhoticized:** A student may pronounce an [r] colored vowel without the [r] coloring, resulting in a schwa-like vowel. The technical name for this is derhoticization.

■ **Lip Rounding:** A student may pronounce an [r] colored vowel with lip rounding, giving the vowel a [w] quality.

Consonant Clusters

Table 9–3 lists word-initial consonant clusters acquired by less than 75% of children preschoolers before they begin school. Some observations about information in this table

■ Students find consonant clusters most challenging when they contain one or more late 8 consonants.

■ Every consonant cluster that 75% of children do not acquire before beginning school contains at least *one* late 8 consonant.

■ Except for [**skw**], every three-member consonant cluster that 75% of children do not acquire before beginning school contains *two* late 8 consonants.

TABLE 9–3. Age of Acquisition (75% Correct) of English Consonant Clusters in Word Initial Positions

Cluster	75%	Cluster	75%
sp	5;0	tr	5;6
st	5;0	dr	6;0
sk	5;0	kr	5;6
sm	5;0	gr	6;0
sn	5;6	fr	6;0
sw	5;6	θr	7;0
sl	7;0	skw	7;0
pl	5;6	spl	7;0
bl	5;0	spr	8;0
kl	5;6	str	8;0
fl	5;6	skr	8;0
pr	6;0		
br	6;0		

Source: Smit, Hand, Frelinger, Bernthal, & Byrd (1990).

Correct Productions

Consonant cluster acquisition in students occurs over several years:

5;0 = two-member [s] clusters

5;6 to 6;0 = two-member liquid clusters

7;0 to 8;0 = three-member clusters

Other Studies, Similar Findings. McLeod's (2002) meta-analysis and McLeod, van Doorn, and Reed (2001a, 2001b) report similar acquisition patterns for consonant clusters. In those reviews, of six consonant clusters not acquired until the school years, two were clusters in which the second consonant is [r], and four were clusters with three consonants.

Speech Errors

Students often adjust late consonant clusters to make them more manageable to say through two different phonological processes:

- **Cluster reduction:** A student deletes one or more consonants in a consonant cluster. For example, they might pronounce *speed* as [pid] or [sid].
- **Epenthesis (ePENthesis):** The insertion of a vowel between consonants in a consonant cluster.

Difficult Words (Vowels, Syllables, and Stress)

In the latter half of grade school, vowels, syllables, and stress may reemerge as speech challenges when students encounter more literary and scientific vocabulary.

Vowels

Morphological alterations requiring vowel changes may challenge a student, as in word pairs such as

divine/divinity

collide/collision

explain/explanation

sane/sanity

serene/serenity

obscene/obscenity

Syllables

As school progresses, vocabulary tends to get longer, challenging a student to say complex strings of syllables in words such as

electronics	(V-CVC-CCV-CVCC)
nomenclature	(CV-CVC-CCV-CV)
iambic pentameter	(V-VC-CVC, CVC-CV-CV-CV)

Stress

What is true of vowels and syllables, also is true of stress. Often, with complex vowel and syllable patterns comes stress patterns atypical in everyday English. This happens especially with scientific vocabulary. To illustrate, *electronics* has primary stress on the third syllable, *nomenclature* has primary stress on the first syllable, and the phrase *iambic pentameter* has primary stress on the second syllable of *iambic* and on either the first or second syllable of *pentameter*, some speakers pronouncing it PENtameter and others penTAmeter.

Similarly, compound words may have stress on the first syllable, while adjective + noun phrases may have stress on the second, as in

Compound Word	Adjective + Noun
RED head	Red HEAD
WHITE house	white HOUSE
GREEN house	green HOUSE
HIGH chair	high CHAIR

Correct Productions

I don't know of any normative studies showing at which ages students learn to pronounce longer and more challenging words they encounter in later grades. Until such information exists, you can fall back on listening to determine whether a speech production is typical or atypical. That is, listen to students in a particular grade to develop a sense of what are "typical" pronunciations in a subject area and determine when problems saying words in that grade and subject are atypical enough to draw attention to the speaker. You can also get the same information by talking with teachers. To illustrate, you might ask at what grade level the teacher expects a student to pronounce vocabulary in such-and-such subject area.

Speech Errors

Speech errors in later grades may can cause a student significant embarrassment. Often, a student feels that their vocal stumble is a chink in their social armor, revealing a person underneath who struggles with learning. My experience is that students who encounter speech challenges with "difficult words" (vowels, syllables, and stress) rely on a variety of communication strategies, including saying words slowly with overemphasis, pausing between syllables, placing the main stress early in a longer word, overemphasizing stressed syllables, and deleting unstressed syllables.

Summary: Speech Development in School

The speech accomplishments and challenges of students in the school years include

- Speech perception difficulties may continue in the school years.
- Students typically acquire the last consonants of English by 6 years old.
- Prominent consonant errors include stopping, gliding, lisping, bladed, and lateralizing.
- Derhotization and lip rounding are prominent speech errors for [r] colored vowels.
- Students master the last consonant clusters by 8 years old.
- Prominent consonant cluster errors include syllable deletion and epenthesis.
- Speech challenges with vowels, syllables, and stress in "difficult words" may emerge in later grades as students encounter more literate and scientific vocabulary.

Sound Communication

School transmits knowledge, ways of thinking, and cultural values from one generation to the next. During the school years, speech supports a student's educational and social development. Topics in sound communication in students include

- What a Student Learns
- How a Student Learns
- Pulling It Together

What a Student Learns

Progression through school both improves and may challenge a student's speech abilities. Table 9–4 offers a simplified depiction of how speech demands change as a student progresses through school.

TABLE 9–4. Changing School Demands

Grades	Changing School Demands
K	Learn outside of an immediate context
1–2	Learn to read and write
3–6	Read and write to learn
7–10	Students assume responsibility for their own learning
11–12	Students become independent learners and process volumes of language information in short periods of time

Kindergarten

In the first school year, a student increasingly learns topics outside an immediate context. For example, a student may speak about continents or types of flowers without traveling to each continent or standing in a bed of daisies. **Phonological awareness** (conscious knowledge of the sound structure of a language) is assessed and trained, typically focusing on dividing words into syllables (**syllable segmentation**), awareness of rhyme and alliteration (**rhyme awareness** and **alliteration awareness**), and isolation of individual sounds in words (**phoneme isolation**). Table 9–5 summarizes typical ages at which students learn aspects of phonological awareness.

First and Second Grade

A student acquires foundations of literacy, including how the language translates such speech elements as consonants, consonant clusters, and vowels into written forms. A student typically learns to segment a word into individual sounds (**phoneme segmentation**).

Third through Sixth Grade

A student increasingly uses reading and writing to learn. Speech makes possible or facilitates—and may cause challenges for—such important social and educational activities as

- Undertaking projects with peers
- Making class presentations and oral reports
- Answering questions in class
- Participating in extracurricular activities such as drama
- Discussing ideas
- Expressing feelings

TABLE 9–5. Development of Phonological Awareness in Late Preschoolers and Students in the Early School Years

Age	Description
4;6–4;11	Syllable segmentation
5;0–5;5	Rhyme awareness
	Alliteration awareness
	Phoneme isolation
6;6–6;11	Phoneme segmentation

Source: Dodd & Gillon (2001).

Seventh through Tenth Grade

A student increasingly assumes responsibility for their learning. Homework becomes an important aspect of education, placing challenging demands on planning and organization. A student reads and speaks fluently on abstract topics and learns to pronounce words encountered in academic reading.

Eleventh and Twelfth Grade

A student becomes an independent learner, processing volumes of language information in a short time. During reading, a student increasingly encounters vocabulary with Greek and Latin roots, requiring mastery of longer sequences of sounds and unfamiliar stress patterns.

How a Student Learns

Though its form may change, what remains the same from infants to adults is the human need to connect with others and to learn in a social context. To illustrate, bonding with a clinician or teacher often helps motivate a student to do the work to succeed, modified speech input may transform phonetic complexities into treatment steps, and familiar routines in clinic and class provide a necessary structure for learning.

Curriculum Matters

A school's curriculum is both a mountain a student must climb and a hand that pulls up a speech student to reach the peak of their potential (Preston, Hull, & Edwards, 2013). Formerly, a clinician often undertook speech treatment in schools largely apart from the curriculum. Schools have changed their perspective on speech, and today, speech services often need to justify themselves by showing their influence on a student's academic and social development.

Incorporating Speech. Incorporating speech into the curriculum is easy because a student typically uses speech for so many daily purposes. Illustrations of ways to include speech in the curriculum include

- **Scientific vocabulary:** Use the student's science book to practice longer scientific vocabulary, practicing them in sentences.
- **Academic unit:** Find out what academic unit is the focus of the class and work on the treatment sound in words encountered in the unit.
- **Spelling words:** Use spelling words to practice speech.
- **Class assignments:** Help the student read books assigned in class, preparing ahead for class discussion to encourage success and generalization.

Benefits

Enormous benefits arise from the tie between speech and the curriculum. A few of them are outlined in the following sections.

Benefits for Students

- Speech treatment is a continuation of activities in the classroom and provides a chance for the student to practice and learn information with another adult.
- The connection bridges the gap between treatment and the classroom.
- The connection incorporates familiar classroom materials and activities into the student's specific treatment goals, so the treatment sessions are more relevant and "real" to the student.

Benefits for Teachers

- The connection provides a way to keep the teacher informed about what the student's speech goals are and what strategies and treatment plans a clinician uses to reach them.
- The teacher can reinforce speech goals and strategies with a student in the classroom during regular lessons.
- The teacher can offer important information and insight about a student's abilities in the classroom setting.

Benefits for Families

- If the activities and materials in speech treatment are the same activities and materials used in the regular classroom setting, families are better equipped to help with their student's speech homework.
- Parents know that their student is not missing important classroom curriculum time while working on their speech goals during the treatment sessions.

Pulling It Together

These are major ideas in sound communication in students:

- Progression through school both improves and may challenge a student's speech abilities.
- Students, like people of all ages, need to connect with others and to learn in a social context.
- For a student with speech challenges, a school's curriculum is both a mountain a student must climb and a hand that pulls them up to reach the peak of their potential.
- Incorporating speech into the curriculum is easy, because a student typically uses speech for so many daily purposes.
- The school's curriculum in speech treatment benefits students, teachers, and families.

CLINIC BOX: Cap and Gown

Though this chapter ends with a student receiving a high school diploma, speech development is lifelong and continues as an adult learns new words, studies a new language, or acquires speech patterns of a new dialect or social group.

Conclusions

Major ideas discussed in this chapter include

1. The speech accomplishments of preschoolers become the foundations of speech development for students.
2. Speech perception difficulties require a clinician to bring a long-standing speech production to a student's awareness.
3. Speech challenges to students may involve the late 8, [r] colored vowels, consonant clusters, and reading-based syllabic shifts and stress patterns.
4. Speech demands change as a student progresses through school.
5. The curriculum plays a central role in speech treatment of students.

Review Questions

1. The first paragraph of this chapter lists what three attainments in speech development during the school years?
2. Do you have examples of misperceptions you have made or heard made as an adult?
3. List the late 8.
4. List three errors that typically affect the late 8.
5. What are the last acquired consonant clusters?
6. What errors typically affect consonant clusters?
7. What vowel is most likely to be in error in students?
8. What speech accomplishments occur in first and second grade?
9. Why may the curriculum both challenge and help a student with speech difficulties?
10. In your own words, how does connecting speech learning to the curriculum benefit a student, teachers, and family?

References

Dodd, B., & Gillon, G. (2001). Exploring the relationship between phonological awareness, speech impairment and literacy. *Advances in Speech-Language Pathology*, 3(2), 139–147.

McLeod, S. (2002). Part I: The plethora of available data on children's speech development. *ACQuiring Knowledge in Speech, Language, and Hearing*, 4, 141–147.

McLeod, S. (2011). Laying the foundations for multilingual acquisition: An international overview of speech acquisition. *Journal of Linguistics and Language Teaching*, *2*, 53–71.

McLeod, S., van Doorn, J., & Reed, V. A. (2001a). Normal acquisition of consonant clusters. *American Journal of Speech-Language Pathology*, *10*, 99–110.

McLeod, S., van Doorn, J., & Reed, V. A. (2001b). Consonant cluster development in two-year-olds: General trends and individual difference. *Journal of Speech, Language, Hearing Research*, *44*, 1144–1171.

Preston, J. L., Hull, M., & Edwards, M. L. (2013). Preschool speech error patterns predict articulation and phonological awareness outcomes in children with histories of speech sound disorders. *American Journal of Speech-Language Pathology*, *22*, 173–184.

Smit, A., Hand, L., Frelinger, J., Bernthal, J., & Byrd, A. (1990). The Iowa articulation norms project and its Nebraska replication. *Journal of Speech and Hearing Disorders*, *55*, 779–798.

CHAPTER 10
SPEECH PUZZLES

This, the second, "learn by doing" chapter contains exercises to prepare you to undertake assessment and treatment of speech sound disorders. The exercises are adapted from classic studies on child phonology. I hope you enjoy the puzzles and find them fun to solve. Topics in this chapter include:

- Communication Strategies
- Exercises

Learning Objectives

I hope on completing the chapter you will

- Appreciate that assimilations can result in unusual pronunciations.
- Understand that sometimes speech improvement results in loss of phonetic accuracy.
- Discover how a child reduces speech complexity through a simple word recipe.
- Identify why a child may add sounds to make a word easier to say.
- Understand how a child may pick-and-choose words to say based on their sounds.

Key Words

Key words you will encounter in this chapter

Communication strategies
Lexical selection (selectivity)
Word-based learning
Favorite sounds and word recipes
Gestalt learning
Regression

Communication Strategies

For convenience, the discussion of communication strategies in Chapter 7, "Toddlers," is included here. See that chapter for more detailed discussion.

Meeting the Challenge

The challenge for toddlers is to find ways to communicate their thoughts and feelings when they can produce only a small number of consonants, vowels, syllables, and stress patterns. A toddler meets this difficulty by developing **communication strategies** that simplify the speaking task. The following is a selection of those strategies.

Lexical Selection

Many children follow a strategy of **lexical selection** (also called **selectivity**), "picking and choosing" words to say based on their ability to pronounce them, which allows a child to ignore the multitude of sounds they cannot pronounce and to communicate instead with words that contain those sounds that lie within their narrow range of speech abilities. First described by Ferguson and Farwell (1975) and studied experimentally by Schwartz and Leonard (1982), lexical selection appears to be a widespread speaking strategy among both typically developing children and those with speech sound disorders (Leonard, 1985).

Word-Based Learning

Word-based learning is another frequently encountered communication strategy. A word-based learner says words just well enough for a listener to understand them, giving little attention to the accuracy of the pronunciation. A word-based learner is somewhat analogous to a person in a foreign country who learns a few words of the language and pronounces them just well enough for someone to understand them. As a result, a word-based learner may pronounce words that contain a word initial **[m]** in the adult language as **[m]** in some words, **[p]** in others, and **[b]** in others.

Favorite Sounds and Word Recipes

While some children "pick and choose" (lexical selection) and others pronounce haphazardly (word-based learning), still others simplify the challenge of speaking through **favorite sounds and word recipes** that allow them to render a wide variety of sounds through a few simple means. To illustrate, a favorite consonant could be **[s]**, which the child uses to begin nearly all words they say (Ferguson & Macken, 1983).

Word recipes are like favorite sounds, though word recipes involve the entire word rather than a single sound. To illustrate, a child's word recipe might be all words he says are CVC and the first consonant is **[b]**, the vowel is lax, and the second consonant is

[m] or [n]. The term *word recipe* conveys that a child, like some inexperienced cooks, repeatedly uses the same few recipes (Menn, 1976; Waterson, 1971). For a novice cook, all meals may end up tasting like spaghetti. For a child with a word recipe strategy, all words may end up sounding like [**di**].

Gestalt Learning

Gestalt learning simplifies speech by bypassing words in favor of phrase and sentence melody. The speech of a child following this strategy may contain phrases with good intonation and relatively poor pronunciation of individual sounds. In a colorful and insightful phrase, Ann Peters has said that such children "learn the tune before the word" (Peters, 1977, 1983).

Exercises

Exercise 1

Assimilations are common in the speech of many younger children. The speech of the following child, aged 1;6 to 1;10, contains two common assimilations that interact with each other in surprising ways (Cruttenden, 1978).

Speech Sample

Intended Words	Child's Words
1. doggie	gʊgi
2. cuddle	kʊku
3. rabbit	babi
4. man	mam
5. crispies	pipi
6. piggy	pɪpi
7. apple	papa
8. about*	bəbaʊ
9. all gone	gʊgʊn
10. acorn*	kɛkʊn

*The child did not say these words, but the pronunciations follow his speech pattern. I added the words to provide additional examples for the exercise.

Questions

1. Words #1 and #2 are examples of a common assimilation. What is the name of the assimilation? (**Hint:** If helpful, review the discussion of phonological processes in Chapter 8, "Preschoolers.")

2. Words #3 and #4 are examples of another common assimilation. What is the name of the assimilation?

3. Now look at the intended words. What is the place of production of the consonants that assimilate in words #1 through #4?

4. Words such as #5 and #6 contain both labial and velar consonants. Does velar assimilation or labial assimilation occur?

5. Develop a hypothesis that summarizes your findings for words #1 through #6. (**Hint:** Describe the assimilations, alveolar consonants, and interactions between labial and velar assimilation.)

6. How does your hypothesis predict that the child will pronounce the consonants in the following words? *Part A of this question is an example.*
   a. dig
   b. bug
   c. pit
   d. tub

7. The words (a phrase in one instance) #7 through #10 begin with vowels in the adult language, but the child produces them with initial consonants. Notice that each word begins with a different consonant. What determines which consonant begins words #7 through #10? (**Hint:** Ignore the [1] in *all gone*, which the child may not have heard because many speakers do not pronounce it.)

8. List two words you could teach the child to determine if your hypothesis is correct. Indicate which sound you think the child will pronounce at the beginning of each word.

Answer Sheet

1. Phonological process:

2. Phonological process:

3. Place of production:

4. Assimilation:

5. Hypothesis:

6. a. *g g*
   b.
   c.
   d.

7. Hypothesis:

8. Possible words:

CLINIC BOX: Individual Differences

Importantly, individual differences in speech development abound, especially among younger children (McLeod, 2003). To illustrate, a comparison of consonant inventories of four 2-year-old children developing typically revealed that their inventories ranged from 5 to 14—impressive variation among children all near the same age and all without speech problems (Bleile, 1996).

Exercise 2

Researchers have known that children sometimes regress in speech development since at least the 1940s, when a German linguist named Leopold described the regression in his daughter's pronunciation of *pretty* over a period of several months (Leopold, 1947). This type of **regression** (loss of phonetic accuracy) is not due to neurological problems, trauma, or an inadequate environment. Rather, it arises from overgeneralization of a regular way of talking. A similar type of overgeneralization occurs later in morphological development when a child (typically, aged about 3 years) who previously said *went* now says *goed*, as in *I goed home.*

This exercise analyzes a famous case of a regression in a child from 1 year, 6 months to 1 year, 8 months (Menn, 1976). The regression affected two previously mastered words and lasted for several months as the child sorted out placement of primary stress in two similar sounding words, *caca* and *cookie*. Ages are listed as year:month:day.

Speech Sample

Age	*Caca**
1;6:27	kaká
1;7:17	gak
1;7:24	káka
1;7:27	káka~ kaká
1;8:22	gʌ́ga-kʌ́ka

Caca* [kaká**] is a Greek word learned from a babysitter that means feces.

Age	*Cookie**
Before 1;6:27	kóki
1;7:10	kʌkí
1;7:24	kʌkí
1 ;7:27	kʌkí
1;8:18	kóki

*The regression also affected *cracker*, which he pronounced the same as *cookie*.

Questions

1. Which syllable in *kaka* receives primary stress before 1;6:27?
2. When does the regression in *kaka* occur?
3. Describe the regression in *kaka* in your own words.
4. Which syllable in *cookie* receives primary stress before 1;6:27?
5. When does the regression in *cookie* begin and end?

6. Describe the regression in *cookie* in your own words.

7. Suppose you taught the child the word *cackle* on 1;7:24. If your hypothesis about the regression that affects *cookie* is correct, which syllable would receive primary stress in *cackle*?

8. The regression in *cookie* is difficult to explain as a physical problem in producing primary stress on the first syllable. Why?

9. *For discussion:* What is your hypothesis for why the child changes the stress patterns in *kaka* and *cookie*?

Answer Sheet

1. Primary stress:

2. Date:

3. Description:

4. Primary stress:

5. Dates:

6. Regression:

7. Cackle:

8. Explanation:

9. *For discussion:*

Exercise 3

Some new cooks attempt different dishes that all end up tasting like spaghetti. Some children do the same thing to words, reducing the vast phonetic complexity of speech to a few word recipes (Menn, 1976). Waterson (1971) was one of the first investigators to describe this phenomenon. This exercise offers an opportunity to reanalyze the speech from Waterson's study of a child approximately 1 year, 6 months.

Speech Sample

Intended Words	Child's Words
1. fish	iʃ-ʊʃ
2. brush	biʃ
3. window	ɲeɲe
4. fetch	iʃ
5. another	ɲaɲa
6. dish	diʃ
7. finger	ɲeɲe~ɲiɲi
8. Randell	ɲaɲe
9. vest	ʊʃ

Questions

1. Describe [ɲ] (the first consonant in the third word) in terms of place, manner, and voicing.
2. The child had two recipes for words on this list, one recipe was to say one-syllable words that end with voiceless friction and the other was for two-syllable words that contain [n] and have primary stress on the first syllable. Indicate by word number which words belong in each recipe.
3. In your own words, describe the child's recipe for the words included in the *fish* recipe. (**Hint:** For this and the following question, focus on the child's pronunciations rather than the intended words.)
4. In your own words, describe the child's recipe for the words included in the *window* recipe.

Answer Sheet

1. [ɲ]:
2. First recipe:

   Second recipe:
3. *Fish* recipe:
4. *Window* recipe:

Exercise 4

Phonological processes such as labial assimilation and velar assimilation describe consonants assimilating to other consonants. Consonants also assimilate to vowels, as is the case with the speech of the child, aged 20 to 23 months, who is the focus of this exercise (Braine, 1974).

Speech Sample

Intended Words	Child's Words
1. ball	bo.ʊ
2. mama	mama
3. pad*	pæ
4. big	dɪʔ
5. boo*	bu
6. milk	nɪʔ
7. bʌbʌbʌbi**	babadi
8. me*	ni
9. pa*	pa
10. "b"	di?

*I added words followed by an asterisk to better illustrate the child's error pattern.
**A nonsense word that the child imitates.

Questions

1. How many speech errors in syllable initial consonants occur in these 10 words? (**Hint:** Remember that each consonant in word #7 is in syllable initial position.) *This is an example.*

2. Describe how the place of production changes in these in these consonants.

3. Consider the consonants produced in error. Which vowels follow these consonants?

4. Develop a hypothesis that describes the errors.

5. How does your hypothesis suggest the child will pronounce the first consonants in *meet*, *bit*, and *battle.*

6. Suppose a colleague believes your hypothesis is incorrect and hypothesizes instead that any close vowel causes the error. Which of the 10 words could you use to argue against this alternative hypothesis? Why?

Answer Sheet

1. Syllable initial consonants: *5*
2. Place of production change:
3. Vowels:
4. Hypothesis:
5. *Meet*, *hit*, and *battle*:
6. Alternative hypothesis:

Exercise 5

This exercise considers two speech errors, one affecting consonants and the other vowels. The exercise comes from the speech of a child named Jacob, the child whose regressions were the subject of Exercise 2. The present example occurred from 1 year, 6 months to 1 year, 9 months (Menn, 1976).

Speech Sample

Intended Words	Jacob's Words*
1. tape	ti
2. duck	dʌ
3. close	doʊ
4. okay	ki
5. gate	gi
6. whee	i
7. cow	kaʊ
8. "a"	i
9. cake	gik~keɪk

*The vowel errors have exceptions, including in the words *away*, *lady*, *Jacob*, and *rain*.

Questions

1. What phonological process affects Jacob's pronunciation of consonants at the end of words?

2. Which of the 10 words is an exception to the above phonological process?

3. List two words that you could teach Jacob to test if your hypothesis about this phonological process is correct.

4. Now, consider Jacob's vowel errors. To begin, use the x y notation (see Chapter 5, "Phonetics Warm-Up") to list Jacob's vowel errors. *The first part of this question is an example.*

5. Based on your answer to the fourth question, which vowel will Jacob pronounce as [i]?

6. Describe Jacob's vowel errors using the distinctive feature system of your choice.

7. If your hypothesis is correct, how will Jacob pronounce the vowels in *hay* and *duke*?

Answer Sheet

1. Phonological process:

2. Exception:

3. Possible words:

4. Words: 1. *tape* eɪ→i

5. Affected vowel:

6. Distinctive features:

7. *hay* and *duke*:

Exercise 6

This exercise focuses on a somewhat unusual sound addition in the speech of a child aged from approximately 1 year, 9 months to 2 years, 2 months (Fey & Gandour, 1982). The sound addition affects consonants in the ends of words.

Speech Sample

Intended Words	Child's Words
1. big	bigŋ̩
2. egg	ɛgŋ̩
3. read	widn̩
4. drop	dap
5. stub	dabm̩
6. eat	ɪt
7. word	wʊdn̩
8. talk	dɔk
9. lightbulb	jaɪtbabm̩
10. fit	vɪt

Questions

1. What is the meaning of the diacritic under the nasal consonant in word #3? The same mark appears after the final consonants in the first and second words, though it is difficult to see. (**Hint:** If the mark seems unfamiliar, see Appendix A, "Special Symbols and Diacritics.")

2. Which class of sounds does the child add to the end of certain words?

3. Sometimes the child adds [m] to a word, other times [n], and other times [ŋ]. Develop a hypothesis that describes which consonant the child adds.

4. Suppose you decide to teach the child some new words. According to your hypothesis, which consonant will the child add to *mud* and *bib*?

5. Notice that the child does not add an additional consonant to certain words. Develop a hypothesis that explains why. (**Hint:** The words are not exceptions.)

6. According to your hypothesis, will the child add a consonant to words ending in [k]? If your answer is yes, indicate which consonant the child will add.

7. **For discussion:** Can you hypothesize what might be a phonetic basis for this speech error?

Answer Sheet

1. Diacritic:

2. Sound class:

3. Hypothesis:

4. *Mud* and *bib*:

5. Hypothesis:

6. Words ending in [**k**]:

7. ***For discussion:***

Exercise 7

Many young children choose to say words that contain stress patterns, syllables, and sounds that they already produce (see discussion of lexical selection in Chapter 7, "Toddlers"). A child, for example, whose expressive vocabulary contains words beginning with [m] is more likely to choose to say new words beginning with that sound. The present exercise focuses on Leslie, the subject of the first study to describe lexical selection (Ferguson, Peizer, & Weeks, 1973). At 11 months, Leslie's expressive vocabulary contained four words. (*Note:* As you perform this exercise, a reasonable thought that may occur to you is that Leslie's parents only taught their daughter words with certain speech characteristics. The authors of the original study thought otherwise, and subsequent research has borne them out.)

Speech Sample

Intended Words	Leslie's Words
1. daddy	dædæ
2. mommy	mama
3. doggie	gaga
4. patty (cake)	bæbæ

Questions

1. Look at the intended words. What do all these words share in terms of stress patterns? (*Hint:* For this exercise, analyze the words Leslie attempted rather than Leslie's pronunciations.)
2. What do all the intended words share in terms of sequence of syllables?
3. The intended words show a restricted range of places of production. What places of production occur in the intended words?
4. The intended words also show a restricted range of manners of production. What manners of production occur in the intended words?
5. What word-final vowel do all the intended words share?
6. Summarize your answers to questions 1 through 5 as a hypothesis regarding the speech characteristics of all the intended words.

Answer Sheet

1. Stress patterns:
2. Sequence of syllables:
3. Place of production:
4. Manner of production:
5. Word-final vowel:
6. Hypothesis:

Exercise 8

The final exercise shows that speech puzzles are not limited to children developing typically.

The exercise focuses on the speech of E, a child whose consonant inventory also appears in Chapter 14, "Phonetic Inventories." E was born prematurely. She received a tracheostomy when she was approximately 3 months old to treat bronchopulmonary dysplasia (BPD), a lung problem sometimes resulting from medical efforts to save children whose immature lungs are too weak to provide the breaths of life (Bleile, Stark, & Silverman McGowan, 1993). The exercise explores E's speech at 2;8, which was 4 months after her tracheostomy was closed. The words are E's entire expressive vocabulary.

Speech Sample

Intended Words	E's Words
1. daddy	dædə
2. hi	haɪ
3. down	da
4. mom	mam
5. hop	bap
6. water	wawa
7. book	bʊk
8. bow	boʊ
9. baby	bʌbʌ
10. up	ʌp
11. please	baɪ
12. bye	baɪ
13. bag	baɪ
14. bubble	bʌ
15. pop	bap
16. ball	bɔ
17. Pop Pop*	pap pap

*Pop Pop is the family name for grandfather.

Questions

1. Of 17 intended words, 16 begin with consonants. Identify how many of these word-initial consonants are bilabial, alveolar, velar, and glottal. (**Hint:** [w] is labio-velar, so place it in both the labial and velar columns.)

2. Divide the number of bilabial consonants by the total number of consonants (17, because [s] is counted twice.) What percentage of the consonants are bilabial?

3. Compare your answer to the expected percentage values for bilabial consonants shown on the answer sheet.

4. In your own words, describe what E is selecting for in the intended words.

5. Is an implication of the results that E will attempt to say words that begin with bilabial consonants more readily than words that begin with other consonants?

Answer Sheet

1. Bilabial:

   Alveolar:

   Velar:

   Glottal:

2. % Bilabial:

3. Expected relative frequency: *17.8%*

4. Lexical selection:

5. Yes or no:

Conclusions

Major topics in this chapter include:

1. A child develops strategies that help them communicate when speech limits their ability to communicate.
2. Well-described communication strategies include lexical selection, word-based learning, favorite sounds and word recipes, and gestalt learning.
3. Regressions in speech accuracy may occur as a child discovers systematic ways to say words.
4. Communication strategies occur in the speech of children both with and without speech sound disorders.

Review Questions

1. How do communication strategies help a child to speak?
2. What is lexical selection?
3. Explain in your own words how a word recipe might help a child communicate.
4. How does gestalt learning help a child communicate?
5. Can vowels cause a consonant to assimilate?
6. If you discover a child selects words beginning with [b], which word (all other things being equal, which they seldom are) will that child most likely attempt to say, *bee* or *pie*?
7. If you discover a child selects two-syllable words with primary stress on the first syllable, which word (again, all other things being equal) will that child most likely attempt to say, *balloon* or *baby*?

References

Bleile, K. (1996). *Articulation and phonological disorders: A book of exercises for students* (2nd ed.). San Diego, CA: Singular.

Bleile, K., Stark, R., & Silverman McGowan, J. (1993). Evidence for the relationship between babbling and later speech development. *Clinical Linguistics and Phonetics, 7,* 319–337.

Braine, M. (1974). On what might constitute learnable. *Phonology Language, 50,* 270–299.

Cruttenden, A. (1978). Assimilation in child language and elsewhere. *Journal of Child Language, 5,* 373–378.

Ferguson, C., & Farwell, C. (1975). Words and sounds in early language acquisition: English initial consonants in the first fifty words. *Language, 51,* 419–439.

Ferguson, C., & Macken, M. (1983). The role of play in phonological development. In K. Nelson (Ed.), *Child language IV* (pp. 256–282). Hillsdale, NJ: Lawrence Erlbaum.

Ferguson, C., Peizer, D., & Weeks, T. (1973). Model-and-replica phonological grammar of a child's first words. *Lingua, 31,* 35–65.

Fey, M., & Gandour, J. (1982). Rule discovery in phonological acquisition. *Journal of Child Language, 9,* 71–81.

Leonard, L. (1985). Unusual and subtle behavior in the speech of phonologically disordered children. *Journal of Speech and Hearing Disorders, 50,* 4–13.

Leopold, W. (1947). *Speech development of a bilingual child, a linguist's record . . . : Grammar and general problems in the first two years.* Evanston, IL: Northwestern University Press.

McLeod, S. (2003). General trends and individual differences: Perspectives on normal speech development. In S. P. Sohov (Ed.), *Advances in psychology research* (Vol. 22, pp. 189–202). New York, NY: Nova Science.

Menn, L. (1976). *Pattern, control and contrast in beginning speech: A case study in the development of word form and word function* (Unpublished doctoral dissertation). University of Illinois, Champagne-Urbana, IL.

Peters, A. (1977). Language learning strategies: Does the whole equal the sum of the parts? *Language, 53,* 560–573.

Peters, A. (1983). *The units of language acquisition.* New York, NY: Cambridge University Press.

Schwartz, R., & Leonard, L. (1982). Do children pick and choose: An examination of phonological selection and avoidance in early lexical acquisition. *Journal of Child Language, 9,* 319–336.

Waterson, N. (1971). Child phonology: A prosodic view. *Journal of Linguistics, 7,* 179–221.

PART III

ASSESSMENT

CHAPTER 11

SPEECH EVALUATION

A speech evaluation is like putting together pieces of a puzzle. This chapter is about a speech evaluation as part of a broader assessment of communication. This is our starting place because the puzzle pieces that go together in a communication assessment—referral, case history, present development, clinical decisions, implementation—are the same as for many other assessments as well. Topics in this chapter include:

- Overview
- Referral
- History
- Present Development
- Clinical Decisions
- Implementation

Assessment of speech sound disorders in bilingual and nonnative speakers of English is the subject of the next chapter, followed by hypothesis testing, and two "learn by doing" chapters on phonetic inventories and phonological processes. The companion website includes Assessment Resources with downloadable materials for assessment of social impact, severity, intelligibility, developmental milestones, informal assessments, and published tests.

Learning Objectives

I hope on completing the chapter you will

- Identify the three questions a speech evaluation answers.
- Understand the reason for each step in a speech evaluation.
- Know the reason for obtaining a child's history.
- Understand the reason for assessing language in a speech evaluation.
- Appreciate the multiple factors in clinical decisions.

Key Words

Key words you will encounter in this chapter

Speech evaluation	Language
Assessment of communication	Speech
	Social impact
Referral	Severity
History	Intelligibility
Early communication history	Developmental level
Medical history	Stimulability
Social history	Voice, resonance, and fluency
Education history	Oral mechanism and hearing
Present development	Clinical decisions
Behavior	Implementation

Overview

By law and good clinical sense, speech treatment begins with a speech evaluation. After all, how do you ask a family to undertake the time and expense of treatment without first determining if a problem exists and the likelihood of it responding to treatment? A **speech evaluation** answers three questions:

1. Does a communication problem exist and, if so, what is its nature?
2. Does the problem warrant treatment?
3. What should treatment focus on?

That is, a clinician's goal is to determine if a communication problem exists sufficient to warrant therapy; discover something about the general nature of the problem (if one exists); and, if a clinician judges a child should receive treatment, provide enough information to plan the first steps in treatment.

A Place to Begin

A speech evaluation gives a place to begin treatment, with the clinician knowing that additional experience with the child will result in a more nuanced and deeper understanding. Notice what a speech evaluation is not: it is not an answer to all possible questions about a child's communication development. A speech evaluation typically lasts from 45 to 90 min, an impossibly short time to answer every question about a child's communication. Better to leave a fuller understanding to a later date, perhaps concurrent with or as part of treatment.

CLINIC BOX: Assessment of Communication

A clinician often performs speech evaluation as part of a broader **assessment of communication** because a child does not produce speech in isolation from language, voice, fluency, resonance, an oral mechanism, or hearing. All those communication areas influence speech, and so, a complete speech evaluation assesses those domains as well.

Steps in a Speech Evaluation

A speech evaluation contains five steps, each focusing on a different clinical question:

1. Referral: *What is the reason for the referral?*
2. History: *How does the past influence present and future communication?*
3. Present development: *How is a child's communication functioning at present?*
4. Clinical decisions: *Does a communication problem exist, what is its nature, and does it warrant treatment?*
5. Implementation: *What plans may improve a child's communication outcome?*

Appendix 11–A provides a checklist of steps in a speech evaluation. The companion website contains the checklist in a downloadable form.

Referral

The first step in a speech evaluation is the **referral**. In a clinic report, referral information typically appears in the section variously called intake, introduction, or referral. Referral questions you may want to ask include:

- Who is the child?
- Who made the referral?
- What is the reason for the referral?
- What does the family see as the problem?
- What does the family see as goals of the assessment?

Logic of the Questions

The questions help you understand the reasons for the referral. To determine what a child's caregivers want the clinician to accomplish, almost always you will do well to ask at the start of the assessment, "How can I help you today?" or "What brings you in today?" Follow-up questions determine the referral source and ask the caregiver to describe what they perceive to be the nature of the child's communication difficulty.

History

A clinician obtains a **history** to determine how a child's past might influence present and future communication development. In a clinical report, this information typically appears in the section variously called case history or background.

Sources of Information

With a younger child, the child typically is present during the history, which also allows you to observe the child and the child-caregiver interactions. Additionally, while you observe the child, the child can observe you and the evaluation setting. With an older child, a clinician typically obtains the history outside of the child's presence, especially if sensitive topics need discussion.

Oftentimes, a clinician obtains a child's history using a questionnaire developed at their clinic setting. While questionnaires may differ in their specific questions, they typically address four aspects of a child's history:

- Early communication history
- Medical history

- Social history
- Education history

The following questions illustrate one way to address these four areas. You can ask questions in a different order or you can move questions from one category to another, if that suits you.

Early Communication History

> ➤ *Goal: Obtain information on babbling, first three words, regular two-word combinations, and short sentences.*

Questions you might ask about a child's **early communication history** include

- When did the child first babble on a regular basis?
- When did the child first speak three different words? What were they?
- When did the child start regularly saying two and three-word sentences?
- When did the child begin to speak in sentences, even though some of the words in the sentence may have been missing?

Logic of the Questions

The communication history helps you decide if a child evidences early communication delay in attaining major communication milestones. Babbling (canonical babbling) is included because research indicates it is important for later speech and language development (Locke & Pearson, 1992; Morris; 2010). Similarly, first words are important because they are a milestone in communication and expressive vocabulary. Development of two and three-word sentences is important because they are the origin of syntax, and speaking in short sentences indicates how syntactic development is progressing (Bates & Goodman, 2013 Brown, 1973; Paul & Jennings, 1992).

Medical History

> ➤ *Goal: Obtain information on pregnancy, delivery, length of stay in hospital after delivery, diagnoses, medical conditions, hospitalizations, ear infections, family history of communication disorders, and present health.*

Medical history questions you might ask include:

- Were there any complications during the pregnancy?
- Was the child born full term?
- How long did the baby remain in the hospital after delivery?
- Has the family ever hospitalized the child?
- Has the child ever had an ear infection?
- Has anyone in the family had a communication disorder?

- Does the child have any diagnosed medical or developmental conditions?
- Does the child take medications on a regular basis?
- How is the child's present health?

Logic of the Questions

The questions explore medical factors that might influence communication development (Bleile & Burda, 2003; Fox, Dodd, & Howard, 2002).

- Were there any complications during the pregnancy?
  Pregnancy complications may point to early difficulties that can influence later communication development.
- Was the child born full term?
  Length of pregnancy is important because infants born premature are at risk for future developmental difficulties, especially if the child also was low birth weight.
- How long did the child remain in the hospital after delivery?
  Length of hospitalization after delivery indicates if a child's medical problems were sufficient to require a hospital stay. Hospitalization for more than two or three days may signal an area that needs further exploration.
- Has the family ever hospitalized the child?
  Hospitalization may suggest potentially serious health problems, perhaps sufficient to influence communication development.
- Has the child ever had an ear infection?
  Research indicates a connection between middle ear problems and communication development (Dhooge, 2003; Shriberg, Friel-Patti, Flipsen, & Brown, 2000; Shriberg, et al., 2003).
- Has anyone in the family had a communication disorder?
  Because communication disorders may "run in a family," it is important to know if members of a child's family have communication disorders (Shriberg, & Austin, 1998; Shriberg, et al., 2005).
- Does the child have any diagnosed medical or developmental conditions?
  Many different medical and developmental conditions influence communication development.
- Does the child take medications on a regular basis?
  Medications can influence a child's communication development as well as their performance in treatment (Gumpper, 2007).
- How is the child's present health?
  A child's present health can influence their performance in the evaluation.

Social History

➤ *Goal: Obtain information on members of family, main persons with whom the child interacts.*

Social history questions you may want to ask include

- Who are the members of the child's family?
- Who are the main people with whom the child interacts?

Logic of the Questions

The social history seeks to determine if a child's environment is sufficiently stable to foster healthy communication development. The question is of stability rather than of composition. For example, many different compositions of people can maintain a stable environment, including a mother and father, a grandparent, same gender couples, or single parents. Examples of questions to help you better understand the make-up of a child's family include, "Who in the immediate family does the child interact with regularly?"; "Does the child play with children outside the immediate family?"; "How many times a week?"

Depending on the results of the medical part of the interview, you might also ask if lengthy hospitalizations occurred in the past. Hospitals, while good places to recover physically, are not well-suited to a child's social and communication needs. To illustrate, pressing obligations of hospital staff may keep them from meeting a child's emotional needs as a family might, which can result in later difficulties in behavior and communication (Fridy & Lemanek, 1993).

Education History

> ➤ *Goal: Obtain information on past and present education placements and any special services (types, amounts and goals).*

Education history questions you may wish to ask include

- Has the child ever attended any type of day care or preschool? Did they receive any special services?
- Is the child currently in any educational program? Did they receive any special services in the past?

Logic of the Questions

The education history helps discover if a child has received formal schooling, including special services. Both types of information may give valuable insights into a child's communication development, or, at the least, keep the evaluator from making recommendations for services that the child may already be receiving.

After Completing the History

After completing the history, you might take the opportunity to let the caregivers know what will happen during the remainder of the assessment. Consider addressing

- Restating the caregiver's concerns
- Explaining to the caregiver how you will assess their child's communication
- Asking if a caregiver prefers to stay in the room or to leave, perhaps to observe

Present Development

This part of an evaluation focuses on a child's **present development** in communication. This information typically appears in the section of a clinic report called current functioning or evaluation results. The following are areas typically addressed:

- How does the child behave?
- How is the child progressing in language?
- How is the child progressing in speech?
- How is the child's voice, resonance quality, and fluency?
- Is the child's oral mechanism and hearing adequate for speech?

This list of questions means you have much to do in less time than an average length movie! Fortunately, you can complete some testing "by ear." To illustrate, when a child speaks you might listen carefully to their vocal quality and fluency to decide if you need to undertake further testing. Since this is a book on speech, the following discussion gives the speech area a central focus, recognizing that other areas may be shortchanged.

Behavior

> *Goal: Determine if the evaluation results reflect the child's knowledge or compliance.*

Questions you might ask about **behavior** include

- Is the child's behavior representative of what they do outside the assessment setting?
- In what ways are the child's behaviors atypical or typical?
- Are there behaviors not occurring in the assessment about which you would like me to know?

Logic of the Questions

If a child is cooperative and compliant, it gives you more confidence in the results of the evaluation. You can confirm this by asking a caregiver something like, "The results we obtain here are only important if they reflect what your child does outside here. So, could you let us know if what we see today is representative of how your child typically communicates?"

If a child is less cooperative or noncompliant compared to similarly aged children, this may raise questions:

1. Most directly, you may reasonably wonder about the reliability of your assessment findings. To illustrate, if an uncooperative child performs poorly on a test, you may

ask if the results are due to lack of cooperation or lack of knowledge (or, of course, lack of cooperation *and* lack of knowledge).

2. Lack of cooperation and compliance could also indicate a behavior problem, which may influence communication development.

3. Lack of cooperation could suggest difficulties in attention and focus, two cognitive functions known to impact communication development.

4. If a child lacks the degree of cooperation and compliance of children of comparable age, it is possible that the child experiences a global developmental delay. That is, a child may behave like a younger child because developmentally the child is in many ways a younger child.

Language

➤ *Goal: Compare a child's language development to speech.*

In a communication assessment with a speech focus, your **language** questions include

- How does the child's language reception compare to similar-age peers?
- How does the child's language expression compare to similar-age peers?
- How does the child's development in language reception compare to their development in language expression?

Logic of the Questions

The first question tells you if the child understands comparably to children of the same age, and the second question tells you the same thing for language expression. The third question compares development of language reception to that of language expression, which tells you if the child is globally delayed (both reception and expression are equally delayed) or if one aspect of language shows greater delay. A very common pattern is for language expression to show greater delay than language reception, meaning the child understands more of language than they can express. The opposite pattern (the child's expression shows more advanced development than their understanding) is more rare but occurs in some children with autism spectrum disorder and some children with hydrocephaly.

Speech

➤ *Goal: Determine how a child's speech development compares to their development in language expression and language reception.*

Questions you may wish to ask about **speech** include

- What is the social impact of the child's speech sound disorder, if one exists?
- What is the child's level of intelligibility?
- What is the severity of the child's speech sound disorder, if one exists?
- What is the child's level of speech development?

Logic of the Questions

Even in a communication assessment with a speech focus, a clinician typically has only 15 to 20 min for speech, so each answer counts, contributing information you need to form your clinical decisions.

- **Social impact** measures concern about a child's speech and is a factor in deciding whether to provide treatment.
- **Severity** measures degree of impairment; it is a primary means to justify providing or refusing clinical treatment.
- **Intelligibility** is the amount of speech a listener understands and is the factor most frequently cited by both clinicians and caregivers in deciding the severity of a child's speech disorder.
- **Developmental level** establishes the age range that most closely approximates a child's speech development, and it is a factor in establishing if a speech sound disorder exists.

Stimulability

In addition to these four areas, you may also wish to undertake specialized assessments. **Stimulability** probably is the most frequently performed specialized assessment.

- Are there stimulable elements in the child's speech?

Stimulability testing determines if a child has any capacity to produce a speech element (consonant, vowel, syllable, stress, etc.) and may be a factor in selecting a treatment sound (see Chapter 17, "Treatment Sounds"). Assessment Resources on the companion website contain downloadable materials for all the above aspects of speech.

Voice, Resonance, and Fluency

> ➤ *Goal: Determine if there are communication challenges in addition to those in speech and language.*

Questions you may wish to address include

- Does the child have difficulties affecting the larynx?
- Does the child have difficulties with coupling between the oral and nasal tracts?
- Does the child's speech contain primary disfluencies and secondary behaviors?

Logic of the Questions

Difficulties in **voice, resonance, and fluency** all can influence a child's speech development. Because of the focus of the chapter, I have reduced these complex topics to a footnote, knowing that sometimes an assessment begins with a speech focus and ends up with a primary focus in voice, resonance, or fluency.

Oral Mechanism and Hearing

➤ *Goal: Determine if the speech and hearing mechanisms contribute to the communication disorder.*

Questions you may wish to ask on these topics include

- Are there abnormalities in the function and structure of the oral mechanism that might interfere with speech production?
- Does a hearing impairment exist that might influence speech development?

Logic of the Questions

Abnormalities in both the **oral mechanism and hearing** can influence speech development. As part of a speech evaluation, you typically screen for disorders in the function and structure of the oral mechanism and for impairments of hearing. Appendix 11–B in this chapter contains a quick 11-step screener to assess oral mechanism structure and function. The companion website contains a downloadable form of the screener.

If you discover a problem, you typically schedule a complete oral mechanism evaluation and make a referral for a hearing assessment with an audiologist. Fortunately, children are flexible and can learn speech with hearing impairments, high palates, small teeth, a small or large tongue, and many other mild to moderate structural and movement problems (Mason & Wickwire, 1978).

Clinical Decisions

With the referral, history, and present development assessments completed, you are ready to answer the following questions: "Does a communication problem exist and, if so, what is its nature?"; "Does the problem warrant treatment?"; and "What should treatment focus on?" **Clinical decisions** usually appear in the clinical diagnosis or clinical impressions section of a clinic report.

Questions you may wish to consider as you reflect on the assessment findings include

- What does the family view as the nature of the child's communication problem?
- What aspects of the child's history may influence communication development?
- What areas of communication (speech, expressive language, receptive language) show developmental delay relative to the child's chronological age?

If, based on the answers to these questions, you recommend a child receive treatment, four additional questions may help answer the question, "What should treatment focus on?"

- What area of communication (speech, expressive language, or language reception) shows the greatest developmental delay?
- What aspects of the child's communication are new and emerging?
- How able is the family to participate in the child's treatment?
- What are the child's daily routines and activities?

Logic of the Questions

The preceding questions influence clinical thinking in the following ways:

- What does the family view as the nature of the child's communication problem? This question influences everything from goal selection to explaining assessment results to the family. To illustrate, if you recommend treatment, you might select a treatment goal that fits the family's perspective on the child's communication problem. Alternately, if you believe a family's perspective contains some misconceptions, you might have a respectful discussion about that with the family.
- What aspects of the child's history may influence communication development? If factors in the child's history place him/her at greater risk for future communication difficulties, you become more likely to recommend treatment. Risk factors for future speech difficulties include an early history of communication delay, significant medical problems, living in an unstable home or in extreme poverty, and absent or minimal improvement in prior developmental services.
- What areas of communication (speech, expressive language, receptive language) show developmental delay relative to the child's chronological age? This question helps decide if a delay in communication exists and in which areas it occurs. A clinician typically bases severity level on extent of delay.
- What area of communication (speech, expressive language, or language reception) shows the greatest developmental delay? This question helps give focus to treatment because a clinician typically gives primary attention to the area of greatest delay.
- What aspects of the child's communication are new and emerging? New and emerging aspects of communication (that is, things a child does occasionally, though not yet frequently) often are goals for treatment.
- How able is the family to participate in the child's treatment? In addition to involvement in treatment being a parent's legal right, generalization is more likely to occur if the family participates in treatment.
- What are the child's daily routines and activities? Incorporating the child's routines and preferred activities in treatment helps promote generalization and are good sources of therapy activities.

Implementation

The final part of an assessment is to develop an **implementation** plan for the child to receive services. This information typically appears in the recommendation section of a clinic report.

Questions you may want to ask include

- Is there additional testing that should be undertaken?
- Where and when will treatment take place?
- What is the initial treatment goal?

Logic of the Questions

Many times, a clinician recommends additional testing to fill in missing assessment information. To illustrate, a young child may have been too distracted to complete a hearing screening, so the clinician recommends retesting. To give a different example, a clinician may believe a child's communication difficulties may be part of broader developmental problems, and so might recommend that the child receive a multidisciplinary developmental evaluation. The answer to the *when* and *where* question identifies the location and time of treatment, and the initial goal provides the first goal of treatment.

Conclusions

Major topics addressed in this chapter include

1. A speech evaluation answers three questions: Does a communication problem exist; and, if so, what is its nature? Does the problem warrant treatment? What should treatment focus on?
2. Best practice is to assess speech as part of an assessment of communication.
3. A speech evaluation contains five steps: referral, history, present development, clinical decisions, and implementation.

Review Questions

1. What three questions does a speech evaluation answer?
2. Why does a clinician typically perform a speech evaluation as part of an assessment of communication?
3. What is the purpose of asking referral questions?
4. What is the purpose of obtaining a child's history?
5. What four areas should you assess in a history?
6. What is the purpose of obtaining information on present development?
7. What might noncompliant behavior signify?
8. What areas do you assess in speech?
9. What is the purpose of reaching clinical decisions?
10. Explain in your own words why you may want to know a child's daily routines.
11. What is the purpose of the final step, implementation, in a speech evaluation?
12. Why is additional testing sometimes recommended?

References

Bleile, K., & Burda, A. (2003). Speech disorders in children: Birth related risk factors. In R. Kent (Ed.), *MIT encyclopaedia of communicative disorders* (pp. 188–190). Boston, MA: MIT Press.

Brown, R. (1973). *A first language: The early stages*. Cambridge, MA: Harvard University Press.

Dhooge, I. J. (2003, July). Risk factors for the development of otitis media. *Current Allergy and Asthma Reports*, *3*(4), 321–325.

Fox, A. V., Dodd, B., & Howard, D. (2002). Risk factors for speech disorders in children. *International Journal of Language and Communication Disorders*, *37*(2), 117–131.

Fridy, J., & Lemanek, K. (1993). Developmental and behavioral issues. In K. Bleile (Ed.), *The care of children with long-term tracheostomies* (pp. 141–166).San Diego, CA: Singular.

Goodman, J. C., & Bates, E. (2013). On the emergence of grammar from the lexicon. In *The emergence of language* (pp. 47–98). London, UK: Psychology Press.

Gumpper, P. (2007). Commonly used medications. In M. Batshaw, L. Pellegrino, & N. Roizen, (Eds.), *Children with disabilities* (6th ed., pp. 699–718). Baltimore, MD: Paul H. Brookes.

Locke, J., & Pearson, D. (1992). Vocal learning and the emergence of phonological capacity: A neurobiological approach. In C. Ferguson, L. Menn, & C. Stoel-Gammon (Eds.), *Phonological development: Models, research, implications* (pp. 91–130). Timonium, MD: York Press.

Mason, R., & Wickwire, N. (1978). Examining for orofacial variations. *Communique*, *8*, 2–26.

Morris, S. R. (2010). Clinical application of the mean babbling level and syllable structure level. *Language, Speech, and Hearing Services in Schools*, *41*, 223–230.

Paul, R., & Jennings, P. (1992). Phonological behavior in toddlers with slow expressive language development. *Journal of Speech, Language, and Hearing Research*, *35*(1), 99-107.

Shriberg, L. D., & Austin, D. (1998). *The speech-language connection*. Baltimore, MD: Paul H. Brookes.

Shriberg, L. D., Friel-Patti, S., Flipsen, P., Jr., & Brown, R. L. (2000). Otitis media, fluctuant hearing loss and speech-language delay: A preliminary structural equation model. *Journal of Speech, Language, and Hearing Research*, *43*(1), 100–120.

Shriberg, L. D., Kent, R. D., Karlsson, H. B., McSweeny, J. L., Nadler, C. J., & Brown, R. L. (2003). A diagnostic marker for speech delay associated with otitis media with effusion: Backing of obstruents. *Clinical Linguistics and Phonetics*, *17*(7), 529–547.

Shriberg, L. D., Lewis, B. A., Tomblin, J. B., McSweeny, J. L., Karlsson, H. B., & Scheer, A. R. (2005). Toward diagnostic and phenotype markers for genetically transmitted speech delay. *Journal of Speech, Language, and Hearing Research*, *48*(4), 834–852.

APPENDIX 11–A
SPEECH EVALUATION CHECKLIST

Referral

_____ Who is the child? *Name and age of client*

_____ Who referred? *Referral source*

_____ Why referred? *Reason for the referral*

_____ What does family see as problem? *Referral source's perception of the problem*

_____ What does family see as purpose of evaluation? *What does the referral source hope the evaluation will accomplish*

History

_____ Who reported history? *Name*

_____ Communication *Babbling, first three words, regular two-word combinations, short sentences, relate stories with four or more events, reading*

_____ Medical *Pregnancy, delivery, length of time in hospital after delivery, diagnosed conditions, hospitalizations, medicines, ear infections, present health*

_____ Social *Members of family, main persons with whom the child interacts*

_____ Education *Past and present education placements, any special services (types, amounts, and goals, if they exist)*

Present Development

_____ Behavior *Degree of cooperation and compliance*

_____ Language *Expressive language, language reception*

_____ Speech *Social impact, severity, intelligibility, developmental level, stimulability*

_____ Voice, Resonance, Fluency *Laryngeal quality, nasality, primary and secondary disfluencies*

_____ Oral Mechanism and Hearing *Structure and function, pure tone and middle ear function*

Clinical Decisions

_____ Family's View

_____ History

____ Areas of delay *(expressive language, language reception, speech)*

____ Greatest delay *(expressive language, language reception, speech)*

____ New and emerging

____ Family participation

____ Daily routines and activities

Implementation

____ Additional testing

____ When and where

____ Initial treatment goal

QUICK 11 STEP SCREENER OF ORAL STRUCTURE AND FUNCTION

Equipment: Gloves, a mirror, a penlight, and a tongue depressor. The evaluator should wear gloves and follow universal health precautions.

___ 1. Face

Sit at eye level across from the child and observe the face. Look for muscle weakness, spasticity, and drooping of one-half of the face.

Pass/No Pass

Comments:

___ 2. Breathing

Observe the child breathing. If mouth breathing observed, ask the child to close mouth and breathe onto a mirror placed under the nose.

Pass/No Pass

Comments:

___ 3. Lips

Observe the child's lips for drooling.

A. Ask the child to say [i] (to test lip spreading).
B. Ask the child to say [u] (to test lip rounding).
C. Ask the child to say [pʌpʌpʌ] (to test rapid movements of the lips).

Pass/No Pass

Comments:

___ 4. Jaw

Turn the child's head to each side and look for gross retrusions or protrusions of the maxilla or mandible.

Pass/No Pass

Comments:

____ **5. Teeth**

Ask the child to open the mouth so you can examine the teeth.

A. Look for missing teeth, especially those in front.
B. Instruct the child to bite down lightly on the back teeth and to open the lips. Look for normal overbite (upper front teeth are about one quarter inch in front of the lower teeth and cover about one third of the top of the lower teeth).
C. Look to see if the child has an excessive overbite or an open bite (i.e., the upper teeth do not cover part of the lower teeth at any point along the dental arch).

Pass/No Pass

Comments:

____ **6. Tongue**

Observe the child's tongue.

A. Look to determine if the tongue is grossly large, small, or shriveled.
B. Ask the child to touch the alveolar ridge with the tongue tip.
C. Instruct the child to move the tongue laterally to test its mobility.

Pass/No Pass

Comments:

____ **7. Hard Palate**

Instruct the child to extend the head back.

A. Observe the child's hard palate for signs of repaired or unrepaired clefts, fistulas, and fissures.
B. Observe the midline of the child's hard palate, using a penlight if needed. If a blue line is found at the midline, gently rub the posterior portion of the hard palate, feeling for a cleft.

Pass/No Pass

Comments:

____ **8. Soft palate**

Instruct the child to open the mouth three quarters of maximum to get the best velar elevation.

A. Observe the soft palate for signs of repaired and unrepaired clefts, fissures, and fistulas.
B. Look for a normal pink and white coloration at the midline.
C. Ask the child to produce a sustained "ah." (A nasal sounding "ah" may indicate difficulty closing the nasal tract.)

Pass/No Pass

Comments:

____ **9. Uvula**

Ask the child to say a sustained "ah" and observe the uvula.

Pass/No Pass

Comments:

____ **10. Fauces**

Ask the child to say a sustained "ah" and look for signs of redness, inflammation, or movement of the faucal pillars.

Pass/No Pass

Comments:

____ **11. Pharynx**

Ask the child to say a sustained "ah" and look at the back of the throat.

Pass/No Pass

Comments:

CHAPTER 12

ASSESSING A BILINGUAL CHILD

Lindsey R. Squires

Presently, only 6% of speech-language pathologists (SLPs) self-identify as being bilingual (ASHA, 2016), and even those who are bilingual may still find themselves diagnosing or treating in an unknown language (Morrow, Goldstein, Gilhool, & Paradis, 2014). When a clinician and a child do not speak the same language, a clinician may struggle to answer, "Does this child have a speech difference, or a speech disorder in addition to a speech difference?" (McLeod, Verdon, IEPMCS, 2017; Oetting, Gregory, & Rivière, 2016; Skahan, Watson, & Lof, 2007). This question can lead to a clinician misdiagnosing a child who is an **English language learner** (ELL) with a speech sound disorder, particularly between the ages of 3 and 6 years (Fabiano-Smith & Goldstein, 2010; Fabiano-Smith & Hoffman, 2018). This chapter focuses on special topics in the speech assessment of bilingual children. Topics include:

- Introduction
- Special Topics in Assessment

Learning Objectives

I hope on completing the chapter you will

- Explain language influences on speech development.
- Describe the distinction between speech differences and speech disorders.
- Understand special assessment issues for bilingual children.

Key Words

Key words you will encounter in this chapter:

Accent

Dialect

Simultaneous bilingual learner

Sequential bilingual learner

Home or heart language

Additive bilingualism

Subtractive bilingualism

English language learner

Interactional Dual Systems Models

Introduction

Let's begin with necessary background information for the assessment of bilingual language learners. Topics include speech variation, accent and dialect, simultaneous and sequential bilingual learners, language systems, and bilingual speech development.

Speech Variations

The title of this section is speech variations. What does that term mean? ASHA guidelines (1993) list various types of speech variations, including those resulting from communication differences and dialects, which is the topic of this chapter. The guidelines define communication difference/dialect as "a variation of a symbol system used by a group of individuals that reflects and is determined by shared regional, social, or cultural/ethnic factors." Importantly, ASHA states that these variations "should *not* be considered a disorder of speech or language" (italics mine).

Accent and Dialect

Accent differs from dialect.

Accent

Accent is a speech variation arising from the influence of the phonology of a home language on the production of a second language. Accents are typical and expected features of second language learning (Flege & Davidian, 1984). In the United States, Spanish is the most commonly spoken language after English; as such, the most common accented speech in the United States is Spanish-influenced English in children whose first language is Spanish (U.S. Census Bureau, 2011). To illustrate this accent, a child may say "eschool" for "school," because s-clusters in Spanish start with a vowel prior to the s-blend (Yavas & Somellian, 2005). The child's use of "eschool" presents a normal variation of how Spanish may influence the pronunciation of English as a second language.

Dialect

While an accent refers to phonological influences from another language, **dialect** is a broader term, referring to *all* the unique aspects of language variation, including the areas of phonology, vocabulary, and morphosyntax. More technically, a dialect is "any language variety that is shared by a group of people" (Oetting & McDonald, 2002).

A dialect often is specific to a given cultural or geographic region (Oetting et al., 2016). To illustrate, you may have noticed dialectal differences in vocabulary referring to the name of a sweet carbonated beverage. In some dialects, the beverage is "soda," in others "pop," and in others "coke." To give another example, you may have heard dialectal morphosyntax differences in English in a child who speaks an Appalachian English dialect that includes sentences such as, *"Did the girl see him a-walkin?"* (Zimmerman, Pond, & Steiner, 2011).

Varieties of Accents and Dialects

As clinicians, we are constantly learning about the unique contributions of a native language accent (phonology) or a language dialect (phonology, vocabulary, morphosyntax). We likely know some common accents and dialects, others less so. For example, many different dialects of Spanish exist, although many people have only heard of two: Mexican and Puerto Rican dialects (Taveras, Namazi, Pazuelo, & Casado, 2015). Appendix C, "Dialect and Accent," at the end of this book lists nine varieties of dialects and accents—a short list, but one that, hopefully, gives some insight into the rich mélange of speech variations you may encounter in your clinical work.

Communication Breakdowns

Although speech differences due to accent and dialects are not speech disorders, they can be sources of a communication breakdown or have a negative social impact (Munro, Derwing, & Sato, 2006). For example, older adult listeners may have more difficulty understanding accented English than those who are younger (Burda, Hageman, Scherz, & Edwards, 2003). In addition to simply asking for help (e.g., "How do you say . . . ?"), these are frequent signs that a bilingual language learner may be struggling to avoid a communication breakdown:

1. The learner may produce parts of a second language and then appeal for help indirectly through a pause or eye contact (Brown, 2000).
2. The learner may use avoidance strategies by leaving a message unfinished.
3. The learner may avoid certain words altogether due to speech differences or mispronunciations (Brown, 2000).

In your clinical practice, you may encounter children who refuse to say certain words because of potential speech differences (confession: with Spanish being my second language, I use synonyms to avoid certain Spanish words in professional settings to escape potential negative misunderstandings). If a child has both a speech difference and a disorder, they might benefit from instruction to repeat a difficult-to-produce word, or you may suggest a synonym for the challenging word.

Simultaneous and Sequential Bilingual Learners

The difference between simultaneous and sequential bilingualism is important in clinical work. A **simultaneous bilingual learner** has initial exposure to both languages at the same time, or dual exposure prior to age 3. Many simultaneous bilinguals grow up with "one-parent one-language" exposure (called an OPOL model) in which one parent uses one language and the other parent uses another (Langdon, 2008).

A **sequential bilingual learner** has exposure to a second language after age 3 (Brice & Brice, 2009; Tabors, 1997). In the United States, many bilingual children follow this stair-step sequential bilingual pattern, where exposure to the **home or heart language** comes before exposure to a second language upon school entrance (Brice & Brice, 2009; Gutierrez-McClellan, 1999).

Diversity in Sequential Bilingual Learners

Sequential learners may show more diversity in their language acquisition than simultaneous bilinguals (Brice & Brice, 2009; Langdon, 2008). To illustrate, in the area of vocabulary, variation is noticeable as children with second language exposure at age 5 may require 1 to 2 years to learn basic communication skills in the second language, and 5 to 7 years to acquire more academic language (Cummins, 1981). Clinically, the implication is that you can expect more variability in the language skills of a child on your caseload who is a sequential bilingual.

Why? Several factors help explain why variability in language acquisition is greater in sequential bilingual children. One reason may be that sequential learners have more variation in language exposure and communication partners (Bridges & Hoff, 2014). Another reason relates to the relative supportiveness of the environment in which a child learns their second language. That is, their environment may support **additive bilingualism** (i.e., honoring and encouraging a child's home language) or **subtractive bilingualism** (i.e., removing, denying, or limiting exposure to a child's home language), both of which may influence a child's learning of their second language (Gutierrez-McClellan, 1999).

One System or Two?

As a clinician, should you think of bilingual language learners having one system or two? For example, does a bilingual speaker of Spanish and English have two separate language systems, one for Spanish and the other for English, or do the two systems somehow interact? Paradis (2001) studied language influence across three groups of 2-year-olds ($n = 18$ English monolinguals, $n = 18$ French monolinguals, $n = 17$ French-English bilinguals). When comparing children's performance on a nonword repetition task (i.e., measuring ability to repeat nonsense words, such as "lapatimoon"), results showed that these young bilinguals had separate phonological systems, but that their systems were interdependent.

The Interactional Dual Systems Model. Paradis' (2001) findings helped to establish the **Interactional Dual Systems Model,** which states that each language contributes to phonological performance, but that they are not autonomous (Genesee, 1989; Goldstein & Gildersleeve-Neumann, 2007). At present, most clinical researchers support that they are two interrelated, nonindependent systems (Gildersleeve-Neumann & Goldstein, 2015; Hambly, Wren, McLeod, & Roulstone, 2013).

Let's Go Dancing. What does it mean that a bilingual's language systems are interrelated? Let's try an analogy to explain how languages may influence one another.

A bilingual's linguistic system is like dancing! (Full disclosure: I like dancing.) For the illustration, imagine a bilingual speaker approximately 4 years old who is more dominant in Spanish than in English for expressive language—dominance meaning the language area in which the child is stronger (Langdon, 2008).

In couples dancing, there are two partners: a lead and a follow. Consider the more dominant language as the "lead," and the less dominant language as the "follow." Dominance or preference for one language is a "typical aspect of early bilingual development" (Paradis, 2001). Each language has an influence on the other. Similarly, a dancer is not independent of the influence of their partner. The "lead" will probably be the most influential because of more exposure and practice; however, if one of the dancers does not maintain a quality connection or sufficient language exposure, then changes in dominance may occur.

Bilingual Speech Development

A common myth is that raising a child bilingually makes them slower to develop their first language. Research negates the myth that bilingualism has a detrimental effect or postpones development (Hambly et al., 2013). Nevertheless, it is important for a clinician to understand that differences exist between monolingual and bilingual children's speech. Two of those differences directly influence speech assessment:

1. Fabiano-Smith and Goldstein (2010) found bilingual preschoolers' speech had lower levels of accuracy in consonant production compared to monolingual preschoolers. As a result, bilingual preschoolers may be at higher risk for misdiagnosis (Fabiano-Smith & Hoffman, 2018).
2. Bilingual children's speech development is more variable than that of monolingual children (Fabiano-Smith & Hoffman, 2018; Hambly et al., 2013). Because a 3-year-old may be more variable in his/her accuracy and productions than his/her monolingual peers, bilingual children are at risk for misdiagnosis (Fabiano-Smith & Hoffman, 2018). The clinical implication is that bilingual children generally warrant careful assessment, sequential bilingual children more so than simultaneous bilingual children.

Speech Acquisition Summary

Much of what is currently known about bilingual speech acquisition is summarized in Hambly et al. (2013), who performed a systematic review of studies that examined multilingual infants' and children's speech. Here are six key findings

1. Limited evidence that multilingual children develop speech slower than monolingual children.
2. More variation occurs in multilingual children's speech than in that of monolingual peers.
3. Interactions occur between a child's two languages, with varied amounts.
4. Children's L1 (1st language) influences L2 (2nd language), and L2 influences their L1.

5. Both increased age and amount of language exposure to L2 facilitate speech production.
6. Research needs to provide more consistency in its description of children's language experience, schooling, and socioeconomic status.

CLINIC BOX: Hello, Late 8; Meet the Final 5

Consonant acquisition varies among languages. English has its late 8, while Spanish has what we might call its final 5. They are [l ð r ɾ s] (Fabiano-Smith & Goldstein, 2010; Leacox, 2018).

Special Topics in Assessment

Grosjean (1998, p. 131) observed, "those who have studied both monolinguals and bilinguals would undoubtedly agree that working with bilinguals is a more difficult and challenging enterprise." One major challenge is distinguishing between speech differences and speech disorders, both of which may exist in the same child. Researchers and clinicians frequently report on challenges associated with making this distinction (McLeod et al., 2017). This section describes special issues that arise in assessing speech in bilingual children, following the steps described in the previous chapter, and is supported by researchers in bilingual education (McLeod et al., 2017; Yavas & Goldstein, 1998). Topics include

- Referral
- History
- Present Development
- Clinical Decisions

Referral

Several important differences exist between referrals for multilingual children and monolingual children.

1. Parent referral rates are lower for multilingual children than for monolingual children (Stow & Dodd, 2005). This suggests that families may need additional opportunities to learn about available services as well as understand the systems of therapy (either educational or medical). Understandably, a language barrier can be a primary source of difficulty. Having interpreters or multilingual professionals available to explain and support services is key.
2. As Kummerer, Lopez-Reyna, and Hughes (2007) noted, mothers who were Mexican immigrants may discuss their child having a communication "delay" or "*retraso*" as an articulation difficulty, even if the child has concomitant language difficulties. A

reasonable clinical precaution is for a clinician to assess language, even if the parent reports the problem results from articulation difficulties.

3. Parents of bilingual children tend to be more concerned about their child's development than parents of monolingual children (Boerma & Blom, 2017). One reason for this may be that families are worried (or misinformed) that being bilingual can somehow cause a communication disorder.

4. Medical and educational professionals may rely too heavily on a "wait and see" model, which could lengthen time for eligibility to services and relates to under-referral rates (Stow & Dodd, 2005).

Taken in conjunction, statements one through four suggest that you may wish to add a prereferral step in the referral process to decrease unwarranted screenings and to answer parent questions regarding their child's development (Langdon, 2008). In my experience, prereferral phone interviews are most successful when conducted by a seasoned clinician with native or near-native proficiency in the language.

CLINIC BOX: Getting Help

The International Expert Panel on Multilingual Children's Speech (IEPMCS) formed in 2012 to examine ways to meet the specific needs of multilingual children. Members of the IEPMCS panel include SLPs, phoneticians, linguists, and speech scientists from 35 different countries. This worldwide collaboration recommends, "Children are supported to communicate effectively and intelligibly in the languages spoken within their families and communities, in the context of developing their cultural identities." The IEPMCS has a tutorial for SLPs who conduct speech assessments with children who speak a language other than English. The tutorial was compiled by 46 researchers and it is a great resource for professionals.

History

The case history is a key tool in evaluation. One challenge to assessment is that bilingual children do not have a static language profile, but typically one that is dynamic as their language exposure shifts between environments and communication partners. For example, a child may experience language loss of the home language upon school entrance, if the school instruction is primarily in the second language.

Estimating Language Exposure

An estimate of language exposure is important because it can predict speech accuracy (Ruiz-Felter, Cooperson, Bedore, & Peña, 2016). Table 12–1 provides a list of evidence-based case history topics to help document language exposure, including age of language exposure, language input–output percentages, older siblings, and dialect. Appendix 12–A in this chapter contains a template for a case history of a bilingual child.

TABLE 12–1. Evidence-Based Case History Questions for Speech Assessment

Language Exposure	Evidence-Support
What Was the **Age of Language Exposure**?	Need to document exposure; earlier exposure may lead to more language influence (Hambly et al., 2013)
What is the **Language Input-Output (%)**?	For early bilinguals, input-output %s appears to be more predictive of phonological accuracy than age of exposure (Ruiz-Felter et al., 2016)
How Many **Older Siblings**?	There is significantly more English vocabulary and greater MLU in English when children have older school-age siblings (Bridges & Hoff, 2014)
What Is the specific **Dialect**?	Bilinguals may use similar dialect density as monolinguals; however, types of dialect features may be different (Fabiano-Smith, Shuriff, Barlow, & Goldstein, 2014)

The Calculation. You or a teacher can estimate language exposure by asking parents to report what language is heard (input) and used (output) by the child on weekdays and weekends (Ruiz-Felter et al., 2016). Next, calculate percentages of input–output in each language. To illustrate, children who are more Spanish dominant may hear and speak 60% to 80% Spanish at home and school, compared to more balanced bilingual children (40%–60% in English and Spanish) or more English dominant children (60%–80% in English) (Ruiz-Felter et al., 2016).

Present Development

Challenging as it may be, a clinician needs to assess a bilingual child in both their languages. Although a greater time commitment, dual speech assessment decreases the chance of later misdiagnosis or inappropriate goal selection. Table 12–2 summarizes both the big picture and specific strategies for assessing the speech of dual language learners (Fabiano-Smith & Goldstein, 2010; Yavas & Goldstein, 1998). Additionally, tutorials exist to help you master this material (McLeod et al., 2017; Yavas & Goldstein, 1998).

What's in the Table

Table 12–2 outlines five specific strategies to consider. Use one or several of the strategies, depending on the needs of the child and resources available. Three strategies involve comparing a child's speech to another speaker (i.e., to a parent, a peer, or an audio recording of a native L1 speaker through a speech archive). Two strategies entail comparing a child's productions to an expected level of mastery (i.e., percent consonants correct) and expected age of acquisition (i.e., early, mid, or late sounds).

TABLE 12–2. Strategies for Assessing Multilingual Children's Speech

Big Picture Strategies (Yavas & Goldstein, 1998)
■ Assess in both languages and choose assessment tools
■ Investigate and contrast phonetic inventory
■ "Describe common and uncommon phonological patterns in L1 and L2" (p. 52)
Specific Strategies
■ Give the parent the same test as the child and compare child-adult productions (Terrell et al., 1992)
■ Compare two children with similar language exposure (McGregor, Williams, Hearst, & Johnson, 1997; McLeod et al., 2017)
■ Listen to speech accent (if available) (McLeod et al., 2017)
■ Calculate percent consonants correct to assess articulation (Fabiano-Smith & Hoffman, 2018)
■ Based on L1 phonetic inventory, consider early, middle, and late developing sounds (Fabiano-Smith & Goldstein, 2010; Fabiano-Smith & Hoffman, 2018)

Speech Assessment Tools

Both formal speech assessment tools and creative informal methods help you assess the speech development of bilingual children.

Formal Speech Assessment Tools. Table 12–3 lists tests in Spanish with the advantages and disadvantages of each. For a more complete discussion of assessment tools available in a language other than in English, see McLeod and Verdon (2014); they reviewed 30 speech assessments across 19 languages other than English, including (in alphabetical order) Cantonese, Danish, Finnish, German, Greek, Japanese, Korean, Maltese-English, Norwegian, Pakistani heritage languages (Mipuri, Punjabi, Urdu), Portuguese, Putonghua (Chinese), Romanian, Slovenian, Spanish-English, Swedish, and Turkish or Turkish-German. The authors found that all tests elicited single word productions, but few tests catered specifically to multilingual speakers (McLeod & Verdon, 2014). McLeod (2012) offers an online resource that provides test descriptions of over 100 tests available in languages other than English.

Informal Measures. Your speech assessment should include both independent analysis (i.e., child's phonetic inventory) and relational analysis (i.e., comparing child's production to correct target words) (Yavas & Goldstein, 1998). See Chapter 7, "Toddlers," and Chapter 8, "Preschoolers," if you want more background on these analyses. Items from tests of single-word productions provide easy and quick ways to obtain a speech sample.

TABLE 12–3. Common Articulation Tests in Spanish

Test	Advantages & Disadvantages
BESA Articulation (Bilingual English Spanish Assessment; Peña, Gutierrez-Clellan, Iglesias, Goldstein, & Bedore, 2014)	**Pros:** Analyzes in both languages (31 English words, 28 Spanish words). Analyzes vowel errors. Ages 5–7 years/ **Cons:** Scaled scoring can be difficult to determine below-average performance.
SAM (Spanish Articulation Measure; Mattes, 1995)	**Pros:** Only 40 test items; similar to GFTA (English). Contains 10-word probe lists of all Spanish sounds for progress monitoring. Appropriate for preschool and/or school-age children (3 years+). **Cons:** No normative data, unless local norms are developed. Items are Spanish only. Black and white lined images.
CPAC-Spanish (Contextual Probes of Articulation Competence; Iglesias & Goldstein, 2006)	**Pros:** Has articulation screener. Helpful for preschool. Online scoring component available. Some analysis for phonological processes. Ages 3;0–8;11 years. Color images. **Cons:** Longer test (81 items). If working with Mexican dialect speakers, test has a few Puerto Rican-influenced dialect targets.
SLAP (Spanish Language Assessment Procedures; Mattes, 1985)	**Pros:** Relatively easy to administer. Provides sentence level probes. **Cons:** Small sample size for criterion-referenced ($n = 54$).
Goldman Fristoe Test of Articulation-Third Edition, Spanish (GFTA-3 Spanish; Goldman & Fristoe, 2017)	**Pros:** Parallel test in English. Normative comparisons. Wide age range for administration. **Cons:** Published recently; spring 2017 (some clinicians may not have purchased yet).
BAPA (Bilingual Articulation and Phonology Assessment; Fernandes, Kester, Buaman, & Prath, 2011)	**Pros:** Standardized scores in English, bilingual English, or Spanish-English. Provides %s of accuracy (63 English words, 48 Spanish words). E-mail or print results. Ages 3;0–10;11 years. **Cons:** Available only on the iPad (could be a pro).

A Clever Method. One clever measure to help assess a bilingual child is to administer the test to a child's parent and then compare productions of the child to those of his/her parent (McLeod et al., 2017). Terrell, Arensberg, and Rosa (1992) used this comparative analysis with a 4-year-old Nigerian-English speaking child and her father, as there were few speakers of the language nearby. Although this child-adult comparison increases testing time for the clinician, accuracy in diagnosis may improve after hearing an adult production, particularly if there are limited linguistic resources.

Plan B. If testing a parent is not feasible, consider listening to a same-age and language-matched peer, or listen to speech archives of speakers with a specific accent of language influence. For example, you can search for specific languages in online speech archives (e.g., http://accent.gmu.edu/browse_native.php), and then listen to adult speakers to identify speech differences of a particular accent. A word of caution: there can be vast differences in speakers based on geographic and/or cultural-linguistic differences. For this reason, use Plan B in tandem with other assessment tools and parent discussion.

Percentage of Consonants Correct. The Percentage of Consonants Correct-Revised (PCC-R) is a well-known speech assessment tool that you may find useful with bilingual children, even when completed in English (Shriberg, 1993; Shriberg & Kwiatkowski, 1982). The companion website for this book contains the PCC-R procedure in Assessment Resources (Severity and Intelligibility).

PCC-R Norms. Fabiano-Smith and Hoffman (2018) used the PCC-R to assess bilingual and monolingual children at the age of 5;0. They found a PCC-R score of 84% or higher indicated a bilingual child was likely developing typically in speech, and a score of less than 84% indicated a bilingual child more likely had a speech sound disorder.

Comparison to Early Acquired Sounds. You can also compare a bilingual child's speech progress on early acquired consonants in English ([m b j n w d p h]). Fabiano-Smith and Hoffman (2018) found a score of less than 90% on early-acquired English consonants (Shriberg, 1993) indicated a bilingual child likely had a speech sound disorder.

Clinical Decisions

There are at least three speech areas unique to assessment of bilingual language learners: distinguishing between accented speech and a speech sound disorder (Oetting et al., 2016), prioritizing developmental speech goals, and selecting a language for treatment.

Speech Accent or Speech Sound Disorder?

One of your most important assessment decisions is to determine if a bilingual child has a speech sound disorder. This is the guideline: bilingual children characterized by difficulties in *both* languages have a speech sound disorder and are eligible for speech-language services (Yavas & Goldstein, 1998).

Accented Speech. Children who present with speech differences due to accent (for example, Spanish-influenced or Chinese-influenced English) do not qualify for speech services under speech-language eligibility criteria. You will encounter teachers, professionals, or parents who request speech modification services for accented speech. Sometimes these requests result from lack of knowledge of speech variation or because a requester wishes for a child to learn to code-switch to more English-sounding pronunciations. In these situations, you may wish to help educate the requester about the difference between accent and speech sound disorder. Additionally, although offering accent modification services to improve intelligibility would not fall under educational speech-language requirements, you might consider intervention as wellness and prevention (ASHA, 2016).

Prioritizing Developmental Speech Goals

You need to write developmental speech goals that support all languages a child speaks, including the home language (Gildersleeve-Neumann & Goldstein, 2015; Guiterrez-Clellan, 1999; Paradis, Genesee, & Crago, 2011). Here is a simple procedure to select developmental speech goals based on their effects on a child's languages (Gildersleeve-Neumann & Goldstein, 2015; Yavas & Goldstein, 1998):

- **Highest priority:** Sounds or phonological processes that occur in both languages.
- **Next highest priority:** Sounds or phonological processes that effect one language more than another language.
- **Third highest priority:** Sounds or phonological processes that are unique to one language.

Selecting a Language for Treatment

If you speak the same non-English language as the child, you may wonder, "Which language should I treat in?" (Goldstein & Fabiano, 2007). You may be glad to learn that research suggests that the choice of a developmental speech goal, based on your understanding of the child's areas of need, is more important than language choice (Goldstein & Fabiano, 2007).

One or Both.　You also have the option to treat speech in both languages. For example, you might select to treat 60% in Spanish and 40% in English. This could translate (pun intended) into one 40-min session in Spanish and a second 20-min session in English. Or, you may treat both languages within one session, where the first part of the session is completed in a home language and the last 10 to 15 min in a second language.

CLINIC BOX: Part of your Job

Part of your clinical job is to combat myths about bilingual language learners. My advice is that clinicians state and restate that "being bilingual cannot cause a disorder." In many of our clinical settings, this myth cannot be overstated to both parents and other professionals on the team.

Conclusions

Major topics addressed in this chapter include

1. Speech variation is dynamic (not static) and comes in many forms: accents and dialects, sequential and simultaneous learners, and additive versus subtractive bilingualism.
2. An evidence-based case history documents age of language exposure, input–ouput (%'s), number of older siblings, and dialect.
3. Special considerations for assessment lead to more accurate identification for bilingual children that includes the "big picture" as well as creative strategies for eligibility and goal selection.

Review Questions

1. What is the difference between an accent and a dialect?
2. Describe the difference between simultaneous or sequential bilingualism.
3. Explain in your own words what might be the clinical implications of additive bilingualism as compared to subtractive bilingualism.
4. In Hambly et al.'s (2013) systematic review, what are three key points about bilingual speech production?
5. List four evidence-based case history questions for a multilingual speech assessment.
6. Explain two "big ideas" for assessing the multilingual child to determine variation versus disorder.
7. Which informal speech strategy do you find most beneficial and/or feasible?
8. How does Fabiano-Smith and Hoffman's (2018) study contribute to your clinical decision making?
9. Explain in your own words the guidelines to determine a speech accent from a speech disorder.
10. How would you go about prioritizing developmental speech goals?

References

American Speech-Language-Hearing Association. (1993). *Definitions of communication disorders and variations* [Relevant paper]. Retrieved from http://www.asha.org/policy

American Speech-Language-Hearing Association. (2016). *Scope of practice in speech-language pathology* [Scope of practice]. Retrieved from http://www.asha.org/policy

Boerma, T., & Blom, E. (2017). Assessment of bilingual children: What if testing both languages is not possible? *Journal of Communication Disorders, 66*, 65–76. https://doi.org/10.1016/j.jcomdis.2017.04.001

Brice, A., & Brice, R. (Eds.). (2009). *Language development: Monolingual and bilingual acquisition.* Upper Saddle River, NJ: Prentice Hall.

Bridges, K., & Hoff, E. (2014). Older sibling influences on the language environment and language development of toddlers in bilingual homes. *Applied Psycholinguistics, 35,* 225–241. https://doi.org/10.1017/S0142716412000379

Brown, D. H., (2000). *Principles of language learning and teaching.* White Plains, NY: Pearson Education.

Burda, A. N., Hageman, C. F., Scherz, J. A., & Edwards, H. T. (2003). Age and understanding speakers with Spanish or Taiwanese accents. *Perceptual and Motor Skills, 97,* 11–20. https://doi.org/10.2466/pms.2003.97.1.11

Cummins, J. (1981). Empirical and theoretical underpinnings of bilingual education. *Journal of Education, 163,* 16–29.

Fabiano-Smith, L., & Goldstein, B. A. (2010). Phonological acquisition in bilingual Spanish-English speaking children. *Journal of Speech, Language, and Hearing Research, 53,* 160–178. https://doi.org/10.1044/1092-4388(2009/07-0064)

Fabiano-Smith, L., & Hoffman, K. (2018). Diagnostic accuracy of traditional measures of phonological ability for bilingual preschoolers and kindergarteners. *Language, Speech, and Hearing Services in Schools, 49,* 121–134. https://doi.org/10.1044/2017_LSHSS-17-0043

Fabiano-Smith, L., Shuriff, R., Barlow, J. A., & Goldstein, B. A. (2014). Dialect density in bilingual Puerto Rican Spanish-English speaking children. *Linguistic Approaches to Bilingualism, 4,* 34–60. https://doi.org/10.1075/lab.4.1.02fab

Flege, J. E., & Davidian, R. D. (1984). Transfer and developmental process in adult foreign language speech production. *Applied Psycholinguistics, 5,* 323–347. https://doi.org/10.1017/S014271640000521X

Genesee, F. (1989). Early bilingual development: One language or two? *Journal of Child Language, 16,* 161–179.

Gildersleeve-Neumann, C., & Goldstein, B. A. (2015). Cross-linguistic generalization in treatment of two sequential Spanish-English bilingual children with speech sound disorders. *International Journal of Speech-Language Pathology, 17,* 26–40. https://doi.org/10.3109/1754907.0214.898093

Goldstein, B., & Gildersleeve-Neumann, C. (2007). Typical phonological acquisition in bilinguals. *Perspectives on Communication Disorders and Sciences in Culturally and Linguistically Diverse Populations, 14*(2), 11–16.

Grosjean, F. (1998). Studying bilinguals: Methodological and conceptual issues. *Bilingualism: Language and cognition, 1*(2), 131–149.

Gutierrez-McClellan, V. F. (1999). Language choice in intervention with bilingual children. *American Journal of Speech Language Pathology, 8,* 291–302.

Hambly, H., Wren, Y., Mcleod, S., & Roulstone, S. (2013) The influence of bilingualism on speech production: A systematic review. *International Journal of Language & Communication Disorders, 48,* 1–24. https://doi.org/10.1111/j.1460-6984.2012.00178.x

Kummerer, S. E., Lopez-Reyna, N. A., Hughes, M. T. (2007). Mexican immigrant mothers' perceptions of their children's communication disabilities, emergent literacy development, and speech language therapy program. *American Journal of Speech-Language Pathology, 16,* 272–282. https://doi.org/10.1044/1058-0360

Langdon, H. W. (2008). *Assessment & intervention for communication disorders in culturally & linguistically diverse populations.* Clifton Park, NY: Thomson Delmar Learning.

Leacox, L.R. (2018). The late eight en español. In K. M. Bleile (Ed.), *The late eight* (3rd ed., pp. 59–91). San Diego, CA: Plural.

McGregor, K. K., Williams, D., Hearst, S., & Johnson, A. C. (1997). The use of contrastive analysis in distinguishing difference from disorder: A tutorial. *American Journal of Speech-Language Pathology, 6*(3), 45–56.

McLeod, S. (2012). *Multilingual speech assessments*. Bathurst, NSW, Australia: Charles Sturt University. Retrieved from http://www.csu.edu.au/research/multilingual-speech/speech-assessments

McLeod, S., & Verdon, S. (2014). A review of 30 speech assessments in 19 languages other than English. *American Journal of Speech-Language Pathology, 23,* 708–723. https://doi.org/10.1044/2014_AJSLP-13-0066

McLeod, S., Verdon, S., & IEPMCS. (2017). Tutorial: Speech assessment for multilingual children who do not speak the same language (s) as the speech-language pathologist. *American Journal of Speech-Language Pathology, 26*(3), 691–708.

Morrow, A., Goldstein, B. A., Gilhool, A., & Paradis, J. (2014). Phonological skills in English language learners. *Language, Speech, and Hearing Services in Schools, 45*(1), 26–39.

Munro, M. J., Derwing, T. M., & Sato, K. (2006). Salient accents, covert attitudes: Consciousness-raising for pre-service second language teachers. *Prospect, 21*(1), 67–79.

Oetting, J. B., Gregory, K. D., & Rivière, A. M. (2016). Changing how speech-language pathologists think and talk about dialect variation. *Perspectives of the ASHA Special Interest Groups, 1*(16), 28–37.

Oetting, J. B., & McDonald, J. L. (2002). Methods for characterizing participants' nonmainstream dialect use in child language research. *Journal of Speech, Language, and Hearing Research, 45*(3), 505–518.

Paradis, J. (2001). Do bilingual two-year-olds have separate phonological systems? *International Journal of Bilingualism, 5,* 19–38. https://doi.org/10.1177/13670069010050010201

Paradis, J., Genesee, F., & Crago, M. B. (2011). *Dual language development and disorders: A handbook on bilingualism and second language learning* (2nd ed.). Baltimore, MD: Brookes.

Ruiz-Felter, R., Cooperson, S. J., Bedore, L. M., & Peña, E. D. (2016). Influence of current input–output and age of first exposure on phonological acquisition in early bilingual Spanish–English-speaking kindergarteners. *International Journal of Language & Communication Disorders, 51*(4), 368–383.

Shriberg, L. D. (1993). Four new speech and prosody-voice measures for genetics research and other studies in developmental phonological disorders. *Journal of Speech and Hearing Research, 36,* 105–140.

Shriberg, L. D., & Kwiatkowski, J. (1982). Phonological disorders III: A procedure for assessing severity of involvement. *Journal of Speech and Hearing Disorders, 47,* 242–256.

Skahan, S. M., Watson, M., & Lof, G. L., (2007). Speech-language pathologists' assessment practices for children with suspected speech sound disorders: Results of a national survey. *American Journal of Speech-Language Pathology, 16,* 246–259. https://doi.org/10.1044/1058-0360(2007/029)

Stow, C., & Dodd, B. (2005). A survey of bilingual children referred for investigation of communication disorders: a comparison with monolingual children referred in one area in England. *Journal of Multilingual Communication Disorders, 3,* 1–23. https://doi.org/10.10.80/14769670400009959

Tabors, P. O. (1997). *One child, two languages: A guide for preschool educators of children learning English as a second language*. Baltimore, MD: Brookes.

Taveras, M., Namazi, M., Pazuelo, L., & Casado, L. (2015). Phonological patterns in Dominican Spanish-English bilingual preschoolers: Implications for assessment. *SIG 16 Perspectives on School-Based Issues, 16*(3), 87–98.

Terrell, S. L., Arensberg, K., & Rosa, M. (1992). Parent-child comparative analysis: A criterion-referenced method for the nondiscriminatory assessment of a child who spoke a relatively uncommon dialect of English. *Language, Speech, and Hearing Services in Schools, 23*(1), 34–42.

U.S. Census Bureau (2011). *Language spoken at home, American Community Survey 1-year estimates*. Retrieved from: https://factfinder.census.gov/faces/tableservices/jsf/pages/product view.xhtml?pid=ACS_16_1YR_S1601&prodType=table

Yavas, M., & Goldstein, B. (1998). Phonological assessment and treatment of bilingual speakers. *American Journal of Speech-Language Pathology, 7,* 49–60. https://doi.org/10.1044/1058-0360.0702.49

Yavaş, M., & Someillan, M. (2005). Patterns of acquisition of/s/-clusters in Spanish-English bilinguals. *Journal of Multilingual Communication Disorders*, *3*(1), 50-55. https://doi.org/10.1080/14769670601110481

Zimmerman, I., Pond, R., & Steiner, V. (2011). *Preschool Language Scale* (3rd ed.). San Antonio, TX: The Psychological Corporation.

APPENDIX 12–A
TEMPLATE FOR EVIDENCE-BASED CASE HISTORY

Name of Student: _____

DOB: _____ Chron Age: _____

Evaluation date(s): _____

Evaluator: _____

Essential Language information:

Language(s) at Home	Language(s) at school
Language(s) spoken in the home: _____	Language(s) spoken at school: _____
Age of home language exposure: _____	Age of English exposure: _____
Dialect: _____	Dialect: _____
# of hours weekdays:	# of hours weekdays:

# of hours weekdays:

	Mon	Tues	Wed	Thurs	Fri
L1:	____	____	____	____	____
L2:	____	____	____	____	____

# of hours weekends:

	Sat	Sun
L1:	____	____
L2:	____	____

# of hours weekdays:

	Mon	Tues	Wed	Thurs	Fri
L1:	____	____	____	____	____
L2:	____	____	____	____	____

Family members: _____

Number of older siblings: _____

CHAPTER 13

HYPOTHESIS TESTING

Speech testing is largely about developing and testing clinical hypotheses. The alternative to hypothesis testing—"one size fits all" clinical solutions—ultimately makes clinic care more difficult, resulting in extra work and frustration through misdiagnosis and unsuccessful treatment. No "right way" exists to undertake hypothesis testing (Bleile, 2002). The discussion in this chapter focuses on clinical tools to support speech testing, offering principles and procedures on which most clinicians would likely agree. Or, if they do not agree (since clinicians hold diverse opinions on most matters), at least provides a place to begin a discussion. Topics in this chapter include:

- Optimal Settings and Otherwise
- Testing Methods
- Speech Samples
- Transcription

Appendix 13–A of this chapter is a resource on preventable harm, and Appendix 13–B is a resource of elicitation activities.

Learning Objectives

I hope on completing the chapter you will

- Understand the value of an ideal setting.
- Weigh the values and limits of informal and standardized testing.
- Explain how sample size changes based on a child's developmental level.
- Describe use of special symbols and diacritics in clinical situations.

Key Words

Key words you will encounter in this chapter:
Spontaneous speech
Naming
Sentence completion
Delayed imitation
Immediate imitation
Labiodental stop
Bilabial fricatives
Unaspirated stops
Glottal stops
[w] coloring of [r]
Lisped sounds
Bladed sounds
Lateral sounds
Wet Sounds

Optimal Settings and Otherwise

Under duress, a clinician can perform speech testing almost anywhere—under a stairwell, in a janitor's closet, outdoors with chickens running around the yard, or in a community clinic with a cement floor without electricity and with a few holes in its roof. The following represents a "gold standard" for an assessment setting.

Ideal Setting

Ideally, the assessment room should be clean, quiet, and free of distractions, but not sterile. A mistake sometimes made when assessing a younger child is to fill the room with toys. Though sometimes a crowded room works well, more often a child becomes so engaged in exploring the toys that little need exists to interact with a clinician. A child may also become grumpy when the nice toys are taken away to be replaced by a far less interesting standardized test. A more useful strategy than filling a room with toys is for you to keep toys nearby, but out of sight, bringing them out as needed and putting them away immediately when the child is finished playing with them.

Another Reason

Another reason to maintain a clean, relatively bare room is that clutter may prove difficult to manage for a child with a neurological impairment, for whom even small distractions may create major problems. To illustrate, a teenager who experienced a head injury or a preschooler with attention deficits may find it distracting to see something as seemingly inconsequential as a clinician's shiny gold necklace or a small nondescript picture on a wall. Because children differ in how well they tolerate distraction, keeping the room bare is the safest decision.

Caregivers

A caregiver typically is present during the assessment with infants, toddler, and some preschoolers. Besides reassuring the child, caregivers often prove good sources of information and, because they know the child so well, may be more adept at elicitation. For example, during the evaluation you might instruct the caregiver, "When you believe your child is calm and paying attention, ask him to pick up a toy truck and give it to you."

As every clinician will testify, asking caregivers to act as elicitors, while useful, is not without problems. To continue the example, if careful instructions are not given (and sometimes when careful instructions *are* given), a parent may point to the truck when asking the child for it, which means you cannot determine if the child's performance results from word knowledge or from a parent's assistance. Despite such challenges, most clinicians find caregivers to be a valuable presence.

Preventable Harm

No clinician wishes to cause harm to a child. You can prevent this from happening by following basic infection control guidelines with all children. Appendix 13–A in this chapter lists those guidelines.

Medical Needs

Assessing a child with medical needs may present the need for additional safety precautions. Often, the best precaution is having the child's parents or professional caregivers either in the room or stationed nearby. If a child has physical limitations or motor problems, it is ideal to undertake the testing with the cooperation of an occupational or physical therapist (Bleile & Miller, 1994).

Help from Others

For a child with a diagnosed medical condition, consider consulting a nurse or other qualified staff member with knowledge of the child's medical status to rule out medical complications that could either interfere with the testing or exacerbate the child's medical difficulties. When assessing a child with medical needs, you should also know red flags that indicate that you should ask for help. Appendix 13–A of this chapter lists red flags (physiological warning signs) for six major medical conditions.

CLINIC BOX: Fair Warning

We're now coming to the part of the chapter where the discussion turns to test methods, speech samples, sample size, recording speech, transcription, and—not to be forgotten—special symbols and diacritics. I suspect you may be thinking, "I don't think those subjects sound very interesting." When you finish the chapter, I believe you will say, "Yup. Not very interesting." However, I hope you also add (whether you say it aloud or not), "But valuable."

Testing Methods

You can undertake speech testing using informal measures, published assessment instruments, or—most typically—a combination of both (Skahan, Watson & Lof, 2007; Williams, McLeod, & McCauley). In previous times, when children seen for speech services generally were less diverse culturally and their disorders tended to be less severe, complete reliance on published tests to collect and analyze speech data was more frequent. Today, over reliance on such tools may ill serve children, especially those from diverse backgrounds or with more severe speech sound disorders.

Strengths and Limitations

Informal measures and published tests both have strengths and limitations.

Informal Measures

Relative strengths and limitations of informal measures are as follows.

Strengths

- Flexible procedures
- Can be used with children who are not testable by other means or when no published test is suitable to the child's needs or developmental level
- Possible in-depth analysis

Limitations

- Requires greater knowledge by the clinician
- Using flexible procedures may impair reliability
- Some procedures require more time than is available

Published Tests

Relative strengths and limitations of published assessment instruments are as follows.

Strengths

- Use of published procedures and speech samples promotes reliability
- Provides an overview of important speech assessment topics
- Often is time efficient
- Insurance companies and other third-party payers more likely to accept results

Limitations

- Not all children have sufficient cognitive and attention skills to perform
- May not analyze speech in sufficient depth

Different Ages

The strengths and limitations of informal and published tests change as children grow.

Infants and Toddlers. Because of their balance of strengths and limitations, informal measures often are the primary or sole assessment procedures with infants and toddlers.

Preschoolers and Students. Even with preschoolers and students, rather than performing an entire published test, a clinician often selects an informal measure.

An Illustration

In addition to the reasons listed above, a clinician often makes this choice because time typically is extremely valuable during an assessment and published tests may be lengthy and contain many irrelevant items. To illustrate, a published test may contain a hundred or more items, many of which test sounds either below or above a specific child's developmental level. For example, testing the oral stops ([**p b t d k g**]) in three different word positions requires 18 items. Completing these items for a child whose speech difficulty may lie with consonant clusters or late acquired fricatives, for example, requires time that does not exist in a busy evaluation. Further, a published test, because it typically attempts to capture a child's performance across a wide array of sounds, may not probe any individual sound in sufficient depth for clinical purposes.

The remainder of this chapter focuses on test options for informal measures. The Assessment Resources on the companion website lists options for selecting published screening tests and completing assessment tests.

Speech Samples

Collecting a speech sample is important because it provides the data for hypothesis making. The hypothesis a clinician formulates is only as good as their data collection procedures. Appendix 13–B in this chapter lists activities to elicit speech.

Types of Speech Samples

One of the most important data collection decisions involves the type of speech sample to collect. Options for collecting speech samples are as follows.

Spontaneous Speech

Spontaneous speech (naturally occurring speech) is the preferred sampling technique because it is most representative of how a child talks (Ingram, 1994; Morrison & Shriberg, 1992; Morrison & Shriberg, 1994). The major limitation of spontaneous speech samples is the length of time it can take to transcribe them, especially if a child speaks in sentences of three or more words. Further, you must record longer utterances to transcribe, which adds additional time to complete the analysis. For this reason, many clinicians prefer to spend a few minutes early in the session listening to a child's spontaneous speech, perhaps making notes about speech errors and estimating the child's severity level and/or intelligibility. The initial impression of a child's spontaneous speech guides the subsequent analysis of the child's elicited speech.

Naming

Naming entails asking a child to name pictures or objects. For example, you might ask, "What is this?" or engage in an object identification game in which the child names objects pulled from a box.

Sentence Completion

Sentence completion entails asking a child to end a sentence begun by the clinician. For example, the clinician might pick up an object or picture and say, "Here/This is a ___." A useful variation of this procedure to test morphological endings is to say, "Here is a ___. Here is another ___. Now I have two ___." One advantage of sentence completion tasks over naming procedures is that sentence completion elicits speech somewhat faster. More importantly, sentence completion tasks direct the child to say the words you want to elicit.

Delayed Imitation

Delayed imitation entails placing a short phrase between the clinician's request to say a word or phrase and a child's response. For example, the clinician might say, "This is a dog. Now you say it." The phrase provides a small space of time during which a child must hold the word in memory, presumably making this task slightly more reflective of cognitive skills than immediate imitation. Delayed imitation is quick and useful when you want to elicit a large number of words.

Immediate Imitation

Immediate imitation entails having a child immediately repeat something said by the clinician. For example, you might say, "Say these words after me . . . " followed by the words. Immediate imitation is the least natural elicitation technique, but it has the advantage of offering a speedy way to elicit large numbers of words.

Sample Size

How many vocalizations or words do you need to obtain a good representation of a child's speech? If too small a sample is collected, you miss important aspects of speech. If a sample is too long, you are swamped with data. Having too much information may not seem a major problem, but it can be, because its analysis requires time a clinician might better spend taking care of other clinic matters.

In general, a sample of between 50 to 100 utterances is ample for a preschooler or school-aged students. Collect smaller samples with toddlers, because their expressive vocabularies contain fewer words. A metric for sample size with a toddler is to collect approximately half the words in a toddler's expressive vocabulary. To illustrate, if a toddler's expressive vocabulary contains 30 words, an adequate speech sample would be approximately 15 words. Whenever possible, obtain two or three productions of the same word, because toddlers often are variable in how they say words.

Recording Speech

If you believe recording speech improves your clinical work, then record, but remember that it takes just as long (and usually much longer!) to listen to an audio recording or watch a video as it did to make the recording, and that transcribing is likely to require much more additional time. Because of the time it takes, extensive recording of children' speech is probably not practical outside of university settings. For this reason, many clinicians restrict their recordings to challenging clinical cases, to educational purposes, and—less often—to document clinical progress.

> **CLINIC BOX: Save Yourself Some Grief**
>
> A suggestion: if recording a child's speech, repeat the word after the child so that you can later identify what the child said. Also say in a quiet voice any characteristics that might be difficult to identify on the tape (e.g., "Oh, I saw your tongue between your teeth").

Transcription

Transcribe speech using the International Phonetic Alphabet (IPA) or an equivalent system. As summarized in Table 13–1, a child's developmental level largely determines whether a clinician transcribes either whole words or isolated sounds.

Infants

Either transcribe the entire vocalization phonetically or use a checklist (see Developmental Milestones on the companion website). Typically, an infant checklist displays

TABLE 13–1. Transcription at Four Levels of Development

Developmental Level	Type of Transcription
Infants	Entire vocalization or checklist
Toddlers	Whole word
Preschoolers	Whole word
School-aged students	Individual sounds or check marks

five developmental levels of vocalizations (vegetative, cooing, vocal play, canonical babbling, variegated babbling) and a clinician checks off the category in which a vocalization belongs.

Toddlers and Preschoolers

Transcribe the whole word, because the presence of a sound in one part of a word can affect the production of another sound elsewhere in the word.

Students

Typically, transcribe isolated sounds or use checkmarks if errors affect individual late acquired sounds.

Special Symbols and Diacritics

Extensive use of special symbols and diacritics consumes time and may lead to transcriptions in which phonetic symbols become lost among the accompanying wiggles, wavy lines, and circles. On the other hand, too few diacritics results in missing clinically significant aspects of speech. The following general rules may help in deciding which diacritics to include in transcriptions:

- Include only clinically relevant diacritics. Do not attempt the nearly impossible task of transcribing all phonetic details in a child's speech.
- Exclude diacritics that describe relatively minor, predictable aspects of speech production. For example, you would not use diacritics to indicate a child produces [s] with lip rounding when preceding [w] in *sweet* or that a student usually produces [r] without voicing when following voiceless consonants in such words as *pride*.
- Exclude diacritics that describe aspects of speech that a child produces in an adult manner. For example, do not use diacritics to indicate stress patterns and syllable boundaries that conform to that of the adult language. To illustrate, do not use a diacritic to indicate stress if the child says *begin* with stress on the second syllable, but do so if the child says the same word with stress on the first syllable.
- If you like, on the top of the first page of the transcription sheet, list the diacritics you are likely to need based on a child's level of speech development.
- While transcribing a child's speech, if you hear a sound pronounced in a way that you cannot readily describe, transcribe the closest approximation you can and place an *X* under it. For example, if you hear something "[s]-like" but somehow different than standard [s], transcribe it as [s] with an *X* underneath. Continue placing *X* under the [s] until you identify how the child is producing the sound.

When this occurs, define the *X*. For example, you might indicate at the bottom of the page that "*X* = voiceless lateral postalveolar fricative."

Common Errors

This section discusses common speech errors and the diacritics and special symbols you use to describe them. See Appendix A in this book for the complete set of the International Phonetic Association's diacritics and special symbols for speech disorders (International Phonetics Association, 2015).

Labiodental Stops

Labiodental Stops typically replace bilabial stops. They sound like bilabial stops, but the upper teeth touch the lower lip, similar or identical to the position for [f] and [v]. The labiodental symbol is a little *m* under the consonant.

Bilabial Fricatives

Bilabial fricatives typically replace labiodental fricatives ([f] and [v]). Bilabial fricatives often sound like a cross between a fricative and a glide. The lips come together as for [p] and [b]. The labiodental symbols for unvoiced and voiced consonants are [φ] and [β].

Unaspirated Stops

Unaspirated Stops typically replace aspirated stops. Voiceless unaspirated stops often are mistaken for voiced stops. For a person who is unfamiliar with voiceless unaspirated stops, the sound often "jumps" between a voiceless and voiced sound. To illustrate, if a [b] "jumps" in perception between [p] and [b], it may be a voiceless unaspirated stop. The symbol for unaspirated stops is a raised little open circle to the right of the consonant [p°].

CLINIC BOX: Some Practice with Voiceless Unaspirated Stops

If you want to learn to hear these sounds, ask a speaker of a language that has voiceless, unaspirated stops to produce [p], [t], or [k]. Alternately, sometimes making a sound facilitates hearing it better. To do this, place your hand in front of your mouth and say [pʰ]. Feel the puff of air on your hand. Now, keep repeating [pʰ], working to reduce the puff of air on your hand. When the puff of air is gone, but the sound is not quite [b], you probably have made a voiceless unaspirated [p].

Glottal Stops

Glottal Stops may replace a variety of consonants. Before a vowel in the same syllable (e.g., replacing [t] in two), a glottal stop may sound like a sudden onset of the vowel.

Between vowels (e.g., replacing [d] in middle), it may sound like someone imitating a Cockney accent. At the end of a syllable following a vowel (e.g., replacing [d] in hid), it may sound like the preceding vowel were suddenly cut off. The symbol for a glottal stop is [ʔ].

[w] Coloring

[w] coloring of [r] replaces consonantal [r]. With rounded lips, [r] sounds like a cross between [w] and [r]. The symbol for [w] coloring of consonantal [r] is a small [w] under the consonant. Alternately, some place a small raised [w] to the right of [r].

Lisped Sounds

Lisped sounds typically replace [s] and [z]. A child can make a lisped sound either with the tongue touching the teeth or protruding slightly between the teeth as for [θ] or [ð]; sometimes the tongue either is more forward or retracted than for [θ] and [ð]. The symbol for lisped [s] or [z] is a small tooth under the affected consonant.

Bladed Sounds

Bladed sounds typically replace [s] and [z]. A bladed consonant is made with the tongue blade raised and may sound like the sound that begins *she* or the consonant in *azure*. The symbol for bladed consonants is a small half oval (like a frown) under the affected consonant.

Lateral Sounds

Lateral sounds typically replace [s] and [z]. A lateral sound is made with one or both sides of the tongue lowered so that, similar to [s], and air flows over the sides of the tongue rather than over its center (Gibbon, 1999; Goozée, Murdoch, Ozanne, Cheng, Hill & Gibbon, 2007). Sometimes you can feel air near the sides of a person's mouth as they make a lateralized sound. A lateralized sound can be voiced or voiceless and sometimes sounds wet. A lateralized sound sometimes is difficult to distinguish from a bladed sound. The symbol for lateral [s] is [ls] and for lateral [s] is [ɬ].

Wet Sounds

Wet sounds may accompany one or several sounds, especially in the speech of a person with oral motor difficulties. Wet sounds sound, well, wet. They also sound slushy and may be accompanied by drooling. Any sound may be made wet. The symbol for wet sounds is a little open circle under the symbol. To illustrate, the symbol for a wet [t] is a small open circle under the [t].

Ages and Symbols

You use different special symbols and diacritics depending on a child's level of speech development.

CLINIC BOX: Infant Vocalizations

Special symbols and diacritics do not describe infant vocalizations well. I don't suggest you use them. However, if you decide to try, you might first read the discussions in Oller (1992), Proctor (1989), and Stark (1980).

Toddlers

Labiodental stops (often produced for bilabial stops), bilabial fricatives (often produced for [f] and [v]), unaspirated voiceless stops (often produced in place of aspirated stops), wet sounds (wet sounding speech often occurs in children with oral motor problems), and glottal stops (often produced replacing between vowels and at the end of syllables).

Preschoolers

The same special symbols and diacritics for toddlers (labiodental stops, unaspirated voiceless stops, wet sounds, and glottal stops) are also useful with preschoolers. Additional diacritics include [w] coloring of [r], as well as lisped, lateralized, and bladed productions of [s] and [z].

Students

The same special symbols and diacritics used for preschoolers can be used for students ([w] coloring of [r] and lisped, lateralized, and bladed production of [s] and [z]).

Conclusions

This chapter discussed the following ideas:

1. Speech testing is largely about developing and testing clinical hypotheses.
2. The ideal assessment room is clean, quiet, and free of distractions, but not sterile.
3. Speech testing relies on informal measures, published assessment instruments, or —most typically—a combination of both.
4. Type of speech sample, sample size, whether to record, and transcription are important considerations in speech testing.

Review Questions

1. What is the problem with "one size fits all" clinical solutions?
2. Explain in your own words why it is especially important that an assessment room to be clean and tidy for children who experienced head injuries.
3. What do many clinicians do rather than collect long samples of spontaneous speech?
4. In your own words, discuss the pros and cons of recording speech.
5. In your own words, list the general rules for including special symbols and diacritics in your transcriptions.
6. Define the term bilabial fricative.
7. What is the definition of an unaspirated stop?
8. What is [w] coloring?
9. Which special symbols and diacritics find use in the transcription of toddlers?

References

Bleile, K. (2002). Evaluating articulation and phonological disorders when the clock is running. *American Journal of Speech-Language Pathology*, *11*, 243–249.

Bleile, K., & Miller, S. (1994). Toddlers with medical needs. In J. Bernthal & N. Bankson (Eds.), *Articulatory and phonological disorders in special populations* (pp. 81–100). New York, NY: Thieme.

Gibbon, F. E. (1999). Undifferentiated lingual gestures in children with articulation/phonological disorders. *Journal of Speech, Language, and Hearing Research*, *42*, 382–397.

Goozée, J. V., Murdoch, B., Ozanne, A., Cheng, Y., Hill, A., & Gibbon, F. (2007). Lingual kinematics and coordination in speech-disordered children exhibiting differentiated versus undifferentiated lingual gestures. *International Journal of Language & Communication Disorders*, *42*, 703–724.

Ingram, D. (1994). Articulation testing versus conversational speech sampling: A response to Morrison and Shriberg (1992). *Journal of Speech and Healing Disorders*, *37*, 935–936.

International Phonetics Association. (2015). *IPA Chart*. Retrieved from http://www.international phoneticassociation.org/content/ipa-chart

Morrison, J., & Shriberg, L. (1992). Articulation testing versus conversational speech sampling. *Journal of Speech and Hearing Disorders*, *35*, 259–273.

Morrison, J., & Shriberg, L. (1994. Response to Ingram letter. *Journal of Speech and Hearing Disorders*, *37*, 936–937.

Oller, K. (1992). Description of infant vocalizations and young child speech: Theoretical and practical tools. *Seminars in Speech and Language*, *13*, 178–192.

Proctor, A. (1989). Stages of normal noncry vocal development in infancy: A protocol for assessment. *Topics in Language Disorders*, *10*, 26–42.

Skahan, S., Watson, M., & Lof, G. (2007). Speech-language pathologists' assessment practices for children with suspected speech sound disorders: Results of a national survey. *American Journal of Speech-Language Pathology*, *16*, 246–259.

Stark, R. (1980). Stages of speech development in the first year of life. In G. Yeni-Komshian, J. Kavanagh, & C. Ferguson (Eds.), *Child phonology. Production* (pp. 73– 92). New York, NY: Academic Press.

L. Williams, S. McLeod, & R. J. McCauley (Eds.), *Interventions for speech sound disorders in children*. Baltimore, MD: Paul H. Brookes.

APPENDIX 13–A
PREVENTABLE HARM

Infection Control Guidelines

Hand Washing

Many persons with medical needs have relatively weak immune systems, and diseases carried by staff are a primary source of infection. The most effective means of reducing the spread of infection is through careful hand washing after each client. Other times to wash hands include when coming on or off duty, when the hands are dirty, after toilet use, after blowing or wiping one's nose, after handling client secretions.

To wash, wet the hands and forearms, apply soap, and wash all areas of the hands and forearms for 20 s, being careful to wash nail beds and between the fingers. Afterward, rinse the soap from your hands and forearms thoroughly. Use an unused paper towel to turn off the faucet, and then discard the paper towel.

Toy Washing

Toys are a possible source of infection for children with medical needs, because children may place toys in their mouths or may put their fingers in their mouths or noses after playing with an infected toy. Wear gloves to clean possibly infected toys. Wipe each toy with warm, soapy water and then rinse. Next, spray or wipe each toy with a disinfectant such as 1:10 solution of household bleach. Finally, rinse the toy well and air dry for 10 min.

Physiological Warning Signs

Children with medical conditions sometimes experience sudden, even life-threatening, changes in their medical status. Clinicians need to recognize and respond appropriately in emergencies, if they occur. The following are the most common physiological warning signs (or red flags) associated with six possibly life-threatening conditions. If the warning signs appear, the clinician should immediately contact the staff member (typically a physician or nurse) designated to handle medical problems.

Mechanical Ventilation

Mechanical ventilation provides breath to a client. The primary indicator for mechanical ventilation in children is bronchopulmonary dysplasia. The physiological warning signs most commonly encountered in clients receiving mechanical ventilation include changes in skin color, exaggerated breathing, coughing, alteration in heart rate or respiratory rate, and either lethargy or irritability.

Tracheostomy

Tracheozstomy is a surgical opening below the larynx on the anterior neck. Persons with tracheotomy assistance breathe through a hole (stoma) placed in the anterior neck. The most common daily hazards associated with tracheotomy care involve blockages that make breathing difficult or impossible. The physiological warning signs of blockage include a blue tint around the lips or nail beds, flared nostrils, fast breathing, a rattling noise during breathing, mucous bubbles around the tracheotomy site, coughing or gagging, clammy skin, restlessness, and either lethargy or irritability.

Seizures

A seizure is a type of abnormal electrical discharge from the neurons in the cortex. Physiological warning signs associated with seizures include pallor, irritability, staring, nystagmus, changes in muscle tone, and vomiting.

Shunt

A shunt is a device that diverts cerebrospinal fluid from a brain ventricle to another part of the body where the fluid is then absorbed. Hydrocephalus often gives rise to the need for a shunt. In children with hydrocephalus, excess fluid causes the ventricles in the brain to enlarge. Physiological warning signs suggesting a shunt malfunction include headaches, vomiting, lethargy, and bulging fontanel (the soft spot on the heads of infants and toddlers).

Gastrointestinal Conditions

Gastrointestinal conditions involve problems in one or more of three areas: controlled movement of food through the body, digestion of food, and absorption of nutrients. If a person cannot receive enough nourishment by mouth (per oral) to sustain life and continued growth, he or she is fed via a gastrostomy or jejunal tube placed into the stomach or small intestine, respectively. Physiological warning signs of problems with a gastrostomy or jejunal tube include the presence of formula leaking from the tube at either the clamp or skin site, in and out movement of the tube, increased irritability, and emesis.

Cardiac Conditions

Cardiac conditions are medical problems affecting the heart. They may occur as isolated medical problems or in conjunction with other disabilities. Physiological warning signs associated with cardiac conditions include changes in skin color, increased heart and/or respiratory rate, chest retractions, nasal flaring, and either lethargy or irritability.

APPENDIX 13–B
ELICITATION

The following are suggestions for speech elicitation ideas for children, students, and adults.

Infants and Toddlers

The optimal elicitation technique is to observe the child interacting with caregivers. You might begin by asking the caregiver, "Will you play with your child a few minutes, so I can get a better idea how your child sounds?" If the caregiver is not available, the clinician should interact with the child. Whether the caregiver or clinician is the elicitor, have the following objects present and introduce and remove them one at a time to avoid overwhelming the child.

Birth to 6 Months

Infants from birth to 6 months old tend to vocalize while shaking a small rattle, listening to a music box start and stop, watching a black and white mobile, holding a handheld or noise-making toy, and playing with a simple busy box.

6 to 12 Months

Infants 6 to 12 months old tend to vocalize while looking in a mirror; watching bubbles; or playing with pop-up toys or toys an infant can manipulate, such as a drum or toy cars.

12 to 18 Months

Toddlers 12 to 18 months old tend to speak while riding a wagon or tricycle, looking at a simple picture book with an adult, putting together and taking apart a Mr. and Mrs. Potato Head, or "talking" on a play telephone.

18 to 24 Months

Toddlers 18 to 24 months old tend to speak while playing with and dressing a doll, looking at a picture book with an adult, playing with building blocks, putting together a big-piece puzzle, or "talking" on a play telephone.

Early Preschoolers (2 to about 3.5 years)

The following ideas may help elicit speech either directly or through the help of a caregiver.

Reading

Read a picture book with the child and have the child name and describe actions in the pictures.

Shopping

Play "shopping" with pretend food, play money, and a cash register.

Tea Party

Have a tea party or make a meal using toy dishes, utensils, and cooking equipment.

Dress a Doll

Help the child dress a doll. The adult holds a doll and the child names the pieces of clothing to put on the doll. Alternately, the adult wears a puppet and the child tells the puppet how to dress the doll.

Puppets

The adult and the child wear finger or hand puppets and have the puppets take turns telling stories such as *Little Red Riding Hood* or *The Three Little Pigs*.

Broken Toy

Present the child with a broken toy that has a missing part and ask the child, "What's wrong?" or "Why won't it work?"

Misnaming

The adult (or a puppet) misnames common objects, saying things like, "This is a dog" while pointing to a toy cat. The hope is that the child will correct the adult by giving the appropriate name for the object.

Late Preschoolers and Students in Early Grades

The following ideas may help to elicit speech from late preschoolers (4 to 5 years of age) and younger grade school students (through third grade).

Spontaneous Speech

Family Photos

If possible, ask the child's caregivers to bring in a family photo album and have the child tell you about the album photos.

Picture Sequence Cards

Lay out picture sequence cards and have the child use the pictures to tell a story.

Most Favorite/Least Favorite

Ask the child to tell you what is his or her favorite/least favorite cartoon, television program, food, animal, and so on. Alternately, ask the child, "What did you have for breakfast?" or "Where's your favorite place to go in the entire world?"

Broken Toy

Present the child with a broken toy and ask him or her to tell you what is wrong and how to fix it.

Tell a Story

Give the child a picture book and ask him or her to tell a story. Alternately, wear finger or hand puppets and either have the child tell a story to the puppet or have the puppet tell the story.

Play Acting

Play act with the child using favorite activities and characters; for example, playing house, going grocery shopping, or pretending to be Bugs Bunny or the Power Rangers.

Explain a Game

Have the child explain a game to you or a puppet; for example, jacks, Cootie, Old Maid, or hide-and-seek.

Funny Clothes

Enter the room wearing something funny (perhaps upside-down toy glasses), hoping the child will notice and discuss it.

Treasure Hunt

Play treasure hunt in which the clinician visually impairs a stuffed animal with sunglasses, so that the child describes where the hidden treasure is in the room.

Bizarre Questions

Ask the child bizarre questions, for example, "Are you married?" or "I like your shoes. Can I have them?"

Single Words

Turn Over the Cards

Play a game in which the child turns over and removes picture cards from a table after naming what is on the card.

Bingo

Play Bingo, allowing the child to pick a picture from a bag, name the picture, and match it to a sheet in front of him or her.

Tossing Games

Play ball or bean bag toss, instructing the child to toss a ball or a beanbag to a board with pictures on it and to name the pictures he or she hits.

Steps

Place picture cards on steps and have the child climb the steps, naming the picture card on each step.

Toy Car

Place cards on a table or the floor and let the child drive a toy car over the cards, naming each card the car rolls over. Alternately, have the child roll a ball and name the card on which the ball stops.

Magic Box

Show the child a "magic box" or a lunch bag. Play a game in which the child reaches into and pulls out and names objects or pictures from the box or bag. Alternately, draw a picture of a cartoon character with a big mouth on a piece of paper; for example, Cookie Monster or a lion. Place the picture over the opening of a cardboard box and instruct the child to reach in and tell you what is in Cookie Monster's (or the lion's) mouth.

Lights Off

Place objects around the treatment room before the child arrives. When the child arrives, turn off the light and have the child shine a flashlight around the room, finding and naming objects.

Play Teacher

Let the child play teacher by wearing glasses and using a pointer to name objects placed around the room.

Adolescents

Ask the student one or more of the following questions.

Blame

Has someone ever blamed you for something you did not do?

Dump Truck

What would you do if someone dropped a dump truck of popcorn in your living room?

Ball on a Roof

Can you tell me how to get a ball off a roof?

Christmas Tree

How do you decorate a Christmas tree?

Sandwich

Can you tell me how you make a peanut butter and jelly sandwich?

Adults

Ask one or more of the following questions.

Today

What were you doing before you came here today?

Store

Would you describe the route from your home to the nearest grocery store?

Kitchen

Would you describe your kitchen for me?

CHAPTER 14

PHONETIC INVENTORIES

Clinicians analyze **phonetic inventories** (a list of speech elements a child can produce) in children in the early stages in speech development, typically toddlers (1 to 2 years) and, less often, early preschoolers (2 years to 3;6). Topics addressed in this chapter include:

- Consonant Inventories
- Exercises

Learning Objectives

I hope on completing the chapter you will

- Recognize that extensive individual differences in speech development are normal.
- Perform phonetic inventory analyzes on different aspects of speech.
- Practice phonetic inventory analyses of consonants.
- Understand limitations of age equivalence scores to measure clinical progress.

Key Words

Key words you will encounter in this chapter

Phonetic inventories
Consonant inventories

Consonant Inventories

Analysis of phonetic inventories does not tell whether a child says the speech element correctly—only that a child produces it. In other words, an inventory analysis describes a child's universe of speech-making abilities, without specifying if the speech is produced correctly relative to the adult language. For convenience, Table 7–1 from Chapter 7, "Toddlers," on **consonant inventories** (a list of a child's consonants that occur in two or more different words) is included here as Table 14–1. For more in-depth discussion of phonetic inventories, refer to that chapter.

TABLE 14–1. Consonant Inventories

Age	Position	Number of Consonants	Typical Consonants
15 months	Initial	3	b d h
	Final	none	—
18 months	Initial	6	b d m n h w
	Final	1	t
24 months	Initial	11	b d g t k m n h w f s
	Final	6	p t k n r s

Source: Stoel-Gammon (1985).

Exercises

Exercise 1

The primary purpose of this exercise is to highlight individual differences in speech development. Its secondary purpose is to put into practice concepts and terminology introduced in Chapter 5, "Phonetics Warm Up." The children are Leslie and Judy, both of whom are 11 months (Ferguson, Peizer, & Weeks, 1973).

Speech Samples

Intended Words	Leslie's Words
1. daddy	dædæ
2. mommy	mama
3. doggie	gaga
4. patty (cake)	bæbæ

Intended Words	Judy's Words
1. mommy	mʌm
2. daddy	da
3. yeah	ja

Questions

1. Which syllable has primary stress in each child's phonetic inventory? (***Two Hints:*** [1] To avoid possible confusion, cover the intended words with your hand and only look at the children's pronunciations. [2] If a transcription does not indicate stress, the word has the same primary stress as in the adult language.). *This is an example.*

2. What syllable sequences occur in each child's phonetic inventory? (***Hint:*** Describe syllable boundaries and sequences of consonants and vowels. For example, the syllable sequence of the nonsense word *mumi* is CV.CV.)

3. What consonants occur in each child's phonetic inventory?

4. What vowels occur in each child's phonetic inventory?

5. Using the descriptive system of your choice, what consonant distinctive features occur in each child's phonetic inventory? *The answer for Leslie is an example.*

6. Using the descriptive system of your choice, what vowel distinctive features occur in each child's phonetic inventory?

7. Summarize your answers by describing major similarities and differences in each child's phonetic inventory in stress, syllable sequence, syllable structure, speech sounds (consonants and vowels), and distinctive features (consonants and vowels).

Answer Sheet

1. Primary stress: *Leslie's words all have primary stress on the first syllable and the second syllable is unstressed. Judy's words are all single syllables (and, therefore, stressed).*

2. Leslie:

   Judy:

3. Leslie:

   Judy:

4. Leslie:

   Judy:

5. Leslie: *voiced (all consonants), bilabial ([m] and [b]), and oral stop ([b], [d], and [g]).*

   Judy:

6. Leslie:

   Judy:

7. Major similarities:

   Major differences:

Exercise 2

Children of approximately the same age can differ markedly in their speech development, yet all may be developing typically and be without speech difficulties. This exercise highlights individual differences in the consonant development of two typically developing children. Davie is 15 months and Child (sorry, the article did not give a name) is 16 months (Branigan, 1976). The speech samples are both children's entire expressive vocabulary.

Speech Samples

Intended Words	Davie's Words
1. book	bʊ
2. binky	bi
3. up	ʌp
4. juice	ʤu
5. that	ʃat
6. momma	momʌ
7. daddy	dadá~dada
8. down	daʊn
9. balloon	jun
10. pop	ap
11. ball	bɔ
12. hot	hat
13. shoe	ʃu
14. cookies	koʊkoʊ
15. baby	beɪbi
16. mine	main
17. apple	apʊ~ápʊ
18. key	ki

Intended Words	Child's Words
1. eye	eɪ
2. goose	gu
3. hi	ha
4. bye	ba
5. kitty	ki
6. button	bʌ
7. mouth	maʊ
8. clock	ta
9. dog	wuwu
10. daddy	dada
11. no-no	nunu
12. popcorn	pap pap

Questions

1. Which consonants occur in word initial position in each child's speech?
2. Which consonants occur in word final position in each child's speech?
3. Which word initial consonants occur in the speech of both children?
4. Which word initial consonants occur in the speech of only one child?
5. Which word final consonants occur in the speech of both children?
6. Which word final consonants occur in the speech of only one child?

Answer Sheet

1. Davie:

   Child:

2. Davie:

   Child:

3. Word initial both children:

4. Word initial one child:

5. Word final both children:

6. Word final one child:

Exercise 3

A phonetic inventory analysis in clinic settings typically focuses on consonants, syllables (sequence and structure), and distinctive features (usually distinctive features of consonants, but sometimes those of vowels). This exercise discusses the speech of Mike, a Korean child adopted by an American couple when he was 2 years, 2 months. Mike is approximately 4 years, 8 months (Pollock, 1983). Cognitive and receptive language testing indicate he is functioning within age-normal limits. The words are Mike's entire expressive vocabulary.

Speech Sample

Intended Words	Mike's Words
1. balls	da
2. dish	dɪ
3. hat	næ
4. fast	dæ
5. got	da
6. mask	næ
7. stand	dæ
8. sun	da~dan
9. right	na
10. tent	dɛ

Questions

1. What syllable sequence occurs most frequently in Mike's speech? *This is an example.*
2. Which word suggests a new syllable sequence may be emerging? What is the new sequence?
3. Which consonants occur in Mike's speech?
4. Which distinctive features occur in all of Mike's consonants?
5. What distinctive feature distinguishes Mike's two consonants?
6. Mike's speech contains four different vowels. What are they?
7. In addition to voicing, what distinctive feature do all the vowels share?

Answer Sheet

1. Syllable sequence: *CV*
2. Word:
3. Consonants:
4. Distinctive features:
5. Distinctive feature:
6. Vowels:
7. Shared feature:

Exercise 4

A primary purpose of obtaining a phonetic inventory as part of a speech evaluation is to determine an age range that best approximates a child's speech development. Because the most complete developmental normative data is for consonants, that area typically is the focus. This exercise focuses on analyzing the consonant inventory in the speech of Johnny, a boy with Down syndrome whose entire expressive vocabulary at 3 years, 11 months consists of eight words.

Speech Sample

Intended Words	Johnny's Words
1. bubble	bʌ
2. baby	bʌ
3. pig	pi
4. dog	gɔ
5. go	gɔ
6. pop	gɔ
7. in	gɔ
8. moo	gɔ

Questions

1. For a consonant inventory to establish a developmental level for speech development, a consonant must occur in two or more different words. Which word initial consonants occur in two or more words?

2. Which word final consonants occur in two or more words?

3. Which distinctive features do all of Johnny's word initial consonants share?

4. How do [b] and [g] differ from each other in terms of distinctive feature(s)?

5. Compare your analysis of Johnny's consonant inventory to Table 14-1 at the beginning of this chapter (the table and a longer discussion also appears in Chapter 14, "Toddlers"). Which age most closely approximates Johnny's consonant inventory?

Answer Sheet

1. Word initial consonants:

2. Word final consonants:

3. Common distinctive features:

4. Different distinctive features:

5. Age equivalence:

Exercise 5

This exercise provides another opportunity to establish an age range for a child's level of consonant development. Additionally, the exercise highlights that two children with similar levels of consonant development can differ in the consonants within their consonant inventories. The first child is Matt, a 2-year, 3-month-old child, whose development appears completely typical except in the speech domain (Carpenter, 1995). The second child is Ethan, a 20-month-old child who was born 2 months prematurely through induced labor because, as Ethan's mother reports, "the fetus had stopped growing in utero" (Lee, 1994).

Speech Samples

Intended Words	Matt's Words
1. mama	mama
2. ball	ba
3. eyes	aɪ
4. bear	bɛ~bɛr
5. bye bye	baɪbaɪ~bʌbʌ
6. dog	da
7. cake	geɪ
8. yeah	jæ
9. bus	bʌ
10. all	aʊ
11. kitty	gigi
12. mine	maɪ
13. babette	bæbə
14. kate	keɪ
15. moo	mun
16. wow	waʊ
17. apple	ʔæʔæ
18. duck	duʔ˞~dʌk
19. up	ʌ
20. yes	ɛs

Intended Words	Ethan's Words
1. balloon	bʌwʊ
2. banana	bʌ
3. bus	bʌ
4. duck	dæ

Intended Words	Ethan's Words
5. dog	gɔ
6. down	dʌm
7. cake	te
8. car	dʌ
9. cookie	tuʔi
10. kite	haɪ
11. sock	tʌ
12. sun	tʌ
13. nose	noʊ
14. eat	di
15. apple	ʌbʌ
16. up	ʌb
17. in	ʌn

Questions

1. In Matt's speech, which word initial consonants occur in two or more words?

2. In Matt's speech, which word final consonants occur in two or more words?

3. In Ethan's speech, which consonants occur in two or more words in word initial position?

4. In Ethan's speech, which consonants occur in two or more words in word final position?

5. What consonants are the same in the speech of both children, which are different?

6. Which age most closely approximates Ethan's consonant inventory?

7. According to the table, which consonants serve as examples of a child's typical consonant inventory at the age you selected?

Answer Sheet

1. Word initial:

2. Word final:

3. Word initial:

4. Word final:

5. Shared:

   Different:

6. Age equivalence:

7. Typical inventory:

Exercise 6

Age equivalence scores have value in helping a clinician establish need for treatment, but they serve less well as a tool to measure clinical progress, especially over short time periods. This exercise highlights an important developmental advance that a clinician may miss by over reliance on an age equivalence score.

The exercise focuses on the speech of E, a child born prematurely and who received a tracheostomy when she was approximately 3 months old due to bronchopulmonary dysplasia (BPD), a lung problem sometimes resulting from medical efforts to save children whose immature lungs are too weak to provide the breaths of life (Bleile, Stark, & Silverman McGowan, 1993). The exercise explores E's speech at two points: at 2;7, which was 3 months after her tracheostomy was closed, and a month later at 2;8. The words are E's entire expressive vocabulary at those ages.

Speech Samples

Intended Words	E's Words
2;7	
1. bottle	baba
2. bubble	baba
3. Pop Pop*	dada
4. daddy	dada
5. mom	mam
6. up	ʌp
2;8	
1. daddy	dædə
2. hi	haɪ
3. down	da
4. mom	mam
5. hop	bap
6. water	wawa
7. book	bʊk
8. bow	boʊ
9. baby	bʌbʌ
10. up	ʌp
11. please	baɪ
12. bye	baɪ
13. bag	baɪ
14. bubble	bʌ

Intended Words	E's Words
15. pop	bap
16. ball	bɔ
17. Pop Pop*	pap pap

Pop Pop is the family name for grandfather.

Questions

1. What consonants occur in word initial position in two or more words at 2;7?
2. What consonants occur in word final position in two or more words at 2;7?
3. What consonants occur in word initial position in two or more words at 2;8?
4. What consonants occur in word final position in two or more words at 2;8?
5. E's word initial consonant inventory shows no developmental advances in one month. What consonant has E added to her word final consonant inventory in one month?
6. E's age equivalence score at 2;7 and a month later remains the same (approximately 15 months). The score fails to capture important consonant developments that occurred during the intervening month. To see this, consider consonants that occurred once in a word. To begin, what consonants occurred in one word at 2;7?
7. What consonants occurred in one word at 2;8?
8. What developmental advances in consonants occurred in one word in one month?
9. *For discussion:* Why may a consonant that occurs in only one word be important clinically?

Answer Sheet

1. Word initial 2;7:
2. Word final 2;7:
3. Word initial 2;8:
4. Word final 2;8:
5. Advances:
6. Emerging word initial 2;7:
   Emerging word final 2;7:
7. Emerging word initial 2;8:
   Emerging word final 2;8:
8. Advances:
9. *For discussion:*

Conclusions

Major ideas in this "learn by doing" chapter include

1. Phonetic inventories list the speech elements a child can produce without regard to correctness relative to the adult language.
2. Phonetic inventories are a primary form of analysis with toddlers and early preschoolers.
3. Individual differences in development are commonplace, especially during the early stages in speech acquisition.
4. Consonant inventory analysis is the most typical type of phonetic inventory analysis in clinical settings.
5. Age equivalence scores do not serve well to measure clinical progress, especially over short time periods.

Review Questions

1. What is the typical age range of children who receive a phonetic inventory analysis?
2. List three types of speech elements that can receive a phonetic inventory analysis.
3. What type of phonetic inventory analysis occurs most frequently in clinical settings?
4. In how many different words must an established consonant occur?

References

Bleile, K., Stark R., & Silverman McGowan, J. (1993). Evidence for the relationship between babbling and later speech development. *Clinical Linguistics and Phonetics*, *7*, 319–337.

Branigan, G. (1976). Syllabic structure and the acquisition of consonants: The great conspiracy in word formation. *Journal of Psycholinguistic Research*, *5*, 117–133.

Carpenter, K. (1995). *Student research project*. Honolulu, HI: University of Hawaii.

Ferguson, C., Peizer, D., & Weeks, T. (1973). Model-and-replica phonological grammar of a child's first words. *Lingua*, *31*, 35–65.

Lee, S. (1994). *Student research project*. Honolulu, HI: University of Hawaii.

Pollock, K. (1983). Individual preferences: Case study of a phonologically delayed child. *Topics in Language Disorders*, *3*, 10–23.

Stoel-Gammon, C. (1985). Phonetic inventories, 15–24 months: A longitudinal study. *Journal of Speech and Hearing Research*, *28*, 505–512.

CHAPTER 15

PHONOLOGICAL PROCESSES

Phonological processes (a child's sound class errors) is a principle analysis in early and late preschoolers and, less often, students in early grades. Distinctive features provide an alternative or complementary means to analyze sound class errors. This book uses a combination of both systems. Topics in this chapter include:

- Definitions
- Exercises

Learning Objectives

I hope on completing the chapter you will

- Know the names of major phonological processes.
- Analyze words with multiple phonological processes.
- Understand the purpose of speech probes.
- Analyze stress patterns.
- Describe speech improvements over time.

Key Words

Key words you will encounter in this chapter

Phonological processes	Cluster reduction
Fronting	Epenthesis
Velar assimilation	Vowel neutralization
Labial assimilation	Vocalization
Backing	Reduplication
Glottal replacement	Syllable deletion
Stopping	Prevocalic voicing
Gliding	Initial consonant deletion
Lateralization	Final consonant devoicing
Affrication	Final consonant deletion
Nasalization	
Denasalization	
Metathesis	

Definitions

For convenience, the phonological processes definitions in Chapter 8, "Preschoolers," are included here. Italics indicate a process occurs less frequently. The resource Informal Assessments on the companion website contains a clinical tool to assess phonological processes.

Consonants

Place Changes

- **Fronting:** Substitution of an alveolar stop for a postalveolar or velar consonant.
- **Velar assimilation:** Consonants assimilate to the place of production of a velar consonant.
- **Labial assimilation:** Consonants assimilate to the place of production of a labial consonant.
- *Backing:* Alveolar (and sometimes postalveolar) consonants are pronounced as velar stops.
- *Glottal replacement:* Replacement of a consonant with a glottal stop.

Manner Changes

- **Stopping:** Substitution of a stop for a fricative or affricate.
- **Gliding:** Substitution of a glide for a liquid.
- **Lateralization:** Sounds typically produced with central air emission (most commonly [s] and [z], but sometimes [ʃ], [ʒ], [ʧ], and [ʤ]) are pronounced with lateral air emission.
- *Affrication:* Stops or fricatives (both usually alveolars) are pronounced as affricates.
- *Nasalization:* Nasal stop replaces nonnasal consonants (usually oral stops).
- *Denasalization:* Oral consonants (usually oral stops) replace nasal consonants.

Sound Reversals

- **Metathesis (meTAthesis):** The reversal of two sounds in a word; for example, saying *pet* as [tɛp].

Consonant Cluster Changes

- **Cluster reduction:** Deletion of a consonant in a consonant cluster.
- **Epenthesis (ePENthesis):** Insertion of a vowel between consonants in a consonant cluster.

Vowels

- **Vowel neutralization:** A neutral vowel (schwa, [ʊ], or [ɪ]) replaces another vowel.
- **Vocalization:** A neutral vowel (schwa, [ʊ], or [ɪ]) replaces a syllabic consonant.

Syllables

Entire Syllable

- **Reduplication:** Repetition of a syllable.
- **Syllable deletion:** Deletion of an unstressed syllable.

Beginning of Syllables

- **Prevocalic voicing:** Consonants before a vowel are voiced.
- ***Initial consonant deletion:*** The initial consonant in the word is deleted.

End of Syllables

- **Final consonant devoicing:** Obstruents are voiceless at the ends of words.
- **Final consonant deletion:** Deletion of a consonant at the end of a syllable or word.

Exercises

Exercise 1

This exercise focuses on a phonological process in the speech of Kylie, a child aged 2 years (Bleile, 1987).

Speech Sample

Intended Words	Kylie's Words
1. lion	jaɪ.ɪn
2. lamby	læmi
3. leg	jɛg
4. lawnmower	jæmaʊ
5. robin	wabɪn
6. read	wi
7. rabbit	wæbɪt
8. rabbits	wæbɪs
9. raccoon	wækun
10. ring	wiŋ
11. rock(n)	wak

Questions

1. Which manner of production includes [l r], but not [w j]?
2. What phonological process affects Kylie's pronunciation of word initial [l r]?
3. One word is an exception to the phonological process affecting [l]. What is the word?
4. Suppose Kylie had pronounced [l] as [w] rather than as [j]. What is the name of that phonological process?
5. Suppose Kylie had pronounced [l] and [r] as [d]. What is the name of that phonological process? (*Hint:* This process does not commonly affect [l].)
6. Sometimes, a special notation provides a convenient means to describe phonological processes. Use the notation x→ y/z (see Chapter 5, "Phonetics Warm-Up") to describe when a child pronounces liquids as glides in word initial position.

Answer Sheet

1. Manner of production:
2. Phonological process:
3. Exception:
4. Phonological process:
5. Phonological process:
6. Notation:

Exercise 2

More than one phonological process may affect the same word. Similarly, multiple phonological processes may affect consonants belonging to the same sound class. This exercise focuses on two phonological processes in the speech of a 2-year-old child named Hildegard (Leopold, 1947).

Speech Sample

Intended Words	Hildegard's Words
1. pillow	bi
2. piece	bis
3. peas	bi
4. piano	ba
5. papa	baba
6. pail	be.a
7. pick	bɪt
8. put	bʊ
9. paper	bubu
10. pudding	bʊ.ɪ
11. push	bʊʃ
12. poor	pu
13. pretty	pɪti
14. please	bis
15. towel	daʊ
16. toast	dok
17. too	du
18. toothbrush	tuʃbaʃ
19. two	tu
20. train	te
21. cover	da
22. candy	da.i
23. kiss	diʃ
24. cold	do
25. comb	do
26. coat	dot~nʊk
27. cake	gek
28. cookies	tutiʃ
29. cry	daɪ
30. crash	daʃ
31. cracker	gaga

Questions

1. What phonological process affects most words that begin with [p] and [t]?
2. Which words beginning with [p] and [t] are exceptions to this phonological process?
3. Prevocalic voicing and fronting affect many words beginning with the initial [k]. What are those words? (**Hint:** Because the processes affect many words, you may find it easier to list the word numbers rather than writing each word.)
4. Which words beginning with [k] show prevocalic voicing, but not fronting?
5. Which word beginning with [k] shows fronting, but not prevocalic voicing?
6. Hildegard's pronunciation of *coat* with a word initial [n] could have resulted from a relatively uncommon phonological process. What is the name of that process? (**Hint:** You can find the process in Appendix B ("Definitions") and on the companion website in Informal Assessments in Assessment Resources.)
7. Use the notation x → y/z (see Chapter 5, "Phonetics Warm-Up") to describe when the child turns voiceless oral stops into voiced oral stops in the beginning of words.

Answer Sheet

1. Phonological process:
2. Exceptions:
3. Word numbers:
4. Words:
5. Word:
6. Phonological process:
7. Notation:

Exercise 3

Exceptions to phonological processes can be as important as phonological processes themselves, because an exception sometimes is a good place to find a treatment sound (see discussion of key words and key environments in Chapter 17, "Treatment Sounds").

The present exercise focuses on the speech of E, a child who was born prematurely, and who received a tracheostomy when she was approximately 3 months due to bronchopulmonary dysplasia (BPD), a lung problem sometimes resulting from medical efforts to save children whose immature lungs are too weak to provide the breaths of life (Bleile, Stark, & Silverman McGowan, 1993). Surgeons removed E's tracheostomy tube when she was 2 years, 4 months. The following words occurred 4 months after decannulation and were E's entire expressive vocabulary at that time.

Speech Sample

Intended Words	E's Words
1. daddy	dædə
2. hi	haɪ
3. down	da
4. mom	mam
5. hop	bap
6. water	wawa
7. book	bʊk
8. bow	boʊ
9. baby	bʌbʌ
10. up	ʌp
11. please	baɪ
12. bye	baɪ
13. bag	ba
14. bubble	bʌ
15. pop	bop
16. ball	bɔ
17. pop pop*	pap pap

Pop Pop is the family name for grandfather.

Questions

1. What common phonological process affects E's pronunciation of voiceless oral stops in word initial position?

2. Which word is an apparent exception to this phonological process?

3. Are there additional words in which E produces [p]? If there are, in what phonetic environment in those words does [p] occur?

4. Correct pronunciation of [p] in *Pop Pop* could be due to chance, or it could be something special about the word itself—if the latter, *Pop Pop* is a key word. Suppose you wait for E to pronounce *please*, *pop*, and *Pop Pop*.

   a. If *Pop Pop* is a key word, will E pronounce [p] in *pop pop* more accurately than in *please* and *pop*?

   b. Suppose your hypothesis that *Pop Pop* being a key word is incorrect and that, instead, it is only due to chance that E pronounced [p] correctly in that word, rather than in the other two words. If *Pop Pop* is not a key word, will E pronounce [p] in *Pop Pop* more accurately than in *please* and *pop*?

Answer Sheet

1. Phonological process:

2. Exception:

3. Phonetic environment:

4. a. Yes/no:

   b. Yes/no:

Exercise 4

Sometimes additional probes help follow up on leads found in a speech sample (see Informal Assessments on the companion website). Informal probes also can serve as treatment pre- and posttests (See Chapter 21, "The Daily Researcher").

The present exercise describes the speech of Tess, a 4-year, 4-month bilingual child (English and Korean) with speech delays in both languages (Kim, 1995). Tess' mother reports a normal prenatal and birth history, but that Tess did not say her first words until 2 years. Tess is an only child and lives in an extended family household in which Korean is the primary language. Tess' exposure to English is primarily through her preschool. A hearing evaluation indicates hearing within normal limits.

Speech Sample

Intended Words	Tess' Words
1. popcorn	patə
2. cannot	tænə
3. cat	tæ-tæt
4. coffee	tapi
5. cookie	tʊti
6. Cookie Monster	tuti montə
7. cow	taʊ
8. crab	dəwæb~tu.æ
9. clown	taʊn
10. because	bita
11. broken	bɔti.ɛn
12. doctor	doktə
13. grandma	dænəma~dæma
14. sticker	tɪtə
15. skate	peɪt
16. chicken	tɪtɛm
17. homework	hɔmwʊ
18. look	jut
19. okay	oʊteɪ

Questions

1. Which phonological process most frequently affects Tess' pronunciation of [k] and [g]? List one affected word.

2. What is the name of the phonological process that affects [f] in *coffee*?

3. What phonological process affects [l] in *look*?

4. Notice that the speech sample does not contain a word beginning with [k] followed by a high back vowel. Because both [k] and high back vowels occur in the velar area, suppose you decide to test whether [k] followed by high back vowel might make it easier for Tess to pronounce [k]. List three words you could use to test your hypothesis.

Answer Sheet

1. Phonological process:

2. Phonological process:

3. Phonological process:

4. Possible words:

Exercise 5

By their third year of life, many children pronounce stops, nasals, and glides correctly in isolated words, although errors may still occur in consonant clusters, longer words, and sentences. Children in their third year may continue to have difficulties pronouncing certain fricatives and liquids in all contexts. This exercise shows a phonological process of a 3-year, 6-month-old child named Rikki (Izuka, 1995).

Speech Sample

Intended Words	Rikki's Words
1. crab	kwæb
2. crayon	kwæn
3. clown	kwaʊn
4. clock	kəlak
5. bridge	bwidʒ
6. broom	bwum
7. drum	dʒwʌm
8. grass	græs
9. glass	glæs~gəlæs
10. french fries	twɛntʃ fwaɪz
11. frog	fwag
12. flag	fwæg
13. strawberry	ʃtrɔbɛwi
14. string	ʃtriŋ
15. sled	slɛd
16. choo choo train	tʃutʃu tʃweɪn
17. radio	weidi.oʊ
18. rose	woʊs
19. rain	wein
20. rocket ship	wɔkɪn ʃip
21. rope	woʊp
22. lamp	læmp
23. lemon	lɛmɪn
24. letter	lɛɾɪ
25. lion	lain
26. lettuce	lɛɾɪs
27. leaf	lif
28. lunch	lʌntʃ

Questions

1. What phonological process affects the greatest number of words beginning with [l] and [r]?

2. Another phonological process affects Rikki's pronunciation of consonant clusters in words #4 and #9. What is the name of that phonological process?

3. The phonological process affecting [r] has exceptions. In which phonetic environment (next to a vowel or in consonant clusters) is Rikki more likely to pronounce [r] correctly?

4. List words in which Rikki pronounces [r] correctly.

5. It seems somewhat surprising that Rikki pronounced [r] correctly in consonant clusters with [g] and [st], but not in other consonant clusters. Although it may be that [g] and [st] are key environments for Rikki (see Chapter 17, "Treatment Sounds"), another possibility is that more complete sampling would reveal other consonant clusters in which Rikki produces [r] correctly. To test these hypotheses, list three words you could use to determine if Rikki can pronounce [r] in [kr] consonant clusters.

6. The phonological process affecting [l] also has exceptions. In which phonetic environment (next to a vowel or in consonant clusters) is Rikki more likely to pronounce [l] correctly?

7. In which consonant clusters does Rikki pronounce [l] correctly?

8. As with [r], although it may be that [gl] and [si] are facilitating contexts for Rikki, another possibility is that more complete sampling would reveal other consonant clusters in which Rikki produces [l]. Illustrate the latter hypothesis by listing three words you could use to determine if Rikki can pronounce [l] in [fl] consonant clusters.

Answer Sheet

1. Phonological process:

2. Phonological process:

3. Phonetic environment:

4. Words:

5. [kr] consonant clusters:

6. Phonetic environment:

7. Consonant clusters:

8. [fl] consonant cluster:

Exercise 6

By 5 years, children's speech errors most often affect individual sounds rather than sound classes. A child whose speech contained gliding when he or she was 3 years, for example, may show [w] coloring of [r] when 5 years. Longer words with relatively unfamiliar stress patterns may also challenge late preschoolers and students alike, as is the case for Ryan, the student who is the focus of this exercise (Izuka, 1995).

Speech Sample

Intended Words	Ryan's Words
1. telescope	tɛləskoʊp
2. refrigerator	frɪdʒɚ.eɪɾɚ
3. alphabet	aʊlfəbɛt
4. astronomy	ʃranami
5. ice skate	aɪs skeɪt
6. iambic	jambɪk
7. barbarian	babeɪri.ɛn
8. hop scotch	hap skatʃ
9. revolutionize	rɛvoʊluʃənaɪz
10. see saw	sisɔ
11. astrological	æʃtroʊlodsɪkl̩
12. concomitant	kəkamɪntɪnt
13. teeter totter	tiɾɚ taɾɚ
14. memory	mɛmɔri
15. vaccination	væksɪneɪʃn̩

Questions

1. List the numbers of those words that contain errors in their initial syllable. (***Hint:*** Ignore apparent errors elsewhere in the words. Note: The postalveolar fricative in *astronomy* and *astrological* was a dialect pattern rather than a speech error, and syllabic [l] and [n] in *astrological* and *vaccination*, respectively, occur normally in conversational speech.)

2. List the numbers of those intended words that typically receive primary stress on the second syllable. (***Hint:*** Remember, for this question, focus on the intended words rather than Ryan's pronunciations.)

3. Describe Ryan's errors based on your answers to the first two questions.

4. Ryan's errors appear to reflect an English bias for a certain type of stress pattern. What is the name of that stress pattern? (***Hint:*** If necessary, review Chapter 5, "Phonetics Warm-Up," Exercise 8.)

5. Of the four speech errors, three involve deletion of syllables, an advanced form of a phonological process found in younger children. What is the name of that phonological process?

Answer Sheet

1. Words:

2. Intended words:

3. Errors:

4. Stress pattern:

5. Phonological process:

Exercise 7

Although occasionally a phonological process is there one day and gone the next, more often its disappearance occurs over weeks, months, and, in some cases, years. This exercise shows how a child named Amahl learns to pronounce two words from between 2 years, 3 months to 3 years, 0 months (Smith, 1973).

Speech Sample

Intended Words	Age
driving	
1. waɪbɪn	2;3
2. daɪvɪn	2;5
3. draɪvɪn	2;7
sauce	
1. dɔd	2;4
2. dɔt	2;5
3. θɔt	2;8
4. tɔt~tsɔts~sɔts	2;11
5. sɔs	3;0

Questions

1. Which two common phonological processes affect pronunciation of word initial [**dr**] in *driving* at 2 years, 3 months?

2. Complete the table showing how Amahl gradually overcame phonological processes affecting his pronunciation of *driving*. (***Hint:*** All the phonological processes are common.)

3. Which two common phonological processes affect the pronunciation of word initial [**s**] in *sauce* at 2 years, 4 months?

4. Two phonological processes affect the pronunciation of [**s**] in word final position at 2 years, 4 months. One is common and the other somewhat unusual. Identify the common phonological process and describe the unusual one. (***Hint:*** Describe it rather than look for its name, because it does not have one.)

5. Complete the table to show how Amahl gradually learns to pronounce *sauce*.

Answer Sheet

1. Phonological processes:

2. driving

Ages	Word Initial Position	Intervocalic Position
1. 2;3		
2. 2;5		
3. 2;7		

3. Word initial phonological processes:

4. Word final phonological processes:

5. sauce

Ages	Word Initial Position	Word Final Position
1. 2;4		
2. 2;5		
3. 2;8		
4. 2;11	(1)	
	(2)	
	(3)	
5. 3;0		

Conclusions

Major ideas in this "learn by doing" chapter include

1. Phonological processes describe a child's sound class errors.
2. Their primary use is with preschoolers and, less often, with students in early grades.
3. Distinctive features provide an alternative, or complimentary, method to describe sound class errors.
4. One or multiple phonological processes can affect the same sound.

Review Questions

1. What do phonological processes describe?
2. What is a descriptive alternative to phonological processes?
3. What is the age range of children who benefit most from phonological process analyses?
4. What is the name of the phonological process in which a consonant assimilates to the place of production of a velar consonant?
5. What is the name of the phonological process that causes *see* [si] to be pronounced as *tee* [ti]?
6. Which two phonological processes result in *creep* [krip] being pronounced as *weep* [wip]?
7. Which three phonological processes result in *sleep* [slip] being pronounced as *tee* [ti]?

References

Bleile, K. (1987). *Regressions in the phonological development of two children.* Iowa City, IA: University of Iowa.

Bleile, K., Stark R., & Silverman McGowan, J. (1993). Evidence for the relationship between babbling and later speech development. *Clinical Linguistics and Phonetics, 7,* 319–337.

Izuka, K. (1995). *Student research paper.* Honolulu, HI: University of Hawaii.

Kim, J. (1995). *Student research paper.* Honolulu, HI: University of Hawaii.

Leopold, W. (1947). *Speech development of a bilingual child, a linguist's record . . . : Grammar and general problems in the first two years.* Evanston, IL: Northwestern University Press.

Smith, N. (1973). *The acquisition of phonology.* London, UK: Cambridge University Press.

PART IV

TREATMENT

CHAPTER 16

DEVELOPMENTAL GOALS

This chapter is a bridge between speech development and speech treatment. The developmental side of the bridge helps us understand what, when, and how a child learns to speak, and the treatment side applies that knowledge to assist a child who needs help with speech learning. Topics in this chapter include:

- The Developmental Logic of Treatment
- Developmental Speech Goals
- Infants
- Toddlers
- Preschoolers
- Students

Other chapters in Part IV, "Treatment," focus on treatment sounds, talking with children, talking about speech, supporting children's speech through alternative and augmentative communication, and the clinician as a daily researcher. The book concludes with a "learn by doing" chapter on sound decisions. On the companion website, Treatment Resources contains useful lists of descriptions and demonstrations, phonetic placement and shaping exercises, and activities for infants through students.

Learning Objectives

I hope on completing the chapter you will

- Understand the connection between speech development and speech treatment.
- Describe the developmental logic of treatment.
- Know how to place a child in a stage of speech development.
- Identify applications of knowledge of speech development clinical care.

Key Words

Key words you encounter in this chapter

Phonological processes
Baby sign
Motherese
Lexical selection (selectivity)
Homonyms
Intraword variability
Interword variability
Facilitative talk
Distinctive features
The late 8

The Developmental Logic of Treatment

Knowledge of speech development is a foundation of speech treatment. To illustrate this relationship, suppose you determine that a child of 3 years has a speech sound disorder. Next, you might ask what I believe is the best question in our profession, "What am I going to do about it?" Consciously or unconsciously, your answer likely entails asking two, maybe three additional questions:

- At 3 years, what does a child without speech difficulties know about speech?
- How does a child of 3 years acquire speech?
- How can I make speech easier to learn for a child with speech challenges?

What and When?

The first question asks *what* and *when* a child learns about speech. For this illustration, suppose your understanding is that a child of 3 years should be 75% intelligible, have a large expressive vocabulary, and speak in short sentences; those might then become possible treatment goals for this potential 3-year-old client. Importantly, another clinician might consult her knowledge base on speech development and decide that elimination of certain **phonological processes** offers this child the best help. Your answers may differ, but both you and the other clinician looked for answers from your knowledge of speech development.

How?

The second question asks *how* a child of 3 years learns about speech. For the sake of illustration, suppose you decide that the child would benefit from decreasing the occurrence of a phonological process—fronting, for example. Next, you might consider—either consciously or not—*how* children typically learn to overcome phonological processes. If you believe in the central role of social relations in speech learning, you will focus your treatment on fostering child-caregiver relationships, and you will likely use treatment techniques that simplify speech input within meaningful social contexts. Alternately, if you believe that children learn speech mainly through reinforcement, then you will build your treatment on those principles.

Developmentalists

Everything in the previous discussion is based on a developmental perspective. There are other perspectives, of course, and there are also important differences between developmental viewpoints. At some point in your career, I hope you have (or already had) the opportunity to sort out your own perspective.

Strict Developmentalists

If you are a strict developmentalist, *what (what is learned?), when (at what age is it learned?),* and *how (how does a child learn it?)* are the only foundations needed for speech treatment. Like many clinicians of my generation, my training was to undertake treatment as a strict developmentalist.

Less Strict Developmentalists

Many clinicians today, myself included, have become less strict developmentalists over time, incorporating ideas and concepts into our clinical work. This "reformist" perspective often came about because a strict developmentalist approach can amount to replicating an environment that had proven unsuccessful for a child with a speech sound disorder. That is, when a child came from a home environment sufficient for speech learning, a strict developmental approach only continues an environment already shown to be insufficient for the child.

Another Type of How?

The third question ("How can I make speech easier to learn for a child with speech challenges?") recognizes that you may wish to include nondevelopmental ideas in your treatment—perhaps hoping to "tweak" an environment to make it an easier place from which to learn. For example, you might decide that our 3-year-old child needs intensive speech production practice, far greater than found in a typical home environment, so you modify the naturalistic family-centered treatment to include more speech production activities.

Developmental Speech Goals

Speech development offers you—literally—hundreds of options to turn into developmental speech goals. As a shortcut, you can also turn to a published treatment approach, most of which contain one to many developmental speech goals. Baker and McLeod's (2011a, 2011b) ontains a wonderfully long list of 134 studies representing 46 different approaches. You can also find an excellent collection of treatment approaches with developmental speech goals in Williams, McLeod, & McCauley (2010).

This section begins with a short review of speech development, followed by a selection of possible developmental speech goals for infants, toddlers, preschoolers, and students (Table 16–1). Each goal begins with a developmental summary, followed by the development goal. The order of developmental goals in a section is not a reflection of their treatment priority. Each section concludes with a list of places in the book and companion website where you can find more discussion and information.

TABLE 16–1. Developmental Speech Goals for Infants, Toddlers, Preschoolers, and Students

Infants	That Wonderful Voice
	Hands Can Mean
	Practicing for Speech
	Clinic Box: Helping Speech Indirectly
Toddlers	Communicate with Words
	Reducing Homonyms
	Reducing Variability
	Breaking It Down
Preschoolers	Mastering Sound Classes
	Ready to Read
	Clinic Box: Slow It Down
Students	Late Sounds
	Difficult Words
	Clinic Box: Social Isolation

Overview

Speech is complex and requires many years for a child to learn. It begins months before a baby is born, when they lie curled in the womb listening to mother's voice, and it continues throughout life. It is convenient to divide this long time into four shorter stages. Table 16–2 summarizes these stages and their hallmarks.

Capsule Summary

During infancy, a child lays the foundations for future speech development, learning such essentials as how to get your mouth to go where you want it to go, that sound can mean, and that conversations entail taking turns with sound. A toddler applies this knowledge to word learning. During the three years that follow, a preschooler acquires complex rules that underlie speech. In the school years, a student applies knowledge of speech to literacy and masters a language's most complex sounds, syllables, and stress patterns.

Developmental Levels

You select developmental goals based on a child's stage in speech development. For many children with speech sound disorders, especially those with milder challenges,

TABLE 16–2. Speech Development: Age Ranges and Hallmarks

Stage	Age Range	Hallmark
Infants	Birth to 12 months	Foundations
Toddlers	12 months to 24 months	Word learning
Preschoolers	24 months to 5 years	Rule learning
Students	5 years to adulthood	Literacy

placing them in a developmental stage is as simple as knowing their chronological age. Other children may show a mismatch between their age and their stage in speech development. For example, a grade school student may have speech that contains phonological processes, or a child of 3 years may speak only in single words. In such situations, consider selecting developmental goals based on their stage in speech development rather than their chronological age.

General Guidelines

Here are general guidelines for placing a child in a stage in speech development:

- **Infant goals:** Child not yet using speech to communicate
- **Toddler goals:** Child speaking primarily in single words
- **Preschooler goals:** Child speaking in sentences that contain phonological processes
- **Student goals:** Student learning the last sounds of the language

Infants

This section describes three possible infant developmental speech goals: That Wonderful Voice, Hands Can Mean, and Practicing for Speech. The topic of the clinic box is Helping Speech Indirectly.

First Infant Goal: That Wonderful Voice

Development

During the third trimester, an unborn child hears their mother's voice. We know this because a newborn will turn toward a recording of her voice when it plays from a speaker on one side while another voice plays on the other side.

Developmental Speech Goal

This goal focuses on mother's voice. You may find it useful with two populations.

First Population. Consider this earliest of interventions for a parent who asks, "Should I talk to my unborn baby?" The objective answer is that a baby hears its mother's voice (and stomach gurgles and coughs and sneezes) without her talking directly to the baby. The developmental answer is that talking to an unborn child creates a link, a bond, between child and parent. The bond of intentional communication is the important benefit of talking to an unborn child.

Second Population. Also, consider this developmental goal for an infant in a neonatal intensive care unit. Talking to and holding an infant is an integral part of skin-on-skin kangaroo care (Milgrom et al., 2013), and, literally, can be as important as life and death, promoting health and well-being for both child and caregivers (Bader, 2014). Parents whose NICU experiences include such care report less posttraumatic stress syndrome than those who do not, and infants who receive this care have better health outcomes both short and long term (Lefkowitz, Baxt, & Evans, 2010). Short-term, touch and voice appear to calm an infant physiologically because it replicates the experience of being in a mother's womb. Long-term, the early experiences of touch and voice may establish bonding between child and parent that creates a foundation for future development (Feldman, Zehava, & Eidelman, 2014).

Second Infant Goal: Hands Can Mean

Development

Sound for meaning is the essential linguistic characteristic of speech. A child as young as 4 to 6 months may turn when they hear their name, and a few months later may look when someone names a family member (for example, "Where is mommy?").

Developmental Speech Goal

While sound can mean, hands can also mean. Consider introducing **baby sign** (a system of gestural communication) for a child and caregiver to support bonding, turn taking, communicating wants and needs, and building an expressive vocabulary. An advantage of baby sign is that it emerges several months earlier than vocal communication because an infant seems to find it easier to gesture with the hand than communicate with the mouth.

When to Begin. An infant is developmentally ready to learn baby sign at about 6 months. If a family wishes, you can introduce baby sign at 4 months to give an infant a first exposure to this form of communication. Some families enjoy having this early start, while others become discouraged if the infant initially appears disinterested or does not use the sign.

Teaching Sign. When teaching a family baby sign, the general guidelines of early intervention remain in place, only the communication modality changes. The difference is that sign input now accompanies speech, so that an infant learns both through the ear and the eye. To promote bonding, baby sign should be enjoyable for both parent and infant, the speech and hand input should reduce the complexities of language to a simple form that holds an infant's attention, and instruction should occur as part of daily routines such as mealtime, diaper changing, and bedtime.

Vocabulary through the Hands. At its heart, teaching baby sign is teaching vocabulary through the hands. As with vocal forms of infant vocabulary learning, progress may seem slow at first, especially if an infant has medical needs that cause fatigue or interfere with attention. Focusing on teaching a few signs at a time often helps; teaching too many signs at once can cause confusion. Frequent repetitions of the sign also help, since an infant tends to learn early what they hear more often. To illustrate the general principle, you might work with a family to introduce the sign for *more* in mealtime, using the sign along with speech throughout the meal.

Questions Parents Ask. Parents have many questions about baby sign. Questions you may hear include

- *Will baby sign slow my child's speech development?*
  The answer is no. Baby sign encourages communication, which is an essential component of speech development (see Chapter 20, Supporting Speech). Further, a parent speaks along with signing, so an infant is learning through both their ears and eyes.
- *Does baby sign mean my child is bilingual?*
  Bilingualism offers an infant many advantages (Ramirez & Kuhl, 2017). Though baby sign offers many benefits, a bilingual advantage probably is not one of them. The reason is that, though baby signs may come from a real language (American Sign Language), baby sign is a vocabulary rather than a rich, complex language.
- *Does baby sign make my child smarter?*
  A common claim is that baby signers grow up to become school students with higher intelligence and better grades. A more accurate claim is that caregivers who select and teach baby sign often are highly motivated and involved with their child. It is the involved motivated caregiver, rather than baby sign itself, which may result in a student with higher intelligence and better school performance.

Third Infant Goal: Practicing for Speech

Development

Infant vocalizations are building blocks that a child later uses to make words. For the first few months, an infant's vocalizations are vegetative noises made as a by-product of breathing in and out. A few months later, cooing appears. A few months after that, an infant's vocalization may consist of raspberries, trills, cooing, and vegetative sounds. By 7 to 8 months, an infant adds babbling (consonants and vowels in syllables) to the mix.

Developmental Speech Goal

Consider this goal for an infant who needs help "practicing their mouth to go where they want it to go."

The Comfort Zone. Infants tend to vocalize more when they are in their comfort zone, a state of well-being that can occur any time of day or night, with or without someone being present. Waking and drifting off to sleep may be preferred vocalization times. To discover if an infant vocalizes when no one is there, suggest a family purchase a baby monitor. If that is not an option, an old school solution is listening behind an open doorway.

Reciprocal Vocalizations. Most infants also find a vocalization comfort zone with familiar people around them. Remember that conversations entail taking turns with sound, which begins as early as 3 to 4 months, when an infant may vocalize when someone speaks to them. At this stage, you can guide a family to begin enjoying reciprocal vocalization games. Soon, an infant and a caregiver may vocalize back and forth, a little conversation consisting of vegetative sounds and cooing instead of words. By 7 or 8 months, infant and caregiver vocal interactions may consist of several turns of reciprocal babbling.

Sound-Gesture Games. You can also encourage vocal interactions through sound-gesture games such as peekaboo and "so big." By 5 months, an infant may be ready to play sound-gesture games, though you may need to explain to families that early on an adult usually plays both turns in the game. For example, in peekaboo, a caregiver may first say their *peekaboo* and then help the child say their *peekaboo*. A child will become a better initiator of the game in the months that follow. As you promote vocalizations between caregivers and their child through reciprocal vocalizations and sound-gesture games, also continue to encourage families to maintain a schedule that allows opportunities for an infant to vocalize on their own.

CLINIC BOX: Helping Speech Indirectly

The goal of early intervention for infants and toddlers is to foster an environment that best promotes a child's development (Britto et al., 2017). You can help speech indirectly by supporting families. To illustrate, reducing a parent's stress level, or finding a babysitter so a parent can work, or helping a family sort through their feelings about their child's medical diagnosis, all may promote better interactions between child and caregiver, which in turn promotes speech development.

Where to Find It

The book and companion website have the following supports to help you treat infants:

- Part II. "Speech Development": Chapter 6, "Infants"
- Chapter 18, "Talking with Children": **Motherese** section
- Chapter 21, "The Daily Researcher": Evaluating Treatment Approaches section
- Companion website: Treatment Resources, Activities

Toddlers

This section describes four developmental speech goals for toddlers: Words to Communicate, Reducing Homonyms, Reducing Variability, and Breaking It Down.

First Toddler Goal: Communicate with Words

Development

Many toddlers (including those with speech sound disorders) "pick and choose" words that contain sounds they already pronounce (Ferguson & Farwell, 1975; Leonard, 1985; Schwartz & Leonard, 1982). **Lexical selection** (originally named **selectivity**) allows a child to ignore the multitude of sounds they cannot pronounce and to communicate instead with words that contain those sounds that lie within their narrow range of speech abilities.

Developmental Speech Goal

Consider this goal with a toddler who has a small expressive vocabulary. Research indicates that a major reason for not using words to communicate is that a child cannot *say* the sounds in words (Miller, 1992; Paul, 1991). That is, expressive vocabulary problems result primarily from a speech difficulty. Approximately 13% of children show difficulty with expressive vocabulary at 2 years.

Think of lexical selection as derailing an unwanted communication cycle. The cycle begins with a child who cannot say sounds in words, and so, says and uses fewer words to communicate. Next, because the child communicates less, people communicate less with him/her. Finally, a child learns less because he/she has fewer opportunities to learn.

Treatment Strategy. Your treatment strategy for lexical selection is to teach words that contain sounds a child already produces, giving special attention to encouraging sounds that open up new places and manners of articulation. To illustrate, if five words in a toddler's expressive vocabulary begin with **[b]** and one begins with **[d]**, you may wish to teach words that begin with **[d]**, since those "**[d]** words" may help "open up" the alveolar region of the mouth. You may wonder how within this strategy a child learns sounds they don't already produce. This happens because a toddler's mouth is small, the tongue is large, and speech is fast, so, as a child says words that contain sounds they know how to make, they "stumble verbally" onto new sounds, which you then can introduce in new words.

Second Toddler Goal: Reducing Homonyms

Development

To communicate, a toddler finds ways to simplify the speaking task. One effective way to achieve this is to pronounce many different words using a few different sounds. These simplifications make it possible for a child to communicate, but come at the cost of making it hard for a listener to understand them.

Developmental Speech Goal

Homonyms are words that sound alike but have different meanings. For example, *red* (the color) and *read* (past tense of read) sound alike but have very different meanings. Consider reducing homonyms for a child who says words using so few sounds and syllables that they are difficult to understand.

Treatment Strategy. Think of the speech of a toddler brimming with homonyms as a knotted string, which is your clinical task is to unknot. The knots are the phonological processes that a child uses to simplify speech. Your clinical strategy is to identify the phonological processes that result in homonyms, and then provide treatment to sounds within those phonological processes. To illustrate, suppose your analysis of a child's speech reveals extensive homonyms because they pronounce many different words as [**di**] through a combination of fronting, stopping, and prevocalic voicing. You then provide speech treatment to sounds affected by those phonological processes, thus reducing homonymy.

Third Toddler Goal: Reducing Variability

Development

The speech of some toddlers shows a great deal of variability. For example, within a few minutes they may pronounce the first consonant in *dog* as [**t**], [**m**], or [**d**]. Or one day may pronounce key as [**ki**], another day as [**ti**], and another day as [**p**]. Some variability is normal in children's speech, especially early on when a child first confronts the challenge of communicating through words.

Developmental Speech Goal

Variability in saying words includes both **intraword variability** (variation in the pronunciation of the same word) and **interword variability** (variation in the pronunciation of the same speech elements in different words). Consider reducing variability as a speech goal for a child whose speech is so variable as to interfere with communication. Approximately 10% of children with speech sound disorders are highly inconsistent in their word attempts (Crosbie, Holm, & Dodd, 2005).

Treatment Strategy. Although variability may interfere with communication, it also suggests that better pronunciation of a sound lies within a child's abilities, even though they cannot yet produce it correctly on all occasions. Your clinical strategy is to encourage a child to produce the most developmentally advanced variant of the sound. Research suggests you obtain better results reducing variability through focusing on a core vocabulary of "functionally powerful words," rather than attempting to reduce variability in all a child's words (Crosbie et al., 2005; Crosbie, Pine, Holm, & Dodd, 2006).

Fourth Toddler Goal: Breaking It Down

Development

One of the clever ways a toddler circumvents a speech challenge is to concentrate on the intonation of a sentence at the expense of its individual sounds. Such a child seems to be talking in sentences, and the individual sounds within the sentence sound like (no offense intended) mush. In a colorful phrase, Ann Peters said such children were "learning the tune before the words." She called them gestalt learners to suggest that they were "learning the whole" (the intonation) before "learning the parts" (the individual sounds).

Developmental Speech Goal

Gestalt learning, like other communication strategies, represents a child's solution to the challenge of learning to talk. Consider breaking down these "sentences" with a child who continues in this strategy to the point where it seriously impairs communication.

Treatment Strategy. Your treatment strategy is to help a child break down a string of speech into its parts. That is, you seek to highlight the individual words within a sentence. Fortunately, many forms of **facilitative talk** help caregivers break down sentences into words, especially modeling, strategic errors, parallel talk, and requests for confirmation or clarification (see Chapter 7, "Toddlers," and Chapter 18, "Talking with Children.").

To illustrate the general idea, suppose a child says a sentence in which you believe you hear the word *ball*. You might follow up, saying: "Ball." (parallel talk); or "Ball. I like this ball. Ball." (modeling); or "I didn't understand. Did you say ball?"; (requests for confirmation of clarification.); or "Yes, I can give you the *small*." (strategic error). You could also include another form of facilitative talk, bombardment, to increase the relative frequency of the treatment word. To illustrate, in the present example you might develop a play activity with lots of opportunities for the child to hear *ball*.

Where to Find It

The book and companion website have the following supports to help you treat toddlers:

- Part II. "Speech Development": Chapter 7, "Toddlers"
- Chapter 8, "Preschoolers": Phonological Processes section

- Chapter 17, "Treatment Sounds": Selecting a Treatment Sound, Establishing a Treatment Sound, and Speech Practice sections
- Chapter 17, "Treatment Sounds": Perception Training section
- Chapter 18, "Talking with Children": Facilitative Talk section
- Chapter 21, "The Daily Researcher": Evaluating Treatment Approaches
- Companion website: Treatment Resources, Activities

Preschoolers

This section describes two options for developmental speech goals for preschoolers: Mastering Sound Classes and Ready to Read. The topic of the clinic box is Slowing It Down.

First Preschooler Goal: Mastering Sound Classes

Development

Mastery of sound classes is a hallmark of speech development in preschoolers. While still a toddler, a child acquires two classes of consonants: those made with the articulators touching (stops and nasals), and those made with the articulators approaching the openness of vowels (glides). During the preschool years, a child masters the less optimal "in between" midpoint sounds, those that stop and start, hiss, and flow—affricates, fricatives, and liquids. Many children begin school with these sound classes completely learned; others may need a longer time to attain that mastery.

Developmental Speech Goal

Consider this developmental goal for preschoolers who have challenges with sound classes. To work on sound class errors, you need a way to describe them. **Distinctive features** and phonological processes can help with this. This book uses a combination of distinctive feature and phonological process terminology, though I gravitate toward the latter because I like its brevity and transparency. If you prefer to use only distinctive features, you can easily translate the following into that system.

Distinctive Features. Distinctive features organize sounds into classes based on shared acoustic and articulatory characteristics; the hoped-for result of treatment is that generalization occurs from the treated sounds to other sounds that share similar features. To illustrate, if a child replaces stop consonants with fricatives, facilitating [f] may facilitate the child's acquisition of other fricatives.

Phonological Processes. Phonological processes organize sounds according to the errors they typically undergo. To continue the previous example, if a child's speech contains a stopping process (fricatives become stops), facilitating [f] may facilitate a child's acquisition of other fricatives.

Which Phonological Process? A preschooler's speech typically contains multiple phonological processes. Which phonological process to select? (This topic of which treatment sound to select *within* a phonological process appears in the next chapter.) The following are two options to consider.

Early Processes. Many clinicians select a phonological process that a child overcomes early in development. Phonological processes typically overcome before 3 years include

- Prevocalic voicing
- Velar assimilation
- Labial assimilation
- Final consonant deletion
- Fronting
- Reduplication
- Syllable deletion

Within this option, treatment gives priority to early disappearing phonological processes, which include a collection of assimilations (prevocalic voicing, velar and labial assimilation), deletion of final consonants, fronting of velar consonants, and repeating or deleting of syllables.

Intelligibility. Another option is to give priority to phonological processes with the greatest impact on a child's intelligibility. Research suggests that listeners are more likely to judge a speaker to be unintelligible as the number of processes increases, deletion and assimilation processes increase, unusual processes occur, processes co-occur, and variability of processes increases (Yavas & Lamprecht, 1988).

Leinone-Davies (1988) lists the relative effect on intelligibility of individual phonological processes

Beginning of Word Most to least effect:	End of Word Most to least effect:
Fronting	Final consonant deletion
Gliding	Fronting
Initial voicing	Word final devoicing
Stopping	
Cluster reduction	

Within this option, your treatment gives priority to phonological processes with the greatest impact on intelligibility. At the beginning of words, these are fronting and gliding; and at the end of words, these are final consonant deletion and fronting.

Second Preschooler Goal: Ready to Read

Development

Few abilities are more important to future school and life success than reading. Preparation for future reading begins in infancy with plastic or cardboard books, and continues in toddlers and preschoolers while a caregiver reads a book and a child points to the pictures.

Developmental Speech Goal

Consider this as a goal to accompany speech treatment with any preschooler that may need help learning to read. Which children are these? Research suggests preschoolers with speech sound disorders, both with and without co-occurring language difficulties, are at increased risk for reading problems (Carroll & Snowling, 2004; Catts, 2001; Gernand, & Moran, 2007; Gillon, 2017; Nathan, Stackhouse, Goulandris, & Snowling, 2004). This means you should consider regularly or always including reading readiness as part of your speech treatment.

Getting Started. Encourage caregivers to read to their child at any age. The primary goal is for reading to be enjoyable, so that both the child and caregiver want to repeat the experience. Early preschoolers (2;0 to 3;6) may benefit from books which include rhyming words as part of their story. During the third year, a preschooler shows increasing awareness of rhyme and syllables.

Around 4 Years. By 4 years, many preschoolers can rhyme words and count syllable beats in words. Around that age, you may wish to introduce an element of direct instruction into your reading activities.

Rhyming. To illustrate a rhyming activity, you might have a "silly puppet" that reads the story but gets the words wrong. A script might look something like this

YOU: Okay, Silly Puppet, it's your turn to read.

PUPPET: Once upon a lime. I mean once a mime. I mean chime, rhyme, dime.

You and the child look at the puppet and shake your heads.

YOU: No, Silly Puppet. It's "Once upon a time."

PUPPET: Oooh. Once upon a *time.*

Syllables. Around the same age (4 years) you might help a preschooler focus on syllables through hand clapping games, such as the following

YOU: Let's count the beats in potato. Po-ta-to. Now let's clap together.

You and the child together clap the syllables po-ta-to.

CLINIC BOX: Slow It Down

There is truth to the parent observation that often begins, "If I could just get him to slow down . . . " Speech rate can have an enormous influence on communication. Although developmental norms exist for speech rate, with a little experience, you soon learn to pick out a preschooler with faster than expected speech. If your caseload includes a preschooler with speech errors and a fast speech rate, consider at least a trial run of working to reduce speech rate to help reduce the speech errors.

Where to Find It

The book has the following supports to help you treat preschoolers:

- Part II. "Speech Development": Chapter 8, "Preschoolers"
- Chapter 17, "Treatment Sounds": Selecting a Treatment Sound, Establishing a Treatment Sound, and Speech Practice sections
- Chapter 17, "Treatment Sounds": Perception Training section
- Chapter 18, "Talking with Children": Facilitative Talk (early preschoolers) section
- Chapter 18, "Talking with Children": Therapy Talk (late preschooler) section
- Chapter 19, "Talking about Speech": Metaphors and Touch Cues sections
- Chapter 19, "Talking about Speech": Descriptions and Demonstrations (late preschoolers) section and companion website: Treatment Resources
- Chapter 19, "Talking about Speech": Phonetic Placement and Shaping (late preschoolers) and companion website: Treatment Resources
- Chapter 21, "The Daily Researcher": Evaluating Treatment Approaches
- Companion website: Treatment Resources, Activities

Students

This section describes two developmental speech goals for students: Late Sounds and Difficult Words. The topic of the clinic box is Social Isolation.

First Student Goal: Late Sounds

Speech Development

Late sounds include consonants, [r] colored vowels, and consonant clusters.

The Late 8. By 5 years old, 50% of students have acquired all the English consonants; by 6 years old, this grows to 75% of students. Collectively, clinicians sometimes call the last acquired English consonants **the late 8** (Bleile, 2017). They include [s ʃ θ ð z ʧ r l].

The Late Vowel. Students complete the acquisition of one type of vowel during the school years, those with [r] coloring. Seventy five percent of students complete their acquisition of such vowels by 5;6.

The Late Clusters. Fifty percent of children acquire all consonant clusters by their 5th birthday. As you would expect, students complete the acquisition of consonant clusters slightly later than individual consonants. By 8 years, 75% of students have acquired all the English consonant clusters.

Developmental Speech Goal

Consider this goal for any student whose speech shows difficulties with later sounds. Your likelihood of placing a student on your caseload will increase if their speech concerns them, their families, or their teachers; the student has developmental or medical conditions; or the student is struggling academically or socially.

When to Begin

If you treat late sounds too early, you will likely treat students who would have self-corrected without your efforts. Alternately, if you wait too long, a student's gains may come slower and treatment success may be less complete. Families have their own perspective on this issue, as do school administrators, who recognize that the decision carries large financial implications. Difficult work place discussions may arise when clinicians, families, and administrators disagree.

Input from Development. Input to your decision from development when it comes to treating speech, is that earlier is generally better. There are two reasons why:

1. Evidence from first and second language acquisition, brain development, and brain disability all suggest that speech is an early-acquired system (Miller, 1999; Stark, Bleile, Brandt, Freeman, & Vining, 1995; Werker, & Hensch, 2015).
2. Research from many sources indicates that speech and language learning slows down considerably during adolescence and afterwards (Johnson, & Newport, 1989; Maurer, 2005; Werker, & Hensch, 2015).

Curriculum Matters

The relationship between speech treatment and the school curriculum has changed remarkably during the last two decades.

Traditional Relationship. Traditionally, a clinician treated speech both literally and figuratively apart from the educational and social life of the school. Literally, the location of speech treatment often was a quiet room. Figuratively, the speech lesson typically consisted of isolated sounds and words in articulation exercises and drills. The quiet room provided (and still provides) a good place for concentrated speech practice. A problem was that the combination of isolation, articulation drills, and use of materials unrelated to school, tended to make it more difficult for a student to generalize treatment successes in the treatment room to outside environments.

Current Relationship. Currently, a clinician typically needs to connect speech treatment to a student's educational and social life to show how speech success contributes to school success and future employment. Fortunately, developmental speech goals for students easily interconnect with the curriculum. To illustrate, in early grade school, you might include a late sound goal with a phonological awareness goal for a student who needs extra assistance mastering this reading foundation. For a student in later grades, you may develop a speech goal focusing on late sounds in pronunciation of longer literary and scientific terminology.

Second Student Goal: Difficult Words

Development

Acquisition of vowels, syllables, and stress begins early in life.

Vowels. Many preschoolers complete acquisition of vowels (except for those [r] colored) by 3 years.

Syllables and Stress. Early on, a child shows a preference for trochaic stress patterns, with stress occurring on the first syllable. Phonological processes like weak syllable deletion prune unstressed syllables, making the word easier to pronounce. By the end of the preschool years, a child typically can pronounce the syllables and stress patterns in the words they encounter in daily life.

Developmental Speech Goal

Consider this speech goal for a student who struggles pronouncing vowels, syllables, and stress patterns in "difficult words."

Problems Reemerge. Challenges with vowels, syllables, and stress may reemerge in third grade as a student transitions from learning to read to using reading to learn. Problems pronouncing longer words may increase in subsequent grades as a student encounter more specialized vocabulary in sciences, humanities, literature, and social studies. Speech difficulties with longer words may cause embarrassment and limit a student's willingness to participate in class.

Treatment Strategies. Two different treatment strategies exist to work on pronunciation of longer words. Both have their advocates.

First Strategy. Practice common syllable and stress patterns found across subgroups of longer words. To illustrate, your speech goal might have a student practice words that contain a specific Latin or Greek root and suffix.

Second Strategy. Practice words that occur in a specific area of study. To illustrate, your goal might include practice of challenging words that arise in an astronomy class.

Your Own Third Strategy. Of course, you may also decide to develop your own hybrid strategy, combining practice with syllable and stress patterns across subgroups of longer words with practice on specific words that arise in a course.

CLINIC BOX: Social Isolation

A student with a speech disorder is at risk for social isolation (McCormack, Harrison, McLeod, & McAllister, 2011). If a student appears isolated, anxious, or depressed, discuss this with the student's family, teachers, and the school counselor. Scheduling treatment around those school activities that a student particularly enjoys, offers a simple means to help a student who feels isolated. Including "speech friends" in treatment also can help a student improve social relations.

Where to Find It

The book has the following supports to help you treat students:

- Part II. "Speech Development": Chapter 9, "Students"
- Chapter 17, "Treatment Sounds": Selecting a Treatment Sound, Establishing a Treatment Sound, and Speech Practice sections
- Chapter 17, "Treatment Sounds": Perception Training section
- Chapter 18, "Talking with Children": Therapy Talk section
- Chapter 19, "Talking about Speech": Metaphors and Touch Cues sections
- Chapter 19, "Talking about Speech": Descriptions and Demonstrations section and companion website: Treatment Resources
- Chapter 19, "Talking about Speech": Phonetic Placement and Shaping and companion website: Treatment Resources
- Chapter 21, "The Daily Researcher": Evaluating Treatment Approaches
- Companion website: Treatment Resources, Activities

Ideas for treating within a school curriculum appear in the Activities section within Treatment Resources on the companion website and include

- Strategies to improve reading comprehension: Reading and Language
- Field trips: Reading and Language
- Classroom books: Reading and Language
- Preschool and grade school: Activities
- School and daily life: Activities

Conclusions

Major ideas discussed in this chapter include

1. Speech development is a cornerstone of speech treatment.
2. The developmental logic of treatment is to determine *what* a child learns about speech, *how* they learn it, and how a clinician can make it easier to learn for a child with speech difficulties.

3. Because speech development occurs over a long number of years, it is convenient to divide it into stages.
4. Simple guidelines help place a child in an appropriate stage in speech development.

Review Questions

1. What two areas does this chapter bridge?
2. In your own words, describe the developmental logic of speech treatment from the perspective of a strict developmentalist.
3. What has led some clinicians away from being strict developmentalists?
4. In your own words, describe the developmental logic of speech treatment from the perspective of a clinician who is not a strict developmentalist.
5. In which stage of speech development do you place a student whose speech contains phonological processes?
6. Why does a clinician promote an expectant mother speaking to their unborn child even though the child hears mother's voice anyway?
7. Why do many toddlers have difficulty developing an expressive vocabulary?
8. In your own words, describe the cycle speech treatment with a toddler attempts to break.
9. What are similarities and differences between phonological processes and distinctive feature approaches for describing sound class errors?
10. In what ways might you help a student with speech problems who seems socially isolated?

References

Bader, L. (2014). Brain-oriented care in the NICU: A case study. *Neonatal Network, 33*(5), 263–267.

Baker, E., & McLeod, S. (2011a). Evidence-based practice for children with speech sound disorders: Part 1 narrative review. *Language, Speech, and Hearing Services in Schools, 42,* 102–139.

Baker, E., & McLeod, S. (2011b). Evidence-based practice for children with speech sound disorders: Part 2 application to clinical practice. *Language, Speech, and Hearing Services in Schools, 42,* 140–151.

Bleile, K. (2017). *The late 8* (3rd ed.). San Diego, CA: Plural.

Britto, P., Lye, S., Proulx, K., Yousafzai, A. Matthews, S., Vaivada, T., . . . Bhutta, S. (2017) Nurturing care: Promoting early childhood development. *Lancet, 389,* 91–102.

Carroll, J. M., & Snowling, M. J. (2004). Language and phonological skills in children at high risk of reading difficulties. *Journal of Child Psychology and Psychiatry, 45,* 631–640.

Catts, H. W. (2001). Speech production/phonological deficits in reading-disordered children. *Journal of Learning Disabilities, 19,* 504–508.

Crosbie, S., Pine, C., Holm, A., & Dodd, B. (2006). Treating Jarrod: A core vocabulary approach. *Advances in Speech-Language Pathology, 8*(3), 316–321.

Crosbie, S., Holm, A., & Dodd, B. (2005). Intervention for children with severe speech disorder: A comparison of two approaches. *International Journal of Language and Communication Disorders*, *40*, 467–491.

Feldman, R., Zehava, R., & Eidelman, A. (2014). Maternal-preterm skin-to-skin contact enhances child physiologic organization and cognitive control across the first 10 years of life. *Biological Psychiatry*, *75*(1), 56–64.

Ferguson, C., & Farwell, C. (1975). Words and sounds in early language acquisition: English initial consonants in the first fifty words. *Language*, *51*, 419–439.

Gernand, K. L., & Moran, M. J. (2007). Phonological awareness abilities of 6-year-old children with mild to moderate phonological impairments. *Communication Disorders Quarterly*, *28*(4), 206–215.

Gillon, G. (2017). *Phonological awareness: From research to practice* (2nd ed.). New York, NY: Guilford.

Ingram, D. (1989). *Phonetic disability in children*. New York, NY: American Elsevier.

Johnson, J., & Newport, E. (1989). Critical period effects in second language learning: The influence of maturational state on the acquisition of English as a second language. *Cognitive Psychology*, *21*, 60–99.

Lefkowitz, D., Baxt, C., & Evans, J. (2010). Prevalence and correlates of posttraumatic stress and postpartum depression in parents of infants in the neonatal intensive care unit (NICU). *Journal of Clinical Psychology in Medical Settings*, *17*, 230–237.

Leinonen-Davies, E. (1988). Assessing the functional adequacy of children's phonological systems. *Clinical Linguistics and Phonetics*, *2*, 257–270.

Leonard, L. (1985). Unusual and subtle behavior in the speech of phonologically disordered children. *Journal of Speech and Hearing Disorders*, *50*, 4–13.

McCormack, J., Harrison, L., McLeod, S., & McAllister, L. (2011). A nationally representative study of the association between communication impairment at 4–5 years and children's life activities at 7–9 years. *Journal of Speech, Language, and Hearing Research*, *54*, 1328–1348.

Maurer, D. (Ed.) (2005). Special issue: Critical periods re-examined: Evidence from human sensory development. *Developmental Psychobiology*, *46*(3), 155–292.

Milgrom, J., Newnham, C., Martin, P. R., Anderson, P. J., Doyle, L. W., Hunt, R. W., & Gemmill, A. W. (2013). Early communication in preterm infants following intervention in the NICU. *Early Human Development*, *89*, 755–762.

Miller, J. (1992). Lexical development in young children with Down syndrome. In R. Chapman (Ed.), *Processes in language acquisition and disorders* (pp. 202–216). Philadelphia, PA: Mosby Year Book.

Miller, J. (1999). *Profiles of language development in children with Down syndrome*. Baltimore, MD: Brookes.

Nathan, L., Stackhouse, J., Goulandris, N., & Snowling, M. J. (2004). The development of early literacy skills among children with speech difficulties: A test of the "Critical Age Hypothesis." *Journal of Speech, Language, and Hearing Research*, *47*, 377–391.

Paul, R. (1991). Profiles of toddlers with slow expressive language. *Topics in Language Disorders*, *11*, 1–13.

Ramirez, N., & Kuhl, P. (2017). Bilingual baby: Foreign language intervention in Madrid's infant education centers. *Mind, Brain, and Education*, *11*, 133–143.

Schwartz, R., & Leonard, L. (1982). Do children pick and choose: An examination of phonological selection and avoidance in early lexical acquisition. *Journal of Child Language*, *9*, 319–336.

Stark, R., Bleile, K., Brandt, J., Freeman, J., & Vining, E. (1995). Speech-language outcomes of hemispherectomy in children and young adults. *Brain and Language*, *51*, 406–421.

Werker, J., & Hensch, T. (2015). Critical periods in speech perception: New directions. *Annual Review of Psychology, 66,* 173–196.

Williams, L., McLeod, S., & McCauley, R. (Eds.). (2010). *Interventions for speech sound disorders in children.* Baltimore, MD: Brookes.

Yavas, M., & Lamprecht, R. (1988). Processes and intelligibility in disordered phonology. *Clinical Linguistics and Phonetics, 2,* 329–345.

CHAPTER 17

TREATMENT SOUNDS

A good subtitle for this chapter could be *decisions, decisions, decisions*. The decisions are about **treatment sounds**, which are the speech elements (vowels, consonants, consonant clusters, syllables, prosody, etc.) through which a clinician facilitates speech change. Another (more widely used) word for treatment sound is treatment target. I prefer treatment sound because target suggests a clinician is shooting something.

In children from toddlers through high school, treatment sounds (or treatment targets, if you prefer) are a pivot on which treatment turns. Infant attention and focus abilities are such that developmental treatment goals seldom benefit from focus on a specific treatment sound. The same may be true for some toddlers and some older children with cognitive disabilities. Topics discussed in this chapter include:

- Selecting a Treatment Sound
- Establishing a Treatment Sound
- Perception Training
- Speech Practice

Learning Objectives

I hope on completing the chapter you will

- Understand the positions on stimulability and on speech knowledge in selecting a treatment sound.
- Be familiar with ways to establish nonstimulable and stimulable treatment sounds.
- Appreciate the distinction between discrimination training and promoting awareness.
- Be knowledgeable about different ways to practice speech.

Key Words

Key words you will encounter in this chapter

Treatment sound
Stimulable
Nonstimulable
Most knowledge method
Least knowledge method
Age of acquisition
Frequency of occurrence
Phonetic placement
Shaping
Discrimination training
Promoting awareness
Key words
Key environments
Therapy talk

Selecting a Treatment Sound

A clinician makes decisions in at least two areas when selecting a **treatment sound**: stimulability and speech knowledge. Additionally, some clinicians figure in age of acquisition and frequency of occurrence in their decision making.

Stimulability

A first question arising in selecting a treatment sound is should you select one that a child demonstrates some capacity to produce or one that a child cannot produce under any circumstance? If you select one a child demonstrates some capacity to pronounce, you have selected a **stimulable** treatment sound. If you select one a child has no capacity to pronounce, you have selected a **nonstimulable** treatment sound. Since at least the last 50 years, researchers have argued the stimulable versus nonstimulable question, sometimes with near religious fervor. I do not think we will resolve the controversy here, but we can strive to achieve the lesser goal of giving the topic a little clarity.

The Logic of the Positions

The logic behind selecting a stimulable treatment sound is that children experience less frustration because they have some capacity to pronounce it. Another reason to select a stimulable sound is that because children can already pronounce it correctly, during treatment they are practicing success. The logic behind selecting a nonstimulable sound is that children already are occasionally pronouncing a stimulable sound correctly and may not require treatment to complete its acquisition.

The reason the stimulable versus nonstimulable debate has continued so long is that research supports both positions. Studies indicate some children self-correct a stimulable sound without treatment, and other studies indicate some children do not self-correct (Dietrich, 1983; Powell, 1991; Powell, Elbert, & Dinnsen, 1991; Shine, 1989). Sometimes in the same study, some children self-correct and others do not.

Usually people groan when they hear the sentence: *Research supports both positions.* The groan is because we want research to answer questions, and we are disappointed when it doesn't. However, in this case, I believe the research, if not giving us an answer, is pointing toward one. The direction it points toward is the need to understand why some children self-correct while others require professional assistance to achieve that goal. That is, children are diverse learners—why should we expect them all to generalize stimulable sounds in the same way?

Stimulable or Nonstimulable?

In the meantime, an element of trial and error exists in stimulability.

Selecting Stimulable Sounds. Relying on experience and intuition, most clinicians select a stimulable treatment sound with a younger child and those with less tolerance for failure. Because capacity to produce the treatment sound already exists, the clinician can more quickly generalize success to other words or phonetic environments, rather than focusing treatment on the possibly frustrating and time-consuming task of teaching a treatment sound that a person shows no capacity to produce in any circumstance.

Selecting Nonstimulable Sounds. Selecting a stimulable sound may not be an option for an older student or an adult learning a second language. In such situations, per force, a clinician selects a nonstimulable sound. With late preschoolers (approximately 3;6 to 5;0) with both stimulable and nonstimulable speech errors, a clinician often first treats a stimulable sound to build a child's confidence and sense of success, and later works on nonstimulable sounds on a trial basis. Techniques also exist to treat nonstimulable treatment sounds with a young preschooler (approximately 2;0 to 3;6). A discussion of these and other techniques for nonstimulable sounds appear later in this chapter under the heading Establishing a Treatment Sound.

Speech Knowledge

The second major question that arises in selecting a treatment sound is how phonetically similar it is compared to other sounds a child makes. If you select a treatment sound only slightly different from other sounds the child produces, you are following a **most knowledge method**. If you select a treatment sound quite different phonetically from sounds the child already produces, you are following a **least knowledge method**.

Most and Least Knowledge

A simple example may help illustrate the logic of the most and least knowledge methods of treatment sound selection.

Example. For the example, imagine a hypothetical child who only can pronounce one consonant, [**b**], and your choices for treatment sound are [**p**] or [**t**]. We can depict the decision this way

b

p?   t?

The question is, which do you select, [**p**] or [**t**]? (Of course, you could always select *both* [**p**] and [**t**], but forget that choice . . . this is just an illustration.)

Choices. If you select [**p**] as a treatment sound, the child learns how to make a voiceless consonant. If you select [**t**], the child learns to make an unvoiced consonant and a new place of production (the alveolar area). The [**p**] selection is the most knowledge method, because [**p**] differs from [**b**] by only one feature (voicing). The selection of [**t**] is the least knowledge method, because [**t**] differs from [**b**] in two features (voicing and place).

Second Example. To clarify the distinction between most and least knowledge, consider the same example, slightly modified:

> b
>
> p?   t?
>
>   s?

Choices. Now you have a choice between three possible treatment sounds, [p], [t], and [s]. [p] remains the most knowledge choice with the child learning one feature, [s] is the least knowledge choice with the child learning three features (voicing, place, and manner), and [t] now is somewhere in the middle with the child learning more features than [p] but less than [s], the least knowledge choice.

Logic of the Positions

The most knowledge method is the traditional way to select a treatment sound. The method ensures that treatment proceeds in small, manageable steps, reducing possible frustrations for the child (Van Riper, 1978). Historically, clinicians followed a most knowledge method when children who received services typically were grade-schoolers whose speech contained one to a handful of consonant errors. Concern arose with the method when clinicians began to treat preschoolers with multiple speech sound errors. Small increments can prove time-consuming with such children. To illustrate, a most knowledge method for oral stops could require six different treatment sounds, one for each oral stop ([p], [b], [t], [d], [k], and [g]).

A least knowledge method speeds speech work by abandoning small incremental steps. To return to our example, rather than devoting the time to teach [p], [t], and [s] individually, a least knowledge method selects [s]. Through learning [s], a child learns —perhaps without being taught—a new place ([t] and [s] both are alveolar) and new voicing ([t] and [s] both are voiceless). Historically, the least knowledge method arose when clinicians began to treat children (typically late preschoolers, 3;6 to 5;0) whose speech contained multiple speech sound errors. The method is a phonological approach to treatment sound selection in the sense that it looks at sounds as belonging to sound classes.

Most or Least Knowledge?

Several considerations may aid in deciding whether a most or least knowledge method best meets your clinical needs:

The Late 8. Little or no difference exists between the methods with students with speech errors affecting a few isolated late 8 consonants. The issue of most or least knowledge only arises when classes of sounds are in error.

Stimulability. The least knowledge method often is associated with selecting non-stimulable treatment sounds. This is because the chief proponents of a least knowledge approach select nonstimulable treatment sounds. However, least knowledge and stimulability are different decisions, and a clinician can use a least knowledge method to select either a stimulable or a nonstimuable treatment sound. To illustrate, in our example the least knowledge choice could have been a stimulable [s] or a nonstimulable one. The essential tenet of a least knowledge method is to select a treatment sound that teaches as many features as possible. Clinicians may find that with youngpreschoolers (2 to 3;6) the least knowledge choices are stimulable sounds, and that the question of nonstimulable choices is more an issue with late preschoolers.

Developmental Norms. If you decide on a least knowledge method, you may find that occasionally the least knowledge choice is a sound that is in advance of a child's level of development compared to developmental norms. To illustrate, the least knowledge choice for a child aged 2;0 might be a stimulable [s], though children typically do not acquire that consonant until several years later. A true developmentalist (which most clinicians—including me—were years ago) would say do not select [s] because the child is not developmentally ready to learn it. I believe time has modified the developmental position. Today, clinicians view developmental norms as the average ages at which children typically stumble on how to make a sound, rather than reflecting developmental steps that they must follow in a strict order. Most would not penalize a child who happened to verbally stumble on [s] at 2;0 by making him wait several years to receive treatment on [s].

Additional Factors

In selecting a treatment sound, you may also want to look at several other factors, including age of acquisition and effect on intelligibility.

Age of Acquisition

Age of acquisition is the average age at which a child without speech difficulties acquires a sound. When I was a student, if the test question was, "How does age of acquisition influence your selection of a treatment target?" your answer had better have been, "You select the sound that children without speech disorders acquire earliest." As mentioned in the preceding section, this was in the days when theorists believed that acquisition of early developing sounds necessarily occurred before that of later sounds. Today, clinicians consider age of acquisition one variable among others in selecting a treatment sound.

Shriberg (1993) provides a useful scheme to categorize consonants as early, mid, or late (the name "the late 8" derives from this system.). Though minor differences between investigators exist regarding placement of individual consonants, most would likely agree on the following general outline:

Early 8: m b j n w d p h

Mid 8:   t ŋ k g f v ʧ dʒ

Late 8: s ʃ θ ð z r l ʒ

Logic of the Position. Following this idea, a clinician would select a treatment sound among the early 8 before selecting one from among the mid 8, and would select one from the mid 8 before selecting one from the late 8.

Frequency of Occurrence

Frequency of occurrence refers to the relative frequency of sounds in the language of the child's community. The hypothesis underlying its use is that, all other matters being equal, sounds with higher relative frequency have greater impact on intelligibility than lower frequency sounds. Relative frequency of English consonants appears in Table 17–1 and on the companion website in Assessment Resources.

Logic of the Position. The most notable finding in Table 17–1 is that oral and nasal stops have the highest frequency of occurrence, followed by liquids. Among fricatives, [s] has the highest frequency of occurrence. The implication of this is

- With younger children, stops make good treatment goals to increase intelligibility.
- The higher relative frequency of [s] compared to other fricatives lends support to the idea of treating [s] as early as a clinician believes reasonable.
- The relatively high frequency of liquids also suggests one reason why problems with [r] and [l] may be noticeable.

TABLE 17–1. Percentage of Occurrence of Consonants

Consonant	Rank	Percentage	Consonant	Rank	Percentage
t ___	1	13.7	p ___	13	3.9
n ___	2	11.7	b ___	14	3.5
s ___	3	7.1	z ___	15	3.0
k ___	4	6.0	ŋ ___	16	2.5
d ___	5	5.8	f ___	17	2.4
m ___	6	5.6	j ___	18	2.2
l ___	7	5.6	ò ___	19	1.5
r ___	8	5.2	v ___	20	1.2
w ___	9	4.8	q ___	21	0.9
h ___	10	4.2	ʧ ___	22	0.7
ð ___	11	4.1	dʒ ___	23	0.6
g ___	12	4.1	ʒ ___	24	0.0

Source: Shriberg and Kwiatkowski (1983).

Establishing a Treatment Sound

After selecting a treatment sound, clinical decision making shifts to establishing it in a child's speech. When you establish a treatment sound, you create a toehold, which you then expand in the next phase of treatment. A clinician establishes nonstimulable and stimulable sounds differently, and so this chapter discusses them separately.

Establishing Nonstimulable Sounds

Traditionally, treatment of nonstimulable sounds was the province of school clinicians. Traditional techniques to establish such sounds reflect the populations they were to serve: they require a degree of maturity and patience, characteristics not typically associated with preschoolers. The advent of least knowledge methods had the good effect of expanding the discussion of nonstimulable sounds to younger children. Today, a clinician has choices to establish nonstimulable sounds for children 2;0 and younger.

Table 17–2 lists 14 treatment tool options to establish nonstimulable treatment sounds. The discussion divides these treatment tools into those appropriate primarily for students and selected late preschoolers, and those more appropriate for early and late preschoolers.

Students and Selected Late Preschoolers

Phonetic placement, shaping descriptions, and demonstrations are primarily for students and selected late preschoolers.

Phonetic Placement and Shaping. **Phonetic placement** and **shaping** help make a nonstimulable sound stimulable (see Chapter 19, "Talking about Speech"). Phonetic placement teaches articulatory postures (typically, tongue, jaw, and lip positions) for speech production. Shaping uses a sound a student already produces (either a speech

TABLE 17–2. Treatment Tools to Establish Nonstimulable Sounds

Phonetic placement	Deletion
Shaping	Self-correction
Descriptions	Old way/new way
Demonstrations	Similar sound
Metaphors	Bombardment
Touch cues	Parallel talk
Minimal pairs	Modeling

error or another sound) to learn a new sound. Both are traditional tools to establish a nonstimulable speech sound with students and selected late preschoolers (approximately 3;6 to 5;0). With both late preschoolers and students in early school grades, you may wish to try simpler phonetic placement and shaping techniques before attempting those with more steps.

Descriptions and Demonstrations. Descriptions and demonstrations, which closely resemble phonetic placement and shaping, often serve an additional supportive role in helping establish a nonstimulable sound. Touch cues, metaphors, and therapy talk techniques can also be useful adjuncts in efforts to establish a nonstimulable treatment sound (see Chapter 18, "Talking with Children," and Chapter 19, "Talking about Speech").

Not as Complicated as it Sounds

The preceding paragraphs probably make establishing a nonstimulable sound seem more complicated than it is. The following example may help reduce any confusion. The brief annotated dialogue shows how you might establish a nonstimulable [s] in the speech of a late preschooler or an early grade school student.

CLINICIAN: Remember the name of our treatment sound? What did we decide to call it?

STUDENT: The snake sound.

Snake sound is the metaphor.

CLINICIAN: That's right. It's a long sound, like this. You do it, too.

Clinician and student each makes a line on their arm while making a hissing noise. The touch cue is the line on the arm.

CLINICIAN: Now I'm going to say a word that starts with our treatment sound, and then say the word with our treatment sound taken away. Raise your hand every time you hear it with our treatment sound beginning the word. Sea. Ea. Sea. Ea.

The deletion is taking away and putting back the treatment sound.

CLINICIAN: You're doing great. Let's both look in this mirror and watch me make the snake sound.

The demonstration is looking in the mirror.

CLINICIAN: Now it's your turn. Place your tongue tip behind your teeth, like we've been practicing, and breath out.

The phonetic placement is placing the tongue behind the teeth and breathing out.

CLINIC BOX: How Many Sounds?

Traditionally, a clinician facilitated one treatment sound per session, the logic being a child might find it confusing to receive treatment on more than one sound at a time. My perspective is more flexible. Instead of an iron rule on how many sounds to teach per session, a short dynamic assessment can help discover what number best fits an individual child (see Chapter 21, "The Daily Researcher"). My experience is that some children become confused with more than one sound per session, while others enjoy the changeup. Interestingly, a recent approach for children aged 2 to 4 years focuses on making nonstimulable sounds stimulable through treating all sounds in every session (Miccio & Williams, 2010).

Toddlers to Late Preschoolers

A second strategy is available for toddlers to late preschoolers not yet ready for phonetic placement, shaping, demonstrations, and descriptions. In this strategy, the goal is to "prime the pump" of a nonstimulable sound, using techniques with limited or no production demands to increase a child's focus and awareness.

- **Late preschoolers:** With late preschoolers (3;6–5;0), try metaphors, touch cues, and therapy talk.
- **Early preschoolers:** With early preschoolers (2;0–3;6), try metaphors, touch cues, and modified facilitative talk.
- **Toddlers:** With toddlers (1;0–2;0), try modified facilitative talk.

If you would like to read about a treatment approach for turning nonstimulable sounds into stimulable sounds in young children, Stimulability Intervention by Miccio and Williams (2010) offers a clever option for children aged 2 to 4 years.

Establishing Stimulable Sounds

A stimulable treatment sound typically establishes itself more easily in a child's speech because the child already knows how to produce it. To illustrate, suppose a child can make a sound in imitation or may say it spontaneously in a few words. With such a stimulable treatment sound, the clinical focus is to help a child make a correct sound more frequently.

Keys

Most often, speech practice techniques (see the following section in this chapter) are sufficient to increase the frequency with which a child says a sound correctly. Additionally, two keys sometime prove beneficial in helping to establish a stimulable treatment sound: key words and key environments.

Key Word. Some children can make a treatment sound in a few special words, but not in others. **Key words** often have a special meaning for the child, perhaps a favorite toy or a beloved movie character. To illustrate, a Star Wars fan might produce a more accurate [v] in Darth Vader than in other words that begin with [v]. A treatment sound established in a key word may give you a place to begin speech practice. Treatment based on a key word seeks to generalize success in producing the sound to other words.

Key Environments. Sometimes it is not a key word, but instead a key phonetic environment that proves a good place to establish a treatment sound. **Key environments** are phonetic contexts (often syllable positions) that may help a child pronounce a sound. Evidence for key environments comes from cross-linguistic phonetics and phonological studies of speech development. If your background is in linguistics, you will probably recognize the influence of Peter Ladefoged behind the idea of key environment. The exercises in the "learn by doing" chapters in this book often deal with phonetic environments that influence the accuracy of a child's speech productions.

Selected Key Environments. Not every child requires a key environment to help establish a treatment sound, but with some children, the right key environment can prove very facilitative. The following is a selection of key environments to consider as places to establish treatment sounds:

- Consider establishing voiced consonants before a vowel as in *bee*.
- Consider establishing voiceless consonants at the end of syllable.
- Consider establishing alveolar consonants before a front vowel as in *tea*, and establishing velar consonants before or after a high back vowel as in *coo* and *duke*.
- Consider establishing consonant clusters in which consonants share the same place of production as in *steep*.

Perception Training

To a greater or lesser extent, perception training is part of most approaches to treatment sounds. The present section offers information to help you make decisions regarding two approaches to perception training: discrimination training and promoting awareness.

Discrimination Training

Discrimination training (helping a child hear the difference between sounds) is the traditional view of perception training. Established by clinical researchers in the 1930s, it remains the dominant perspective today. Discrimination training addresses the well-known phenomenon that some children do not appear to hear their own speech errors. Sometimes called "the rabbit kids," these are children who pronounce *rabbit* as *wabbit*, but who, when asked if they say *rabbit* as *wabbit*, may reply, "No. I say wabbit as wabbit." In addition to making a good story, the reply of "the rabbit kids" suggests they do not hear their speech error.

Something Broken

The presumed explanation for failure of children to hear their own errors is that their speech discrimination mechanism has sustained damage. The intervention is to repair the mechanism through discrimination training. The most typical training activity within this approach is identification. To illustrate, the clinician instructs, "I'm going to read a list of words. When you hear our treatment sound, I'd like you to raise your hand." Of course, instead of a list, the activity could involve a story, pointing to objects, and so forth. After you establish discrimination (that is, once the child can discriminate the treatment sound from other sounds), treatment moves to production practice.

Promoting Awareness

Promoting awareness (promoting a child's awareness of the difference between sounds) offers a more cognitively oriented perspective on perception training. Promoting awareness begins by noting that it is highly unlikely that "the rabbit kids" fall down the wabbit hole because they have a broken discrimination mechanism. Speech perception, in common with other sensory systems, develops and matures months before an infant's first birthday (see Chapter 6, "Infants"). Like all parts of the body, damage can affect speech perception. However, because it is a critical foundation for speech learning, the outcome would be catastrophic and not limited to one or several late acquired sounds.

Something Normal

If perception problems are not the result of an immature or broken speech perception system, what *is* the problem? And, equally importantly, what can we as clinicians do about it? The answer may be that when children speak, their attention is on their intention, not the sounds tumbling out of their mouth.

Fast Fading Memories. This attention on intention is true for children with and without speech disorders, and for adults as well. In many ways, our perceptual system makes it difficult to monitor speech sounds. To illustrate, echoic memory lasts only milliseconds and then fades. Short-term memory lasts slightly longer, from 10 to 15 seconds up to a minute.

Just Like Adults. Adults—including highly trained speech-language pathologists—find it difficult to pay attention to small differences in their own speech. To illustrate, even an experienced clinician may not realize that their [r] in *ride* is voiced and their [r] in *pride* is voiceless, that [k] in *key* is made much more forward in the mouth than

[k] in *cool*, and that [p] is aspirated in *pie* but is unaspirated in *spy*. In other words, a child with a speech sound disorder does what everyone else does: not pay attention to the actual sounds coming out of their mouth. The difference between children with and without speech disorders is that we notice the child with the speech disorder because their intended production differs so markedly from their actual production.

Treatment Goal

Within this perspective, the goal of promoting awareness is to focus a student's attention on their speech. Promoting awareness also helps to promote generalization of treatment sounds to persons and settings outside the clinic. Almost all children and students need this assistance and so almost all receive ongoing help promoting awareness integrated with speech production practice (Anthony et al, 2011).

Awareness Activities. A clinician has a wide range of clinical tools to turn into awareness activities. Table 17–3 lists nine options.

These options are useful with any child whose development is sufficiently advanced to allow them to reflect on their speech, typically late preschoolers and older. The following brief annotated dialogue illustrates promoting awareness with a late preschooler receiving speech work on [s].

CLINICIAN: Do you remember what we call our treatment sound?

CHILD: The snake sound.

The metaphor reminds the child that [s] is continuant.

CLINICIAN: Do you remember how you used to say [s]?

CHILD: I said ta.

CLINICIAN: Now you're a big kid and say [s]. I know. Can you say [s] the big kid way, the little kid way, and then the big kid way again.

CHILD: sa ta sa.

Old way/new way focuses the child on the difference between [t] and [s] while building self-esteem through demonstration of progress.

TABLE 17–3. Clinical Options to Promote Awareness

Metaphors	Deletion
Touch cues	Self-correction
Descriptions	Old way/new way
Demonstrations	Similar sound
Minimal pairs	

> **CLINICIAN:** And now can you say sa three times in a row, listening to yourself, without me saying anything?
>
> **CHILD:** sa sa sa.
>
> **CLINICIAN:** How do you think you did?
>
> *Self-correction promotes self-monitoring, which the child needs to do to generalize treatment success.*

Distraction Activities. When a child leaves speech treatment, the world is full of distractions that may push his awareness of speech right out the window. You may find that including some distractions during speech tasks helps maintain hard won speech gains outside the treatment session. Children enjoy—and may find it challenging—to say words with treatment sounds while hopping on one foot, or rolling a ball in miniature bowling, or—for a student—practicing a class speech that contains the treatment sound.

Speech Practice

You have many different options to practice speech, ranging from quick and unnatural ("Say after me ___.") to slower and more language centered ("Retell the story of ___.") Of course, the various types of speech practice are not mutually exclusive. You might decide to employ different practice techniques both within the same session and as a child progresses in treatment. Table 17–4 lists 12 major speech practice techniques, each with their own advantages and disadvantages. Many times, if you are aware of a technique's limitations, the only needed adjustment is to use it in conjunction with speech practice that balances it.

Imitation

Imitation entails a child immediately repeating the clinician. This form of speech practice makes up with speed of elicitation what it lacks in naturalness, allowing a clinician to obtain copious productions in a short time. Clinicians tend to use imitation at the

TABLE 17–4. Speech Practice Techniques

Imitation	Spontaneous speech
Delayed imitation	Therapy talk
Picture or object naming	Minimal pairs
Sentence completion	Deletion
Story retelling	Self-correction
	Old way/new way
Short descriptions	Similar sound

beginning of treatment when a treatment sound is newly established and near the end of treatment to provide mass practice for a well-established sound.

Advantages and Disadvantages

An additional advantage of imitation is most children of any age can imitate. You may find its major limitation is that a child does not process speech, only repeats, and that what a child says in imitation may not be representative of his typical speech, and so may not generalize to words or to places outside the treatment setting.

CLINIC BOX: Time

What does a clinician do if a child is too young developmentally to "stick with a treatment sound" (practice) from beginning to end? The clever answer of a cycles approach is to stay with a treatment sounds for a certain amount of time rather than until a child reaches a certain percentage of correctness. Within a cycles approach, a clinician devotes a certain amount of treatment time (typically, 60 min) to a treatment sound affected by a phonological process (Hodson, 2007). After that time, treatment shifts to a treatment sound affected by a second and, perhaps, a third phonological process. After a clinician completes treatment for all phonological processes (called a cycle), the clinician cycles back through the phonological processes again (a second cycle). Cycles repeat until a clinician has remediated all the treatment sounds affected by the phonological processes, typically requiring from three to four cycles (approximately one year of treatment).

Delayed Imitation

Delayed imitation is imitation with a small break between what a clinician says and what a child repeats. To illustrate, a clinician says, "Say dog. Now you say it". The child then says "dog." The small break is "Now you say it" between the clinician and the child's speech. The logic of delayed imitation is the delay moves a child's response from echoic memory (which lasts only milliseconds) to a slightly longer-term memory. Theoretically, this makes delayed imitation slightly more natural than immediate imitation, though I am not familiar with research that shows delayed imitation is more representative of a child's natural speech or that treatment successes in delayed imitate generalize better than immediate imitation. Delayed imitation has similar advantages and limitations as immediate imitation.

Picture or Object Naming

In picture naming or object naming, a clinician shows a picture or an object for the child to name. This is a favorite practice technique for many clinicians because naming approaches the speed of imitation, but requires linguistic processing of real words, making it more likely that results of speech practice will generalize to other words, persons, and settings.

Advantages and Disadvantages

Naming also offers the advantage of being extremely flexible. If mass production practice is a clinician's purpose, the pictures and objects can come quickly, one after another. If the purpose is less mass practice and more to promote linguistic processing, a clinician can intersperse naming pictures or object with opportunities for therapy talk and saying the words in a sentence. A potential limitation of picture or object naming is that people typically do not speak in isolated words, so, while more natural than imitation, it is less natural than some other speech practice options.

Sentence Completion

Sentence completion is a stepping-stone toward a child using a treatment sound in a sentence. To illustrate sentence completion, a clinician may tape pictures of snakes of different color around a treatment room to elicit [sn] clusters that a child can make at the word level. The clinician then turns off the lights, shines a flashlight, and says, "I see a ___." A child then completes the sentence ("a yellow snake!" or "a blue snake!"). An easy alternate, one requiring slightly greater linguistic ability, is for a clinician (or the child, of course) to shine the flashlight and for a child to say a full sentence ("I see a yellow snake!").

Advantages and Disadvantages

The clinical place of sentence completion is when you are working with a child who has learned to make a treatment sound in words, but who needs a bridge between words and sentences. Its limitations as a speech practice technique are those you might expect: fewer productions result than with imitation or naming, and the sentences are semi-rote.

Story Retell

Story retell entails a clinician reading a short story that contains a treatment sound, and the child then retells the story. To illustrate, a clinician may present a three to six sentence story about a dog at the beach and then ask a child to retell the story. The clinician may add aides to help a child organize their thoughts, including a series of pictures depicting the story for the child to organize in the correct order. For example, after completing the story, a clinician may say, "Now it's your turn to tell the story back to me. But, first, let's put the pictures in order and tell me some things because I forgot." The clinician then asks a series of questions such as: "Who was the story about? What happened first? What happened next? What was the most surprising thing that happened in the story?" The props in place, the child then retells the story.

Advantages and Disadvantages

Story retell provides a way to practice a well-established treatment sound in sentences that a child processes and assembles into a story discourse structure, an activity that promotes generalization because it practices speech in contexts found in school and home. If the story you select for retell fits into the curriculum of a child's preschool or school, so much the better. A limitation of story retell is that it is not a good fit if a child still struggles with a treatment sound at the word level. It also does not provide mass practice with a treatment sound, though interspersed imitation, word naming, and therapy talk may provide concentrated practice, if you feel a child needs that.

Short Descriptions

Short descriptions entail a clinician presenting a situation that requires a child to say a treatment sound to describe. To illustrate, the situation could be an arrangement of objects in a barrier game, a picture, or an answer to a question ("What did you have for breakfast this morning?"), and so forth.

Advantages and Disadvantages

The advantages of short descriptions are like those for story retells: practicing a well-established treatment sound in sentences while creating a discourse structure. I am not sure which speech practice is more challenging for a child, story retell or short descriptions; I suppose it differs depending on the story a child retells and the complexity of the description. The limitations of short descriptions are comparable to those for story retell.

Spontaneous Speech

To produce a treatment sound correctly in spontaneous speech is the goal of speech practice. To illustrate this form of practice, a child (typically a student or a selected late preschooler) engages in natural conversation with a clinician or another person. After a natural or previously determined interval, the student stops, and the student and clinician review, discuss, and perhaps practice the treatment sound.

Advantages and Disadvantages

You may find the advantages and limitations of speech practice in spontaneous speech are opposite of imitation. Whereas imitation makes up with speed what it lacks in naturalness, spontaneous speech makes up with naturalness what it lacks in speed.

Therapy Talk

The last way to practice speech, **therapy talk**, is a distillation of therapeutic ways to talk about speech with children, typically those who are late preschoolers or older. Therapy talk includes minimal pairs, deletions, self-corrections, old way/new way, and similar sounds. With no production demands, therapy talk promotes speech awareness. With production requirements, it facilitates speech practice while promoting phonological and literacy development.

Advantages and Disadvantages

You can use therapy talk by itself or in conjunction with other speech practice options. Limitations of therapy talk are that a child needs to be developmentally ready to reflect on speech and that the techniques elicit fewer productions than imitation and naming.

Dialogue Variations

The following variations of a dialogue showing speech practice with [r] in *race* illustrate the functions and forms of different types of therapy talk (see Chapter 18, "Talking with Children," for a fuller discussion).

Minimal Pairs. Alternates production of a treatment sound with rhyming sounds, providing speech practice and promoting phonological awareness.

> CLINICIAN: Race starts with treatment sound. Can you say race and three words that rhyme with race?
>
> CHILD: Race, lace, face, case.

Deletions. Adds and removes a treatment sound from a word, providing speech practice and promoting phonological awareness

> CLINICIAN: And if you take the [r] sound away from race, what word do you have?
>
> CHILD: Ace.
>
> CLINICIAN: Can you say ace with the [r] sound and then without the [r] sound? Do it three times.
>
> CHILD: Race, ace. Race, ace. Race, ace.

Self-Corrections. Repeats words with treatment sound at least three times without clinician feedback, providing speech practice and promoting self-monitoring and generalization

> CLINICIAN: Now can you say race three times, without me saying anything? Just listen to yourself and then tell me how you did.
>
> CHILD: Race, race, race.

Old Way/New Way. Alternates former and present pronunciation of a treatment sound, providing speech practice and promoting self-awareness and positive feelings about speech progress.

CLINICIAN: Do you remember when you were a little kid how you said the [r] sound in race?

CHILD: Wace.

CLINICIAN: Why don't you say race the old way you used to say it and the new big kid way you say it now, then the old way, and then the new way big kid way?

CHILD: Wace. Race, wace, race.

Similar Sounds. Alternates between a treatment sound and a similar sound in a child's phonetic repertoire, providing speech practice differentiating between two similar sounds.

This is similar sound: *

CLINICIAN: You know what sound is really a lot like [r]? [w], the sound you used to say instead of [r]. Can you say race, wace three times?

CHILD: Race, wace. Race, wace, Race, wace.

*In the illustration, [w] is the same in the practice of old way/new way and similar sound. This is not always the case. To illustrate, a child who, when younger, pronounced [s] as [t], would have [t] as the old sound, and a clinician might decide to make [ʃ] the similar sound for [s].

Conclusions

Major ideas in this chapter include:

1. Treatment sounds are the speech elements (vowels, consonants, consonant clusters, syllables, prosody, etc.) through which a clinician facilitates speech change.
2. Selection of a treatment sound entails a clinician making decisions about stimulability and speech knowledge, and, less often, about age of acquisition and frequency of occurrence.
3. Many ways exist to establish nonstimulable and stimulable sounds in a child's speech.
4. Discrimination training and promoting awareness are alternate views on speech perception training.
5. Speech practice options range from imitation to spontaneous speech. Therapy talk promotes speech along with literacy and language.

Review Questions

1. What is the logic of selecting a stimulable treatment sound? What is the logical of selecting a nonstimulable treatment sound?
2. What are the differences between most knowledge and least knowledge as ways to select a treatment sound?

3. How might you establish a nonstimulable sound in the speech of an early preschooler?
4. List five ways you could establish a nonstimulable sound in the speech of a 3rd grade student.
5. What is a key word and how might it assist in establishing a treatment sound?
6. What are key environments? How might they assist in establishing a treatment sound? What are possible key environments for [s]?
7. Compare advantages and limitations of imitation and word naming as ways to practice speech.
8. Develop a sentence completion activity for speech practice.
9. What are advantages and disadvantages of story retell to practice speech?
10. Create an example of short descriptions interspersed with delayed imitation and deletions.

References

Anthony, J. L., Aghara, R. G., Solari, E. J., Dunkelberger, M. J., Williams, J. M., & Liang, L. (2011). Quantifying phonological representation abilities in Spanish-speaking preschool children. *Applied Psycholinguistics, 32*(1), 19-49

Diedrich, W. (1983). Stimulability and articulation disorders. *Seminars in Speech and Language, 4*.

Hodson, B. (2007). *Evaluating and enhancing children's phonological systems: Research and theory to practice.* Greenville, SC: Thinking Publications/Super Duper.

Miccio, M. W., & Williams, A. L. (2010). Stimulability intervention. *Interventions for Speech Sound Disorders in Children (CLI), 179*–202.

Powell, T. (1991). Planning for phonological generalization: An approach to treatment target selection. *American Journal of Speech-Language Pathology, 1*, 21–27.

Powell, T., Elbert, M., & Dinnsen, D. (1991). Stimulability as a factor in phonological generalization of misarticulating preschool children. *Journal of Speech and Hearing Research, 34*, 1318–1328.

Shine, R. (1989). Articulatory production training: A sensory-motor approach. In N. Creag-head, P. Newman, & W. Secord (Eds.), *Assessment and remediation of articulatory and phonological disorders* (pp. 355–359). Columbus, OH: Charles E. Merrill.

Shriberg, L. (1993). Four new speech and voice-prosody measures for genetics research and other studies in developmental phonological disorders. *Journal of Speech, Language, and Hearing Research, 36*, 105–140.

Shriberg, L., & Kwiatkowski, J. (1983). Computer-assisted natural process analysis (NPA): Recent issues and data. *Seminars in Speech and Language, 4*, 397.

Van Riper, C. (1978). *Speech correction: Principles and methods* (6th ed.). Englewood Cliffs, NJ: Prentice-Hall.

CHAPTER 18

TALKING WITH CHILDREN

Adult speech has the power to transform the noise in a child's world into a ladder for learning. Speech that facilitates learning holds a child's interest, changes in response to a child's shifts in attention, and adjusts to accommodate a child's experiences and developmental level (Gleitman, Newport, & Gleitman, 1984; Goldstein & Schwade, 2008; Kuhl, 2004, 2007; Masataka, 1992). For an infant, toddler, or an early preschooler not yet possessing sufficient attention skills for more structured treatment, these speech modifications form a core of treatment. For a late preschooler or a student, therapeutic speech modifications are an important part of a clinician's repertoire. Topics in this chapter include

- Motherese
- Facilitative Talk
- Therapy Talk

Learning Objectives

I hope on completing the chapter you will

- Understand the importance of Motherese.
- Have advice to offer families about talking with their child.
- Appreciate the difference between Motherese and facilitative talk.
- Know the difference between facilitative talk and modified facilitative talk.
- Identify different types of therapy talk.

Key Words

Key words you will encounter in this chapter

Motherese
Facilitative talk
Strategic errors
Modeling
Bombardment
Requests for confirmation or clarification
Parallel talk
Expansions
Modified facilitative talk
Therapy talk
Minimal pairs
Deletions
Self-corrections
Old way/new way
Similar sounds

Motherese

Motherese is a primary way that caregivers teach an infant about speech and language. This section explores what Motherese is and how it helps an infant learn. Topics include

- What Is Motherese?
- Motherese and Families
- Talking with Infants

What Is Motherese?

Motherese is an essential part of almost all treatment approaches with infants and young children (Camarata, 2010; Miccio, 2005; Scherer, & Kaiser, 2010; Warren et al., 2006). Motherese answers a caregiver question that is probably old as Homo sapiens: how do I get and keep an infant's attention? Attention is needed for a child to learn, and often is difficult to obtain and maintain given an infant's cognitive limitations (Chang & Thompson, 2011; Dore, 1986; Snow, 1984).

Technically Speaking

Technically, Motherese is a specialized speech register, one of many ways that people modify speech in response to situation and person. Importantly, in addition to Motherese there also is fatherese and siblingese, although they have a smaller research base and their contribution to infant learning is less clear (Soderstrom, 2007). Parentese is a more recent term, though it has not yet become standard. For this reason, with apologies to fathers and siblings, the present discussion focuses on Motherese.

Capturing an Infant's Attention

Altering speech is a normal aspect of language use. Consider how your own speech changes depending on if you are speaking with family or strangers, with a younger or older person, at a baseball game or in a bank, or with people you respect and those you do not. Verbal tricks of Motherese that caregivers use to capture and hold an infant's flickering attention include

- Higher than usual pitch
- Talking about shared perceptions
- Exaggerated intonation
- Use of repetitions
- Calling attention to objects

Motherese requires an adult to know a child well enough to anticipate and respond to their needs and wants. The conversation topics of Motherese are those that interest a child and modifications in intonation, syntax and vocabulary are those needed to keep the child's attention. Thus, a caregiver shapes the vast complexities of language into a lesson from which a child can learn. Motherese changes as a child develops, adjusting to fit a child's cognitive level and greater experience with language. To illustrate, Motherese appropriate to a child of 3 months would seem silly and immature if directed to a toddler or preschooler.

Motherese and Families

Families are the principal users of Motherese (which is why we call it Motherese rather than clinicianese). Motherese comes naturally to most caregivers. However, situations arise when a family may have difficulties using Motherese spontaneously. In the following sections, I've described three that I have encountered frequently.

Baby Talk

Some families confuse Motherese with baby talk. When this occurs, every time a clinician says Motherese, they picture you asking them to say *gee gee* and *gaa gaa* to their child, and that you are asking them to talk in a way they find embarrassing. They may also hold the belief that an infant will benefit more from an adult speaking to them in full, complete sentences.

The Silent Infant

A different challenge may arise if an infant is silent, perhaps unable to vocalize or interact extensively for medical reasons or developmental delay. Families may limit their interactions with a silent infant, even in the face of encouragement from hospital staff, believing the child does not benefit from the contact.

Family Stress

A family under severe chronic stress may limit their time with an infant, or may be too distracted to interact in a way that promotes learning. Chronic severe stress can have neurological consequences for both caregivers and infants, as well as being a risk factor for future educational and social challenges (Harden, 2015; National Scientific Council on the Developing Child, 2014).

Talking with Infants

Regardless of the specific reason that inhibits a family's use of Motherese, the general clinical advice is to encourage families to talk to their child in ways that they and the child find enjoyable and natural. A child who has fun communicating is more likely to want to communicate again.

Eye on the Prize

It may help to ask caregivers to keep the following questions in mind as they interact with their child:

■ Does your child appear interested?
■ Is your child paying attention?

Encourage caregivers to speak in whatever way maximizes the chance that they answer "yes" to both questions. For most infants, "yes" occurs more often if an adult speaks in short sentences and single words, talks about the "here and now," and focuses the conversation on what appears to interest the child. That is, "yes" occurs more often if a caregiver uses Motherese, although a clinician may elect not to use that word to describe their speech. For a silent infant, interest and attention may take the form of eye widening, smiling, movement of the extremities, or imitative oral motor movements.

Talking Points

When discussing Motherese with families, the following four points may help summarize the essential ideas about talking with an infant:

1. Talk about what you and your baby are doing and seeing.
2. Talk in a way that seems natural to you and that holds your baby's attention.
3. Daily routines such as eating meals, preparing for bedtime, and changing diapers provide excellent opportunities to help your baby learn.
4. Avoid extensive use of electronic teachers (videos, tapes, and television) because they do not change based on your baby's response.

Facilitative Talk

Facilitative talk is an advanced form of Motherese for use with a toddler or an early preschooler (2;0 to approximately 3;6) too young to benefit from direct instruction. A preschooler midway in development between facilitative talk and direct instruction may benefit from a combination of both. Facilitative talk topics include

■ What Is Facilitative Talk?
■ Facilitative Talk and Families
■ Forms of Facilitative Talk
■ Modified Facilitative Talk

What Is Facilitative Talk?

Facilitative talk is Motherese for an older child. This book employs the term *facilitative talk* to differentiate it from Motherese with infants. If you prefer the term toddler Motherese, advanced Motherese, or simply Motherese, please feel free to use them. The exact term matters less than the fact that facilitative talk (however it is called) offers a means to facilitate speech and language for a child not yet old enough to benefit from direct instruction (Camarata, 2010; Soloman-Rice & Soto, 2009; Tsybina, Girolametto, Weitzman, & Greenberg, 2006). Facilitative talk includes

- Strategic errors
- Modeling
- Bombardment
- Requests for confirmation or clarification
- Parallel talk
- Expansions

Facilitative talk comes from studies of how families naturally teach language to their children. In this book, they are adapted into tools to promote speech development.

Therapy Ingredients

Think of forms of facilitative talk as therapy ingredients that you select from and alter to fit a specific child's needs. To illustrate, one child may benefit from a combination of parallel talk and strategic errors, while another may respond better to expansions. To continue the cooking analogy, some ingredients find more general use than other ingredients. Forms of facilitative talk with wide use include modeling, bombardment, expansions, and parallel talk.

Facilitative Talk and Families

As with infant Motherese, many families use facilitative talk naturally, without need of any instruction. If a family requests assistance, work together to discover which techniques seem most compatible with their interactive styles, and then practice facilitative talk together with the child. If a family's request is for general suggestions about talking with a toddler, you might offer the following:

1. Interact often and, when you do, talk about what you and your child are doing and seeing.
2. Focus more on what your child says than how they say it.
3. Speak in short simple sentences about the here and now.
4. Talk about what seems to interest your child.
5. Encourage your child to communicate through "using your words."
6. Have fun. Stay away from drills and rote memorization.
7. Avoid extensive use of electronic teachers (videos, movies, and television), which do not change their messages based on your child's response.

Forms of Facilitative Talk

Strategic Error

A **strategic error** focuses a child on speech—not something easy to achieve in a toddler or early preschooler who seldom seems aware of speech matters. Strategic errors, as adapted here for speech treatment, do this by mimicking aspects of a child's speech sound disorder. If, for example, a child pronounces word-initial [t] as [d], a clinician might point to a toy and say, "doy." The hoped-for response is that the child looks confused or laughs. Sometimes, along with a confused look or laugh, a strategic error elicits a speech production.

FATHER: This is my favorite doy.

Child smiles.

FATHER: I love my doy.

CHILD: Toy.

Modeling

Modeling, as the name suggests, provides a child an example of a speech element. For example, an adult might model [t] in *tea* while they play with a toy kitchen set.

ADULT: Would you like some more tea?

CHILD: Yes, please.

ADULT: Tea is good. Do you like tea?

CHILD: Yes.

ADULT: Would you like toast with your tea?

CHILD: Yes.

ADULT: Mmm. This is good toast. Toast and tea taste so good together.

Bombardment

Bombardment increases the relative frequency of a treatment sound. The logic behind this form of facilitative talk is that a child tends to learn earlier what they heard more often (Maye, Weiss, & Aslin, 2008). Bombardment places no production demands on a child. Bombardment is like preparing the soil for future planting—providing exposure to a treatment sound in meaningful naturalistic contexts, readying a child to say it when the time is right. The following brief dialogue demonstrates bombardment of words ending in nasal consonants while an adult and child eat lunch.

ADULT: This peanut butter is so yum. So *yum*.

Child nods.

ADULT: Sandwiches are so *fun*. Aren't they *fun*?

Child nods.

ADULT: What other *fun* things *can* we do? Would you like to play out in the *sun*?

Child smiles.

ADULT: Let's do it. The *sun* is so *warm* today. This will be *fun*.

Requests for Confirmation or Clarification

Requests for confirmation or clarification focus a child's attention on speech for communication. The following dialogue demonstrates a request for clarification for a child who pronounces [k] as [t] as an adult shows a child a small box with a lock.

ADULT: I bet there are fun things inside the box. Think so?

CHILD: Maybe.

ADULT: How do you open a locked box?

CHILD: With a tea.

ADULT: With a tea? I thought you drank tea.

Child laughs.

Requests for confirmations and clarifications require some care, since, if overused, a child may "shut down" and either speak less or resort to pointing. A possible sidestep around this is for a puppet or doll to ask questions, as in the following slight alternation of the preceding dialogue.

ADULT: I bet there are fun things inside the box. Think so?

CHILD: Maybe.

ADULT: Puppet, how do you open a locked box?

PUPPET: With a tea.

ADULT: With a tea? I thought you drank tea.

PUPPET: I meant a key.

ADULT: That's right. With a key.

Parallel Talk

Parallel talk narrates a child's activities and interests, providing a verbal description of what captures the child's attention for the moment. Parallel talk supports the well-known truth that a child acquires words that refer to things and actions they find interesting. The following sequence demonstrates the adaptation of parallel talk to facilitate [d] in *dog*.

The child picks up a toy dog.

CLINICIAN: Doggy.

The child pets the dog.

CLINICIAN: Nice doggy. So cuddly.

The child kisses the toy dog.

CLINICIAN: Ohhh . . . Sweet dog.

Expansions

As adapted here for speech treatment, **expansions** "fill in the missing speech parts." The following brief dialogue shows its use to facilitate word final consonants as a child picks up a book and hands it to the adult.

CHILD: Boo.

ADULT: Book.

The child opens the book and points to a picture of a pig.

CHILD: Pi.

ADULT: Pig. Yes. It's a pig.

Modified Facilitative Talk

Modified facilitative talk is facilitative talk with a gentle speech production nudge provided by occasional questions, sentence completions, and requests to imitate. Whereas facilitative talk occurs naturally in families, modified facilitative talk is a clinician's therapy tools.

The following three dialogue variations show modifications of a request for confirmation or clarification to encourage a speech production.

Modification with a question:

ADULT: I bet there are fun things inside this locked box. Think so?

CHILD: Maybe.

ADULT: Puppet, how do you open a locked box?

PUPPET: With a tea.

ADULT: With a tea? I thought you drank tea.

Adults looks at child.

ADULT: How do you open a locked box?

CHILD: Key.

Modification with an imitation:

ADULT: With a tea? I thought you drank tea.

Adults looks at child.

ADULT: Say, *key.*

CHILD: Key.

Modification with a sentence completion:

ADULT: With a tea? I thought you drank tea.

Adults looks at child.

ADULT: You open a locked box with a . . .

CHILD: Key.

Therapy Talk

Therapy talk is a compilation of treatment techniques to promote speech and speech awareness in late preschoolers through adults. Some individual techniques are relatively new and unexplored (deletions, similar sounds), while others have been clinical mainstays for many years (old way/new way, minimal pairs). Therapy talk topics include

- What Is Therapy Talk?
- Forms of Therapy Talk

What Is Therapy Talk?

Think of therapy talk as the basic kitchen equipment of the clinical craft—it's spoons, forks, knives, and ladles. They are compatible with almost any treatment approach for late preschoolers and students, and are useful for introducing a treatment sound, promoting speech awareness, reminding a child of a correct pronunciation, practicing a motor skill, and encouraging generalization. Therapy talk includes

- Minimal pairs
- Deletion
- Self-correction
- Old way/new way
- Similar sound

Unlike Motherese and facilitative talk, both of which mirror what caregivers do naturally, clinicians developed therapy talk. That is, therapy talk comes from observing what clinicians do well. Nothing in principle prevents a clinician teaching therapy talk techniques to families as part of a home program.

Forms of Therapy Talk

Minimal Pairs

Minimal pairs highlight the communicative value of speech. Minimal pairs typically entail a clinician or child saying a word that contains the treatment sound, and then replacing the treatment sound to create a rhyming word. The following brief dialogue demonstrates minimal pairs to encourage phonological awareness through a reading game with an adult, child, and puppet.

Puppet:　Once upon a lime . . . I mean once upon a mime. No, a crime. A chime. A dime.

Adult:　No, silly puppet. It's not, Once upon a lime. A lime is green and sour tasting. Not a mine, not a crime, not a chime, not a dime. It's, Once upon a time.

Puppet:　Oh. Sorry. I'll start again. Once upon a time . . .

Adult:　That's right. Once upon a time.

The following dialogue shows minimal pairs with a production activity in which an adult sets out three picture cards, pictures down.

Adult:　Please turn over a card.

Child turns over a picture of cat.

Adult:　Cat starts with [k], our treatment sound. Can you think of three words that rhyme with cat?

Child:　Rat. Mat. Bat.

Adult:　That's right. Rat, mat, and bat all rhyme with cat, and by changing out the treatment sound from [k] we get words that mean different things.

Deletion

Deletions are like minimal pairs, except in deletions a clinician demonstrates the communicative value of a treatment sound through deleting it from a word. The following dialogue demonstrates this technique in a production activity for [z] in a game with a toy train.

Adult:　A train has cars. This train has an engine, a passenger car, and a caboose.

The child and adult assemble the cars.

Adult:　We can also take cars away.

The adult removes the engine car.

Adult:　Words are like trains. You can add and take away parts of words. Zoom is like a train with three parts: "z-oo-m." Let's take away the first sound. That leaves only two cars, the vowel and [m]. Can you say zoom without the first sound?

Child:　Oom

Adult:　Now say it with the first sound.

Child:　Zoom.

Adult:　Now try it with and without the first sound.

Child:　Um. Zoom. Um Zoom.

You can use deletions and other forms of therapy talk either alone or in conjunction with each other, providing the option of multiple avenues to explore a treatment sound. The following dialogue pairs minimal pairs and deletions in a production activity focusing on the voiceless interdental.

Minimal Pairs:

ADULT: Can you think of a word that begins with our treatment sound?

CHILD: Thin.

ADULT: Good. Can you think of two words that rhyme with thin?

CHILD: Win. Fin.

Deletions:

ADULT: Good. Suppose you take the first sound away from thin. How would you say the word?

CHILD: In.

ADULT: Can you say thin with and without the first sound two times?

CHILD: Thin. In. Thin. In.

Self-Correction

Self-corrections help a child learn to self-monitor speech to promote generalization of a treatment sound to other settings. This technique typically proves most useful after a child demonstrates some ability to successfully pronounce a treatment sound. Interestingly, sometimes successful use of self-correction proves easier for the child than the clinician, because it requires the clinician not to provide feedback on the child's success or failure. The following dialogue demonstrates self-correction in a production activity focusing on the final consonant in *bush*.

ADULT: I want you to say bush three times. Listen carefully to yourself each time you say it and change how you say it if it doesn't sound quite right.

CHILD: bus.

The child looks at the clinician, who, carefully, does not indicate if the sound was pronounced correctly or not.

CHILD: Bush. Bush.

ADULT: What do you think? Did you pronounce our treatment sound correctly?

CHILD: I thought it got better as I went along.

Self-corrections combine well with other therapy talk techniques as illustrated in the modification of the previous dialogue.

With Deletions:

ADULT: Can you say bush without the final sound?

CHILD: Bu.

ADULT: Now, please say bush without the final sound, then with the final sound, then without the final sound.

CHILD: Bu. Bush. Bu.

With Self-Correction:

Adult: Very good. Now say bush three times, listening to yourself to hear if you are saying it correctly.

Child: Bu. Bush. Bush.

Adult: What do you think?

Old Way/New Way

Old way/new way helps a child feel and hear the difference between two ways to pronounce a treatment sound, promotes self-monitoring, and encourages positive self-esteem. This form of therapy talk asks a child to alternate between old and new ways of saying a treatment sound. "Younger kid way" and "bigger kid way" sometimes replaces old way/new. Avoid wrong way/right way in the interest of promoting a child's positive self-image. The following dialogue demonstrates this therapy talk form in a treatment activity focusing on [r] in *race*.

Adult: You are really making lots of progress. Do you remember how you used to say [r]?

Child: As a double u.

Adult: That's right. I'd like you to say *race* the old way, then the new way, and then the old way again. Okay?

Child: Wace. Race. Wace.

Similar Sound

Similar sounds, like the much more familiar old way/new way, promote self-monitoring and help a child feel and hear the difference between a treatment sound and another sound. Differing from old way/new way, the contrast in similar sounds is with a sound phonetically close to the treatment sound, rather than to a child's previous pronunciation. The following dialogue demonstrates use of similar sounds in an activity focusing on [s] in the beginning of words.

Adult: Our treatment sound is [s] in *see*, and the sound we are comparing it to is the sound that begins *she*. Say *see*, then *she*, then *see*, listening to yourself and feeling the difference between [s] and the other sound.

Child: See. She. See.

The following examples use similar sounds in conjunction with deletions and self-corrections.

With Deletions:

Adult: First, can you say *see* without our treatment sound?

Child: ee.

ADULT: Good. Now can you say it with our treatment sound, without it, and then with it?

CHILD: See. Ee. See.

ADULT: Now say *see* and then *she, see, she, see,* listening to yourself and feeling the difference between [s] and the other sound.

CHILD: See. She. See.

With Self-Correction:

ADULT: Now say *see* and then *she, see, she, see,* listening to yourself and feeling the difference between [s] and the other sound.

CHILD: See. She. See.

ADULT: Now can you say *see* three times, listening carefully to yourself?

CHILD: *See. See. See.*

Conclusions

Major ideas in this chapter include

1. Adult speech has the power to transform the noise in a child's world into a ladder for learning.
2. Motherese is the name of the speech register that caregivers use to encourage infant learning.
3. Facilitative talk is an advanced form of Motherese for use with toddlers.
4. Modified facilitative talk is facilitative talk with the addition of a speech component.
5. Therapy talk is a collection of clinician-developed techniques for use with late pre-schoolers and students.

Review Questions

1. What is Motherese and why is it important developmentally?
2. What is a speech register?
3. In your own words, explain how you might encourage a family to use Motherese if they confuse Motherese with baby talk.
4. What advice about speaking to their child might you offer a family of a silent infant or a family under severe chronic stress?
5. What is facilitative talk and what is its purpose?
6. List three suggestions to offer a family on talking with a toddler.
7. Create an adult/child dialogue of parallel talk.
8. What is modified facilitative talk?
9. Create an adult/child dialogue for expansions and sentence completion.
10. What is therapy talk?
11. What are the names of the five types of therapy talk?

References

Camarata, S. (2010). Naturalistic intervention for speech intelligibility and speech accuracy. In L. Williams, S. McLeod, & R. McCauley (Eds.), *Interventions for speech sound disorders in children* (pp. 381–405). Baltimore, MD: Brookes.

Chang, R., & Thompson, N. (2011). Whines, cries, and motherese: Their relative power to distract. *Journal of Social, Evolutionary, and Cultural Psychology*, *5*, 131–141.

Dore, J. (1986). The development of conversational competence. In R. Schiefelbusch (Ed.), *Language competence: Assessment and intervention* (pp. 3–59). San Diego, CA: College-Hill Press.

Gleitman, L., Newport, E., & Gleitman, H. (1984). The current status of the motherese hypothesis. *Journal of Child Language*, *11*, 43–79.

Goldstein, M., & Schwade, J. (2008). Social feedback to infants' babbling facilitates rapid phonological learning. *Psychological Science*, *19*(5), 515–523.

Harden, B. J. (2015). *Services for families of infants and toddlers experiencing trauma. A research-to-practice brief* (OPRE Report 2015-14). Washington, DC: Administration for Children & Families.

Kuhl, P. (2004). Early language acquisition: Cracking the speech code. *Nature Reviews: Neuroscience*, *5*, 831–843.

Kuhl, P. (2007). Is speech learning "gated" by the social brain? *Developmental Science*, *10*, 110–120.

Masataka, N. (1992). Motherese in a signed language. *Infant Behavior and Development*, *15*, 453–460.

Maye, J., Weiss, D., & Aslin, R., (2008). Statistical phonetic learning in infants: Facilitation and feature generalization. *Developmental Science*, *11*, 122–134.

Miccio, A. W. (2005). A treatment program for enhancing stimulability. In A. G. Kamhi & K. E. Pollock (Eds.), *Phonological disorders in children: Clinical decision making in assessment and intervention* (pp. 163–173). Baltimore, MD: Brookes.

National Scientific Council on the Developing Child. (2014). *Excessive stress disrupts the architecture of the developing brain* (Working paper 3). Retrieved from http://developingchild .harvard.edu/resources/reports_and_working_papers/working_papers/wp3/

Scherer, N., & Kaiser, A. (2010). Enhanced milieu teaching with phonological emphasis for children with cleft lip and palate. In L. Williams, S. McLeod, & R. McCauley (Eds.), *Interventions for speech sound disorders in children* (pp. 427–452). Baltimore, MD: Brookes.

Snow, C. (1984). Parent-child interaction and the development of communicative ability. In R. Schiefelbusch & J. Pickar (Eds.), *The Acquisition of communication competence* (pp. 69–108). Baltimore, MD: University Park Press.

Soderstrom, M. (2007). Beyond babytalk: Re-evaluating the nature and content of speech input to preverbal infants. *Developmental Review*, *27*, 501–532.

Soloman-Rice, P., & Soto, G. (2009). Language modeling as an efficacious early language intervention approach with young children demonstrating complex communication needs. *Perspectives on Augmentative and Alternative Communication 18*, 21–27.

Tsybina, I., Girolametto, L., Weitzman, E., & Greenberg, J. (2006). Recasts used with preschoolers learning English as their second language. *Early Childhood Education Journal*, *4*(2), 177–185.

Warren, S., Bredin-Oja, M. Escalante, M., Finestack, L., Fey, M., & Brady, N. (2006). Responsivity education/prelinguistic milieu teaching. In R. McCauley & M. Fey (Eds.), *Treatment of language disorders in children* (pp. 47–76). Baltimore, MD: Brookes.

CHAPTER 19

TALKING ABOUT SPEECH

As speech-language pathologists, we know [s] is an alveolar consonant produced with the folds of the larynx apart, the air flowing over the tongue, and the tongue tip either raised or lowered behind the front teeth. Our challenge is how to convey that and other speech information to a child? Or to someone with intellectual challenges? Or, really, *anyone* who hasn't received an advanced degree in communication disorders? Fortunately, our profession has developed ways to meet this necessary challenge. Organized from simplest to most complex, ways to talk about speech with a child include:

- Metaphors
- Touch Cues
- Descriptions and Demonstrations
- Phonetic Placement and Shaping

Learning Objectives

I hope on completing the chapter you will

- Understand the importance of talking about speech in treatment.
- Know the value and limits of metaphors.
- Recognize why clinicians use touch cues.
- Locate lists of instructions for descriptions and demonstrations.
- Recognize that newer, higher technology options exist for descriptions and demonstrations.
- Understand the purpose of phonetic placement and shaping.

Key Words

Key words you encounter in this chapter

Metaphors
Touch cues
Tactile cues
Visual phonics
Descriptions
Demonstrations
Electropalatography (EPG)
Spectography
Visi-Pitch
Ultrasound
Phonetic placement
Shaping

Metaphors

Metaphors compare some aspect of speech to something with which the child is familiar. To illustrate, a metaphor for [s] may be "the snake sound," and a metaphor for any fricative may be "the long sound."

Purpose

Metaphors are a simple way to talk to a child about a treatment sound. Tables 19–1 to 19–3 show metaphors for place (Table 19–1), manner (Table 19–2), and syllable and word position (Table 19–3). The source for many of these tables is Blodgett and Miller (1989) and Flowers (1990).

Who May Benefit

Metaphors find their greatest use with children 3 years and older, though some children younger than 3 also find them beneficial as prompts for them to say a sound in a way that a clinician praises. Grade school students typically enjoy metaphors, while students in junior high school or older often find them too childish.

Suggestions

A few simple guidelines may help you make the most of this very useful clinical tool:

1. Vary your metaphors based on a child's speech challenge. A useful metaphor helps a child focus on the aspect of a sound that challenges them. This can change by

TABLE 19–1. Examples of Possible Metaphors for Places of Production

Place of Production	Metaphors
Bilabial	Lip sounds
Labiodental	Biting lip sounds or biting sounds
Interdental	Tongue tip sounds, tongue sandwich sounds
Alveolar	Bump sounds, hill sounds
Postalveolar	Back of the hill sounds
Palatal	Middle sound
Velar	Back sounds
Glottal	Throat sound

TABLE 19–2. Examples of Possible Metaphors for Manners of Production

Manner of Production	Metaphors
Fricatives	Long sounds, hissing sounds
Glides and liquids (approximants)	Flowing sounds
Lateral	Side sound
Affricates	Engine chugging sounds
Nasals	Nose sounds
Stops	Short sounds, dripping sounds, and popping sounds
Voiced	Motor on, voice on, buzzing sound, hand buzzer sound, noisy sounds, buzzing voice box, and voice box on
Voiceless	Motor off, voice off, not a buzzing sound, not a hand buzzer sound, quiet sounds, no buzzing voice box, and voice box off

TABLE 19–3. Examples of Possible Metaphors for Consonant Clusters, Syllables, and Words

Sound Units	Metaphors
End of word	End sound
Multisyllabic words	Words with parts
Single syllable words	Words with one part
Initial consonants	Starting sounds
Consonant clusters	Sound friends

Source: Adapted from *Easy Does It for Phonology*, by E. Blodgett and V. Miller, 1989, East Moline, IL: LinguiSystems.

individual child. For example, two children may have [s] difficulties, the first because the tongue tip is in the wrong position and the second because of difficulties maintaining frication. For the first child, "the tongue tip sound" might prove useful, and for the second, "the long sound" might work better.

2. Whenever possible, let a child help select the metaphor (Dean, Howell, Hill, & Waters, 1990). The best metaphor is the one a child "buys into." For example, you might offer a child a choice between two metaphors, both focusing on the child's challenge with the treatment sound.

3. Provide a little practice to help cement the association between the metaphor and the treatment sound. If, for example, the metaphor for [s] is the snake sound, you

might say, "Raise your hand when I say our snake sound. Is it [ʃ]? Is it [f]? Is it [s]?" If the child has difficulty associating the metaphor with the treatment sound, try increasing the number of distinctive features between the treatment sound and its foils. For example, if the child raises their hand when you ask if the snake sound is [f], try contrasting [s] with [m] (nasal) or [t] (oral stop).

Annotated Dialogue

The following annotated dialogue illustrates one of a multitude of ways to establish a metaphor.

> *The student is in an early grade and the activity is reading about a lion.*

CLINICIAN: We're going to work on the sound that begins "lion." Hmm . . . we should think of a name for our sound. Let's see . . . It's a side sound because it's made with the air coming over the sides of the tongue, its's a long sound because you can make it last a long time . . . What do you think we should call it?

CHILD: Wong wion sound.

CLINICIAN: Long lion sound? I like that. Ok. The long lion sound it is. I'm going to say two words. You raise your hand when I say the word that begins with the long lion sound. Lip. Sun.

> *The addition of a deletion (see Chapter 18, "Talking with Children") offers an easy means to strengthen the lesson.*

CLINICIAN: Now I'm going to say a word that begins with our long lion sound. Sometimes I'm going to say the word with our long lion sound and sometimes without it. You raise your hand when I say it with our treatment sound. The word is *low*. Ready? O.

Child frowns, keeps hand down.

CLINICIAN: Low.

Child raises hand.

Touch Cues

Touch cues (also called **tactile cues** or **visual phonics**) use sight or touch to draw a child's attention to treatment sounds (typically, their place of production). For example, a clinician and child might touch the lips for bilabial oral stops, touch above the upper lip for alveolar stops, and touch under the back of the chin for velar stops.

Purpose

The clever clinical trick of touch cues is to make the treatment sound a multimodal experience, coming to a child through the ear, eye, and touch. Possible touch cues for consonants and voicing appear in Table 19–4.

Who May Benefit

Designed originally for children with oral-motor challenges, touch cues now enjoy wide clinical use. Most children 3 years and older benefit from touch cues. As with metaphors, even toddlers may respond well to them, perhaps because touch cues serve as prompts to produce a sound in a way that the clinician praises.

TABLE 19–4. Examples of Possible Touch Cues for Consonants and Voicing

Sound Class	Sound	Touch Cue
Nasals	[m]	Fingers and thumb hold lips together
	[n]	Lay finger over front of cheek bone
	[ŋ]	Lay finger on back of check bone
Oral Stops	[p] [b]	Lay finger in front of lips
	[t] [d]	Lay finger above top lip
	[k] [g]	Lay finger at uppermost part of neck
Fricatives	[f] [v]	Lay finger below bottom lip
	[θ] [ð]	Place finger horizontally in front of lips
	[s] [z]	Point to the corner of the mouth (to indicate spread) and remind child of the teeth being together
	[ʃ]	Lay finger in front of lips as if saying shhh
Liquid	[l]	Lay tip of finger on middle of upper lip
	[r]	Lay thumb and index finger on cheek, pull away like twirling hair
Voiced		First and second finger together or ask child to feel vibration on neck
Voiceless		First and second finger apart

Annotated Dialogue

Touch cues work best paired with other ways of talking about speech, especially metaphors.

> *This brief dialogue adds a touch cue to the "long lion sound" from the previous dialogue.*

CLINICIAN: You know what might help us to say words that have our long lion sound?

Clinician lays tip of finger on the middle of the clinician's upper lip.

CLINICIAN: Now you do it.

Child lays tip of finger on the middle of their upper lip.

Descriptions and Demonstrations

Descriptions and **demonstrations** provide another way to heighten a child's speech awareness, either with or without production demands. A possible description of [p], for example, may draw the child's attention to the closing lips, the build-up of air behind the lips, and the sudden release of air. A demonstration accompanying the description might involve placing a piece of paper in front of the child's lips to show the sudden release of air or gently pressing the child's lips together to show lip closure.

Purpose

Descriptions and demonstrations provide a lesson on how to say a treatment sound. Occasionally, a description or demonstration successfully converts a nonstimulable sound into a stimulable one, removing the need to perform phonetic placement and shaping. Treatment Resources on the companion website contain bare bones descriptions and demonstrations for voicing and all the English consonants.

Who May Benefit

Consider this form of talking about speech for

- Students and second language learners
- Grade school students in conjunction with metaphors and touch cues
- Late preschooler with intact attention and cognitive skills

Suggestion

If in doubt about whether a child is ready for this type of speech talk, a dynamic assessment can determine how a preschooler or student responds to this technique (see Chapter 21, "The Daily Researcher").

First Annotated Dialogue

Here are three options for descriptions and demonstrations of voicing from the Treatment Resources on the companion website, followed by an annotated dialogue.

Voicing Options

1. Instruct the child to listen to and identify the difference between a voiceless and voiced [ɑ].
2. Place the child's hands over his/her ears and instruct the child to hum, which heightens the sensation of vocal cord vibration.
3. If the child can produce a voiced and voiceless fricative, ask the child to cover their ears and make these sounds. Alternatively, ask the child to make [h] and [ɑ].

Annotated Dialogue

The child is a late preschooler whose treatment sound is [s] and who pronounces voiceless fricatives as voiced fricatives in the beginning of words.

CLINICIAN: Remember what we call sounds like [s]?

CHILD: Hissing sounds.

Hissing is the metaphor for [s] to help focus the child on the treatment sound.

CLINICIAN: And what do we call sounds like [z]?

CHILD: Buzzing sounds.

Buzzing sound is the metaphor for [z].

CLINICIAN: Right. [z] is a buzzing sound. I'm going to say some words that rhyme—clap your hands one time when you hear a word that starts with a hissing sound, and clap your hands two times when you hear a word that starts with [z], our buzzing sound.

Minimal pairs help focus the child.

CLINICIAN: See, zee. zoo, Sue. zap, sap.

The child claps.

CLINICIAN: Excellent. Now, first, we're going to cover our ears, and then, we're going to say a long [s]. Cover your ears and we'll both say a long [s].

Now that the child is focused, the clinician demonstrates the voicing contrast by placing the hands over the ears and humming, which heightens the sensation of vocal cord vibration.

CHILD AND CLINICIAN: sssssssss.

CLINICIAN: Now, with our hands over our ears, let's both say a long [z], a buzzing sound.

CHILD AND CLINICIAN: ZZZZZZZZ.

CLINICIAN: Hear the difference bertween sssss and zzzz? [s] is kind of a hiss, and [z] is more like a buzzing bee sound. Let's say both sounds with our hands over our ears, first [s], then [z]. Let's do it three times.

CHILD AND CLINICIAN: sss zzz sss zzz sss zzz.

The repetitions solidify the lesson.

CLINICIAN: Hear the difference?

Child nods.

CLINICIAN: Now let's practice saying *see, zee. zoo, Sue. zap, sap*, remembering to say [s] as a hissing sound and [z] as a buzzing sound.

The lesson shifts to speech practice.

Second Annotated Dialogue

Here is a demonstration of tongue placement from the Treatment Resources on the companion website, followed by an annotated dialogue.

Tongue Placement

Description. Draw attention to the hissing sound and the position of the tongue tip (behind the front upper or lower teeth).

Demonstrations: Place (Alveolar)

First method: Ask the child to feel the bump on the roof of his or her mouth just behind the two front teeth.

Second method: Place a little peanut butter or a favored food on a Q-tip, touch the Q-tip to the alveolar ridge, and ask the child to remove the food with the tongue tip.

Annotated Dialogue

This grade school student pronounces [s] as [θ]. The clinician determined previously that the student found [s] easier to make with the tongue tip raised.

CLINICIAN: Remember what we call the sound we're working on?

STUDENT: The hissy sound.

The metaphor reminds the student [s] has a hissing quality.

CLINICIAN: And what's the sound made with the tongue between the teeth?

STUDENT: The leaking tire sound.

The leaking tire sound is the metaphor for [θ], the sound the student makes in place of [s]. The clinician is contrasting the treatment sound with the error.

CLINICIAN: Right. Now, I'm going to say some words and you raise your right hand when you hear the cage sound and raise your left hand when you hear the leaking tire sound. Some of these may be made up words. Sun, [θ]un. Thick, sick. Think, sink. See, [θi].

The cage sound is the metaphor for [s] (the cage is the front teeth) and the leaking tire sound is metaphor for [θ]. The minimal pairs activity contrasts the treatment sound with the error.

CLINICIAN: Here, I brought a mirror to help us today. Please look in the mirror and stick your tongue out for a leaking tire sound.

The student looks in the mirror and sticks out his tongue.

CLINICIAN: Your front teeth are like a cage for your tongue. For the hissy sound, we want the tongue behind the cage. Can you put your tongue behind the cage?

The student follows the description and draws the tongue tip behind the front teeth.

CLINICIAN: Remember where we put the peanut butter on that bump last time? Raise your tongue tip up just a little bit to that spot.

The final description places the tongue tip at the alveolar ridge.

Higher Technology Options

Electropalatography, spectrography, Visi-Pitch, and ultrasound offer exciting advances in how you can help a child to see and place the articulators. Williams (2010) contains an excellent chapter on electropalatography (Gibbon & Wood, 2010) and another fine chapter on ultrasound (Bernhardt, Stemberger, & Bacffalvi, 2010).

Electropalatography

Electropalatography (EPG) measures contact between the tongue and roof of the mouth and is useful for describing and demonstrating sounds made with extensive closure in the mid region of the mouth, including such sometimes challenging sounds as [r], [s], [ʃ], and [ʧ]. Hitchcock, Byun, and Lazarus (2017) describe how EPG can successfully treat misarticulation of [r] in grade school students with age-appropriate language and hearing.

CLINIC BOX: What about Computer Applications?

Anyone reading this who is under 30 years old probably knows far more about computer apps than I do, which is why they are not discussed here.

Spectography and Visi-Pitch

Spectography displays speech in terms of frequency, amplitude, and time, and is potentially useful with all sound classes. **Visi-Pitch** displays intonation and prosody.

Ultrasound

With **ultrasound**, a hand-held transducer held at the mouth allows tongue position and movements to be displayed on a screen, which provides valuable feedback about sound errors affecting sounds in which articulators do not come in contact, including glides, liquids, and vowels. Researchers have used biofeedback through ultrasound to successfully treat children with childhood apraxia and students with speech errors affecting late acquired sound (Byun & Hitchcock, 2012; Preston, Leece, McNamara, & Maas, 2017).

Phonetic Placement and Shaping

Phonetic placement teaches articulatory postures (typically, tongue, jaw, and lip positions) for speech production. A phonetic placement technique to teach [t], for example, may ask a student to raise the tongue tip, touch the tongue tip to the alveolar ridge, and then quickly draw the tongue tip down again. **Shaping** uses a sound a student already produces (either a speech error or another sound) to learn a new sound. A shaping technique, for example, may provide a series of steps through which a student who says [w] learns to say [r]. Phonetic placement and shaping were a clinician's stock-and-trade throughout much of the 20th century (Fairbanks, 1960; Nemoy & Davis, 1954), though their use declined as clinical populations shifted downward in age and increased in severity (Bleile, 2017).

Purpose

Think of phonetic placement and shaping as multipurpose tools. Their primary function is to transform a nonstimulable sound into a stimulable one. After that, treatment proceeds as for a stimulable sound. Their related function is to increase awareness of speech, acting in much the same way as their close cousins, descriptions and demonstrations. The same higher technology options for those methods can also assist in phonetic placement and shaping. Treatment Resources on the companion website contains, I believe, the largest collection of phonetic placement and shaping techniques, listing over 100 different methods.

Who May Benefit

Phonetic placement and shaping often proves effective with grade school through high school students, and with selected late preschoolers. They also may assist adults learning English as a second language (Müller, Guendouzi, & Ball, 2000).

Suggestion

Dynamic assessment offers the most reliable method to determine if an individual child or student is a candidate for these methods (see Chapter 21, "The Daily Researcher").

CLINIC BOX: Pumping Iron

Phonetic placement and shaping is sometimes confused with nonspeech exercises. Phonetic placement and shaping rely on phonetic knowledge to convert a nonstimulable sound into a stimulable one. Stated simply: the techniques place and shape the articulators for speech. Nonspeech exercises seek to improve speech through building the strength and flexibility of the speech musculature—for example, blowing bubbles through a straw, touching the nose with the tongue, or filling the cheeks with air. Researchers have observed three problems with using nonspeech exercises to improve speech: (1) speech uses oral structures differently than nonspeech exercises; (2) the strength requirements for speech differ from those for nonspeech exercises; and (3) speech uses different brain areas than nonspeech exercises (Chapter 3, "Speech Production" (Bohnenkamp); Clark, 2003; Lass & Pannbacker, 2008; Lof, 2009; McCauley, Strand, Lof, Schooling, & Frymark, 2009; Muttiah, Georges, & Brackenbury, 2011; Powell, 2009; Ruscello, 2008). Stated simply: building muscles and flexibility through nonspeech exercises probably is not a reasonable way to improve speech.

Annotated Dialogue

The following section provides a phonetic placement and shaping technique for [s] from the Treatment Resources on the companion website, followed by an annotated dialogue.

Phonetic Placement and Shaping of [s]

Phonetic Placement

1. Place a tongue depressor just behind the student's upper or lower front teeth and ask the student to use his or her tongue tip to hold it there.
2. Next, ask the student to keep his or her tongue still while the clinician carefully removes the tongue depressor.
3. Ask the student to breathe out, resulting in [s].

Shaping: [θ] to [s] Lisping

1. Instruct the student to protrude his or her tongue between the teeth and to say [θ].
2. As student says [θ], instruct him or her to bring the tongue back into the mouth and behind the upper or lower front teeth, depending on which variety of [s] you facilitate. An alternate method is to ask the student to scrape his or her tongue tip

back along the back of the front teeth. (If needed, push the tip of the student's tongue inward with a tongue depressor.)

3. Next, ask the student to either raise or lower the tongue tip slightly, depending on which type of [s] you are teaching.
4. Ask the student to blow air through the mouth, which typically results in [s].

Annotated Dialogue

This is same grade school student in the dialogue for descriptions and demonstrations. The dialogue occurs in the middle of the session following the description of [s].

CLINICIAN: Let's work some more on the hissy sound.

The student, who just came in from recess, looks out the window.

CLINICIAN: Can you think of a few words that begin with our sound?

STUDENT: Um, sing.

CLINICIAN: That's right. And, remember, when we take the hissy sound away from sing, what is left?

STUDENT: ing.

CLINICIAN: And when we bring it back?

STUDENT: sing.

Deletion focuses the student.

CLINICIAN: Let's look in the mirror. Put your tongue between your teeth like you're going to say the first sound in *thin*. Now, pretend there is a string at the back of your head that I'm going to pull on to bring your tongue back.

The clinician pretends to pull string back and the student pulls the tongue back behind the front teeth. This is shaping.

CLINICIAN: I brought some suckers. We're going to practice saying the hissy sound with a sucker stick to help us keep the tongue from touching the back of the teeth. Do you get to eat the sucker at the end of therapy today? Absolutely.

Student smiles. They carefully place the sucker stick in place, gently remove it, and breathe out.

STUDENT: sssss.

Then he eats the sucker. This is phonetic placement.

> **CLINIC BOX: Summing it Up: Clever Ways**
>
> Our clinical work often has us talking about speech, typically as a step to producing treatment sounds. The challenge is to reduce the complexities of speech to an explanation that a child or student can understand. Fortunately, our profession has clever ways to do this. Some methods (metaphors and touch cues) a child grasps easily, while others (descriptions and demonstrations) require more self-reflection and focus, and still others (phonetic placement and shaping) require a child to possess perseverance and well-developed attention skills. All these ways of talking about speech, simple or complex, alone or in conjunction, have their place in the clinical repertoire, and all are tools that a clinician uses daily.

Conclusions

Major ideas discussed in this chapter include

1. Clinical work often requires us to talk to children about speech.
2. Metaphors, touch cues, descriptions and demonstrations, and phonetic placement and shaping all are useful tools to talk about speech.
3. New, higher technology options exist for descriptions and demonstrations.
4. The primary clinical purpose of phonetic placement and shaping is to convert a nonstimulable sound into a stimulable sound.

Review Questions

1. What is the clinical purpose of metaphors?
2. What is the age range of children most likely to benefit from metaphors?
3. What do touch cues attempt to do for a child?
4. Why might children under 3 years of age benefit from touch cues?
5. What is the clinical purpose of descriptions and demonstrations?
6. For which ages are descriptions and demonstrations most useful?
7. What does electropalatography (EPG) measure?
8. How does phonetic placement differ from shaping?
9. What is the primary purpose of phonetic placement and shaping? What is a secondary purpose?

References

Bernhardt, B., Stemberger, J., & Bacsfalvi, P. (2010). Vowel intervention. In L. Williams, S. McLeod, & R. McCauley (Eds.), *Interventions for speech sound disorders in children* (pp. 537–556). Baltimore, MD: Brookes.

Bleile, K. (2017). *The late eight* (3rd ed.). San Diego, CA: Plural.

Blodgett, E., & Miller, V. (1989). *Easy does it for phonology*. East Moline, IL: LinguiSystems.

Byun, T., & Hitchcock, E. (2012). Investigating the use of traditional and spectral biofeedback approaches to intervention for /r/ misarticulation. *American Journal of Speech-Language Pathology*, *21*, 207–221.

Clark, H. M. (2003). Neuromuscular treatments for speech and swallowing: A tutorial. *American Journal of Speech-Language Pathology*, *12*, 400–415.

Dean, E., Howell, J., Hill, A., & Waters, D. (1990). *Metaphon resource pack*. Windsor, UK: NFER-Nelson.

Fairbanks, G. (1960). *Voice and articulation drill book*. New York, NY: Harper & Row.

Flowers, A. (1990). *The big book of sounds*. Austin, TX: Pro-Ed.

Gibbon, F., & Wood, S. (2010). Visual feedback therapy with electropalatography. In L. Williams, S. McLeod, & R. McCauley (Eds.), *Interventions for speech sound disorders in children* (pp. 509–536). Baltimore, MD: Brookes.

Hitchcock, E. R., Byun, T. M., Swartz, M., & Lazarus, R. (2017). Efficacy of Electropalatography for Treating Misarticulation of/r. *American Journal of Speech-Language Pathology*, *26*(4), 1141-1158.

Lass, N., & Pannbacker, M. (2008). The application of evidence-based practice to nonspeech oral motor treatments. *Language, Speech, and Hearing Services in the Schools*, *39*, 408–421.

Lof, G. L. (2009). The nonspeech-oral motor exercise phenomenon in speech pathology practice. In C. Bowen (Ed.), *Children's speech sound disorders* (pp. 181–184). Oxford, UK: Wiley-Blackwell.

McCauley, R. J., Strand, E., Lof, G. L., Schooling, T., & Frymark, T. (2009). Evidence-based systematic review: Effects of nonspeech oral motor exercises on speech. *American Journal of Speech-Language Pathology*, *18*, 343–360.

Müller, N., Guendouzi, J., & Ball, M. J. (2000). Accent modification, pronunciation training, communication enhancement: The need for definitions, delimitations, and research. *Advances in Speech-Language Pathology*, *2*, 151–154.

Muttiah, N., Georges, K., & Brackenbury, T. (2011). Clinical and research perspectives on nonspeech oral motor treatments and evidence-based practice. *American Journal of Speech Language Pathology*, *20*(1), 47–59.

Nemoy, E., & Davis, S. (1954). *The correction of defective consonant sounds*. Magnolia, MA: Expression.

Powell, T. W. (2009). Non-speech oral motor exercises: An ethical challenge. In C. Bowen (Ed.), *Children's speech sound disorders* (pp. 199–202). Oxford, UK: Wiley-Blackwell.

Preston, J., Leece, M., McNamara, K., & Maas, E. (2017). Variable practice to enhance speech learning in ultrasound biofeedback treatment for childhood apraxia of speech: A single case experimental study. *American Journal of Speech-Language Pathology*, *26*, 840–852.

Ruscello, D. M. (2008). Nonspeech oral motor treatment issues in children with developmental speech sound disorders. *Language, Speech, and Hearing Services in Schools*, *39*, 380–391.

Williams, A. L. (2010). Multiple oppositions intervention. In L. Williams, S. McLeod, & R. McCauley (Eds.), *Interventions for speech sound disorders in children* (pp. 73–94). Baltimore, MD: Brookes.

CHAPTER 20

SUPPORTING COMMUNICATION

Evette Edmister

If you are reading this book, you most likely have a passion to support someone who has difficulty expressing themselves with natural speech. You already know that there are times when this person has much to say, but communication partners struggle to understand their messages. For some children, this breakdown in communication may occur for only a few words during a long conversation, and for others, a larger portion of what they try to express may be left unresolved.

One way for you to assist someone who has difficulty expressing themselves with speech is to focus on ways to improve their sound production. This book provides a resource for such strategies. The present chapter discusses an additional consideration: augmentative and alternative communication (AAC) to provide support for a child with significant speech difficulties. The intended audience for this chapter is a preservice student or clinician providing speech intervention for a child with AAC or struggling to make themselves understood. Topics include:

- What Is AAC?
- Benefits of AAC
- Treatment Strategies

Learning Objectives

I hope on completing the chapter you will

- Define augmentative and alternative communication (AAC).
- Describe what research says about AAC and speech development.
- Describe how AAC can assist language development.
- Define strategies to support the use of AAC.

Key Words

Key words you will encounter in this chapter

Augmentative and alternative communication (AAC)
Unaided (unaided symbols)
Aided (aided symbols)
AAC device
AAC system
Feature matching
Remnant book
Aided input
Wait time

What Is AAC?

AAC stands for **augmentative and alternative communication (AAC)**. AAC is described as any form of communication a person uses to supplement or replace natural speech either permanently or temporarily (ASHA, 2018a). As the definition suggests, for some children, AAC use is short term. For others, AAC use is more consistent. The use may be more compartmentalized with heavier use in certain settings and less use in others, or used steadily across a person's day and throughout his/her life.

Aided and Unaided AAC

You are so familiar with some forms of AAC that you may be surprised to find out they actually are AAC and that you use them from time to time throughout your day. Daily forms of AAC can include gestures, facial expressions, and vocalizations (e.g., ahhh). You create these forms of AAC with your own body; their formal name is **unaided** forms of AAC (Beukelman & Miranda, 2013). Unaided forms of AAC include symbols (called **unaided symbols**) that represent words and ideas (Beukelman & Miranda, 2013). For example, imagine a person waving at a familiar person walking down the street. The wave is an unaided form of AAC you create with your body that represents (symbolizes) a greeting, hello.

Aided forms of AAC require an additional tool to relay a message (Beukelman & Miranda, 2013). For example, a computer that can speak a novel message out loud is a form of aided AAC. Aided forms of AAC have **aided symbols** that represent words or ideas (Beukelman & Miranda, 2013). To illustrate this, consider a tablet and an app with a library of pictures somewhat similar to emojis. The tablet could be an aided form of AAC (or device), and the pictures such as a smiley face representing the feeling of like or happy would be aided symbols.

Devices and Systems

It is important to distinguish between the terms **AAC device** and **AAC system**. An AAC device (an aid) is the physical something the individual uses to assist their communication (United States Society of Augmentative and Alternative Communication [USSAAC], 2018). In contrast, an AAC system is everything that person uses to communicate, including the AAC device (ASHA, 2018b). For instance, an AAC system would include unaided symbols like speech, speech approximations, vocalizations, facial expressions, gestures, and so forth, as well as the AAC device(s) with aided symbols like line-drawn pictures and photos.

Technology Level

The types of AAC devices available range from low tech to high tech (ASHA, 2018b; USSAAC, 2018).

Low Tech

As the name implies, low-tech AAC requires no external source of power. Examples of low-tech AAC include objects (i.e., cup, book, etc.), a piece of paper with the alphabet on it, a page of paper with line-drawn pictures set in rows and columns, a page with photos representing language rich events (i.e., from a birthday party), a book containing many pages of pictures forming a communication book, or any combination of these choices.

High Tech

High-tech devices include items like computers, tablets, and iPads. They are usually devices that use batteries or are plugged in to be recharged. They frequently have touch screens as well as additional options for access like eye gaze or switches that can be used when it is not possible for the individual to touch the screen directly. Often, high-tech devices have commercially available premade sets of vocabulary that contain hundreds of pages of possible vocabulary to get started with and customize to meet the individual's preferences and needs. The additional pages are all accessible from one master page with the selection of a button.

Voice output from the device is also an option. The voice output may use computer-generated voices, recordings of natural speech, or computer-generated voices developed from samples of natural speech (a technique called voice banking). There are a range of computer-generated voices available that vary in pitch (representing child, adult, male, or female) and accents for numerous languages. The natural speech may be recorded by another child of similar age and pitch of the individual using AAC. Voice banking as well as recordings of one's own messages (called message banking) can be used when someone is losing or will lose their natural speech (Costello, 2016).

CLINIC BOX: What's in a Name?

Some variance exists regarding "tech" names and groupings of AAC devices. For example, "mid tech" is sometimes found on websites or in descriptions of AAC to describe AAC devices that need batteries (generally alkaline) and allow for the programming of one, two, or multiple messages (possibly as many as in the 30s) (Desch, Gaebler-Spira & the Council on Children with Disabilities, 2008). Programming for mid-tech devices usually includes recordings of natural speech. The clinician typically prints the symbols from the computer and cuts them to fit the surface of the device or inserts them just below a protective surface. In other instances, mid tech is absorbed into the high-tech category, making two groups: low tech without batteries and high tech with batteries (ASHA, 2018b; USSAAC, 2018). Adding to the number of terms, sometimes an author may use "light tech" in place of "low tech" (Gulens & AAC Mentor Project Team, 2000). Lastly, no tech may be used to refer to supports produced by one's own body like gestures (ASHA, 2018b). Being aware that there is some variance is helpful, as it will give you additional tools and knowledge when reviewing websites and literature or talking about technology with team members.

Feature Matching

The form of AAC the person uses is determined individually through matching the needs of the person with the features of the AAC system. This process is referred to as **feature matching** (Costello, Shane, & Crane, 2013). Clinicians have used this process for years and have found it an effective means of selecting AAC (Clarke, 2016; Costello, Shane, & Crane, 2013). Analyzing the tasks or events the person completes during the day is an important part of the process as this is where one can see where the individual is using natural speech to effectively convey a message, and where support might be beneficial (e.g., pointing to pictures along with speech attempts) to share their message (Soto, 2009). Tools exist that can assist teams in the feature matching process. For example, the Student, Environments, Tasks, and Tools (SETT) framework (Zabala, 2005) can assist a team's ability to identify the needs of the child, systematically review possible technology relevant to that individual's needs, and navigate the decision-making process, especially when considering when and for what tasks to use AAC.

CLINIC BOX: Where Can I Look for More Help?

This chapter is meant to be an introduction to AAC. For additional supports and resources, see

- The American Speech-Language-Hearing Association (ASHA) hosts a variety of informational web-based AAC resources for professionals and families.
- The International Society of Augmentative and Alternative Communication (ISAAC) provides definitions, information, and a professional journal dedicated to AAC topics available via a website with links to affiliate chapter organizations by country. The United States chapter offers webinars throughout the year.
- The Rehabilitation Engineering Research Center on Augmentative and Alternative Communication (RERC-AAC) provides a range information online about research including, but not limited to, information about current research, presentations, proceedings, and publications.

Benefits of AAC

Benefits of AAC include promoting language, reducing frustration and anxiety, and supporting speech.

Promoting Language

AAC promotes language development through increasing a child's ability to express himself/herself (ASHA, 2018b; Oommen & McCarthy, 2015). Expressive communication influences all facets of our everyday lives, such as developing relationships, advocating for ourselves or others, finding out information, understanding another's point of view, gaining access to academic curriculums, and developing job skills. AAC can keep these avenues of opportunity open to assist with language development when the student is not able to use their natural speech (Cress & Marvin, 2003; Romski, Sevick, Barton-Husley, & Whitmore, 2015).

To illustrate this process, imagine pairing AAC with words to assist in making longer utterances and expressing more sophisticated language skills (Binger & Light, 2007). For example, if a child is unable to verbally express two-word utterances, they may use the device to say one word to add to the one word they said verbally. Or to give another example, the child could use the device to express morphemes like "-ed" to mark regular past tense or "-s" to mark plural or possession, if they are not able to verbally articulate this linguistic information (Binger, Maguire-Marshall, & Kent-Walsh, 2011).

How Young Can You Go?

Studies have demonstrated that very young children can successfully learn from and benefit from AAC (Romski et al., 2015). Branson and Demchak (2009) completed a systematic review of studies that included children from 16 months to 36 months who had a variety of diagnoses that presented with a risk for communication difficulties. The review included 12 studies (seven with a total of 158 participants that showed "conclusive evidence"). The findings indicated that after intervention, young children not only exhibited the ability to learn to use an AAC system at such a young age, but they also increased their expressive communication (language) skills.

CLINIC BOX: A Window into Language Development

When a child you are supporting is having trouble producing speech it can be difficult to determine their current language skills from their verbal output alone. In addition to assisting with expressive and receptive language development, AAC can also provide a window into expressive language skills not verbalized (Cress & Marvin, 2003; Romski et al., 2015). For example, when a child independently selects a symbol that represents the desired word, they are also showing some of their knowledge about their expressive and receptive language abilities. That is, they may be expressing their understanding of how and when to use that word or string of words to convey a message. To give another illustration, if the child says "me" and points to the symbol of a "cookie" to combine the two to indicate the desire for a cookie, the child has expressed the pragmatic functions of both requesting and expressed the semantic functions of existence and state of being. With speech alone, we would have missed this linguistic information the device brought to the interaction by adding a second word.

Reducing Frustration and Anxiety

AAC may reduce frustration and anxiety in a child who struggles with expressive communication skills (Baumann Leech & Cress, 2011). Imagine or remember the last time you were trying to express a word that didn't come out correctly. Have you had that experience—had a word you couldn't say? Have you had a time you needed to communicate but no one understood you? Perhaps you were in a foreign country where you did not speak the language. Now imagine a message tied to a time demand like finding out what time the next bus is coming, having an idea it is very soon. Perhaps you can put yourself in that situation to experience some of the frustration and anxiety the child may feel. Now imagine this happens regularly. You may become anxious entering similar scenarios with a fear of "here we go again." You may say, "I wonder if they will understand me?" In all these situations, having another alternative to assist your communication could be helpful.

A benefit of AAC is that it can reduce frustration (Baumann Leech & Cress, 2011). If the person is not understood, AAC tools can add cues or the words to assist in successfully relaying the message. AAC may also relieve some of the anxiety that may be present when initiating speech after previous unsuccessful attempts. If a child knows that a symbol is present to assist in conveying the message or repairing communication breakdowns, the stress of speaking may be reduced (Binger & Light, 2007, Cumley & Swanson, 1999; Oommen & McCarthy, 2015). For some, reduced anxiety fosters more willingness to practice speech (Oommen & McCarthy, 2015).

Supporting Speech

Clinically, the choice is not between AAC and speech. AAC assists with conveying a message and does not interfere with speech therapy. Nor is AAC just for someone with no speech. A child can use AAC while they work on their speech production and a child's natural speech can be incorporated into the AAC system (ASHA, 2018b). To illustrate, using input from a child and family as well as other team members that support the individual throughout the day, you could develop an AAC system that supports a child who struggles with speech intelligibility (ASHA, 2008; Cress & Marvin, 2003; Individuals with Disabilities Education Improvement Act, 2004; Romski et al., 2015).

Are You Giving Up on Speech?

One of the most common questions I hear from families regarding AAC is, will the child lose speech or not produce as much speech if they use AAC? This question is understandable, especially if a child's communication difficulty focuses on speech. The use of AAC has not been found to reduce speech production (Baumann Leech & Cress 2011; King, Hengst, & DeThrone, 2013; Millar, Light, & Schlosser 2006; Oommen & McCarthy, 2015; Romski et al., 2010; Schlosser & Wendt, 2008). Systematic reviews and individual studies with dates spanning from 1975 to 2013 have examined the question of the influence of AAC on speech development. The findings indicate (1) that speech did not decrease when AAC is part of the intervention, and (2) some children who use AAC improve in speech (Millar et al., 2006; Schlosser & Wendt 2008).

Systematic Reviews. Schlosser and Wendt (2008) completed a systematic review of studies published from 1975 to 2007 investigating interventions with a focus on natural speech production along with AAC intervention. The studies selected by Schlosser and Wendt (2008) focused on individuals who had a diagnosis of autism or pervasive developmental disorder. Results indicated that speech production was not observed to decrease when interventions included AAC. Instead, some individuals (though not all) exhibited an increase in their speech production. Millar, Light, and Schlosser (2006) also completed a systematic review, focusing on individuals with intellectual disabilities or a diagnosis of autism. As with Schlosser and Wendt (2008), most children exhibited gains in speech production; no child exhibited a decrease in his/her speech production.

Individual Studies. King, Hengst, and DeThrone (2013) investigated the use of AAC for three individuals with significant speech delays and a diagnosis of childhood apraxia of speech. All three exhibited an increase in the quantity of speech production in single words and in connected conversation while also using AAC. Baumann Leech and Cress (2011) indirectly investigated speech production while using AAC in a single participant design to teach words used during natural play. All the children increased their speech production. Lastly, Romski et al. (2010) focused their research on 62 children with a speech and language delay. Results indicated that children who used AAC produced more speech than the randomly assigned speech intervention group.

CLINIC BOX: Planes, Cars, and Bicycles

Here is an analogy to show how AAC assists in communication: when we think of getting from one point to the next, we consider what is the most efficient means of transportation. Sometimes that is a plane, sometimes a car, sometimes a bike, sometimes our feet, and sometimes we use something that assists our movement like a cane, walker, or wheelchair. We choose a form of transportation because it is the most efficient one available. For example, I would not choose to take a plane, car, or bike to a neighbor's house that is just 100 feet from my own. Also, I, and most other people, won't walk from the southern portion of the United States to Canada.

The point is that, while one form of transportation may be way easier and more efficient in the moment, I do not give up using other forms of transportation. That is, I can both walk *and* take a plane sometimes, depending on which seems most appropriate. Similarly, a child may use AAC when it is more effective than their speech. If their speech is more effective, they will use that.

Treatment Strategies

There are two vantage points you should consider when approaching AAC strategies. One view is from the child's perspective to increase their success communicating. The second view is from that of the communication partner to create an environment tailored to encourage the child's successful use of the tools. In this section, I will discuss AAC strategies from both viewpoints.

Child's Viewpoint

There are several ways for a child to use AAC to clarify what they are trying to say verbally. As mentioned earlier, feature matching is the technical name for the process of matching a form of AAC to a particular child (Costello, Shane, & Crane, 2013; Zabala, 2005). A range of AAC options are available from no tech to high tech, and there are clarifying strategies available to support speech across the AAC options. Some examples of strategies are as follows:

1. A child can use an unaided or no tech form of AAC by pairing a gesture with a verbal approximation and possibly a facial expression to clarify a word or phrase not understood. When you have identified the target word or phrase, implement other strategies to assist in shaping the verbal speech.
2. Develop a record in a diary or dictionary documenting what each gesture means (Hunt Berg & Loncke, 2000). This is especially useful if some of the child's gestures are not conventional and may be hard to recognize by less familiar communication partners in the community (Beukelman & Mirenda, 2013).
3. If gestures and vocalizations are not enough for a communication partner to determine a child's message, line-drawn pictures or photos may support emerging language skills, providing an opportunity where the child can independently select a picture or photo that represents the word they are trying to say. This can be completed with low- or high-tech devices.
4. **Remnant books** (a scrapbook containing mementos from previous events) are another option to help a child establish a topic of conversation or clarify a word (Cumley & Swanson, 1999). You can represent past events with objects like a movie stub, wedding invitation, business card, portion of a to-go menu, or photo(s) of the event. To illustrate, the child points to the movie stub when talking about a movie they saw.
5. You might also consider selecting the topic/category to which the word belongs. For example, an individual with literacy skills could select a letter to represent the first letter of the word they are trying to say. This works because, when the communication partner knows the letter cue or topic context, they often are better able to guess or understand the verbal attempt (Hanson, 2014; Hanson, Yorkston, Beukelman, 2004).

Communication Partner's Viewpoint

It is rare that simply placing a device in front of a child results in the child knowing exactly how to use it to express themselves, especially if symbols are to assist in their speech and language development. For the child to benefit from AAC, you will need time for the child to become familiar with the AAC system, learn how to independently use the system in conversations, and understand the symbols housed in the device.

While teaching could include some direct instruction of device operation or of symbol meaning, it is important to include learning experiences during naturally-occurring meaningful interactions with others. Useful natural learning strategies include *modeling* the use of the device, providing *wait time* for a child to match symbols to their message on their own, *creating communication opportunities*, and offering *gentle feedback* to help a child when a listener does not understand them.

Modeling

When modeling AAC, an important strategy, you use the device while talking to the child (Binger & Light, 2007; Blackstone, 2006). One technical name for this is aided language stimulation (Goossens, Elder, & Crain, 1992). A more general term for modeling is **aided input** or aided language input. Modeling serves the purpose of showing how to use symbols to express oneself in a natural context. You can use it to demonstrate the location of vocabulary and to give opportunities to learn what additional vocabulary to add, because if you can't say it, neither can they. Modeling can also serve as a multimodal way to support teaching language structures, such as putting two words together (Binger & Light, 2007) or teaching how to add "-ed" when using regular forms of past tense (Binger et al., 2011).

You may find modeling challenging if a child does not need to use AAC all the time; because they can use their natural speech, they may only use the device when they run across things they can't say verbally. The challenge arises because in this situation communication partners sometimes feel less motivated to model if the child is not using the device. However, if modeling stops, the child is at risk for not learning how to find the words they need. During such times, you may need to remind conversation partners of the future benefits of modeling. The symbols may also provide the added receptive input to support what is being said by the adult.

Wait Time

Another important strategy for success is **"wait time"** (Light & Drager, 2012; Mathis, Sutherland, & McAuliffe, 2011). Remember, it can take time for a child learning language to process both what you say and what they wish to contribute to the conversation. Additionally, a child using AAC may need to consider what words to say verbally, how to orally create the words, synonyms that might be easier to say if they can't say that word, and/or where those symbols might be in their AAC system. All this takes time, so pausing after a question or comment creates more opportunity for thinking, composing a message, and contributing.

Creating Communication Opportunities

Creating opportunities for participation in the conversation is another important AAC strategy (Light & Drager, 2012). For example, if the communication partner provides a long string of communication (think lecture or monologue) without providing pauses for the child to contribute, the child will not have many opportunities to practice. Your clinical strategy should include setting up opportunities to encourage a range of language structures. To illustrate the need for this strategy, imagine a communication partner who only asks yes/no questions. The expected response of the child will be limited to yes/no answers. On the other hand, if a communication partner balances their comments and questions, tries to use open-ended questions, and provides wait time for an answer or comment, the child will have an opportunity for a wider range of possible words and increased number of language structures.

Gentle Feedback

Sometimes a child may not realize his/her speech is unintelligible, which can result in the child not attempting to repair communication breakdowns. In this situation, it is important for the communication partner to let the child know when they understand and (gently) when they do not understand the child. A clinician's responsibilities may include helping the child develop a plan to recognize when problems in understanding arise and how to clarify the message (Garcia, 2012).

The plan for repairing communication breakdowns in an individualized plan toward independence may or may not include AAC. For example, you as the communication partner can signal a misunderstanding either indirectly through a facial expression indicating confusion and simply saying "what?" or directly through saying something like, "I didn't understand. What is the first step in your communication repair plan you want to try?" You can provide instruction teaching the child to identify the signal and then to follow the next step in the plan, which could be just to repeat the attempt or to point to a symbol. Individual differences for each person requires a case-by-case decision on what works best for that person (Oommen & McCarthy, 2015).

Conclusions

These are major points in this chapter

1. AAC is any form of communication a person uses to supplement or replace natural speech either permanently or temporarily.
2. AAC supports language development and may reduce a child's frustrations and communication anxieties.
3. Research indicates that a child's use of AAC does not interfere with their speech development.
4. Easy to implement treatment strategies exist to foster a child's use of AAC.

Review Questions

1. What does the acronym AAC stand for and what does it mean?
2. What is a way you can determine what the child is trying to say when they are verbally unintelligible?
3. What can you as a communication partner do to support AAC use?
4. What is aided input?
5. What is the difference between an AAC system and AAC device?
6. Why is feature matching important?
7.. How can you monitor language development when speech is unintelligible?
8.. What would you say to a parent or colleague concerned about speech development and introduction to AAC?

References

American Speech-Language-Hearing Association (ASHA). (2008). *Roles and responsibilities of speech-language pathologists in early intervention: Guidelines*. Retrieved from http://www.asha.org/policy

American Speech-Language-Hearing Association (ASHA). (2018a). *Augmentative and alternative communication overview*. Retrieved from https://www.asha.org/PRPSpecificTopic.aspx?folderid=8589942773&section=Overview

American Speech-Language-Hearing Association (ASHA). (2018b). *Augmentative and alternative communication key issues*. Retrieved from https://www.asha.org/PRPSpecificTopic.aspx?folderid=8589942773&section=Key_Issues#AAC_Myths_and_Realities

Baumann Leech, E. R., & Cress, C. J. (2011). Indirect facilitation of speech in a late talking child by prompted production of picture symbols or signs. *Augmentative and Alternative Communication, 27*, 40–52. doi:10.3109/07434618.2010.550062

Binger, C., & Light, J. (2007). The effect of aided AAC modeling on the expression of multisymbol messages by preschoolers who use AAC. *Augmentative and Alternative Communication, 23*(1), 30–43.

Binger, C., Maguire-Marshall, M., & Kent-Walsh, J. (2011). Using aided AAC models, recasts, and contrastive targets to teach grammatical morphemes to children who use AAC. *Journal of Speech, Language, and Hearing Research, 54*, 160–176.

Beukelman, D., & Mirenda, P. (2013). Symbol and rate enhancement. In D. Beukelman & P. Mirenda (Eds.), *Augmentative and alternative communication: Supporting children and adults with complex communication needs* (4th ed.). Baltimore, MD: Brookes.

Blackstone, S. (2006). The role of modeling in AAC. *Augmentative Communication News, 18*(3), 3–4.

Branson, D., & Demchak, M. (2009). The use of augmentative and alternative communication methods with infants and toddlers with disabilities: A research review. *Augmentative and Alternative Communication, 25*(4), 274–286. doi:10.3109/07434610903384529

Clarke, V. (2016). *AAC assessment corner by Vicki Clarke: Is AAC feature matching still relevant?* Retrieved from http://praacticalaac.org/?s=feature+matching

Costello, J. M. (2016). *Message banking, voice banking and legacy messages*. Boston, MA: Boston Children's Hospital.

Costello, J. M., Shane, H. C., & Crane, J. (2013). *AAC, mobile devices and apps: Growing pains with evidence based practice*. Boston, MA: Boston Children's Hospital.

Cress, C. J., & Marvin, C. A. (2003). Common questions about AAC services in early intervention. *Augmentative and Alternative Communication, 19*(4), 254–272, doi:10.1080/0743461 0310001598242

Cumley, C., & Swanson, S. (1999). Augmentative and alternative communication options for children with developmental apraxia of speech: Three case studies. *Augmentative and Alternative Communication, 15*(2), 110–125. doi:10.1080/07434619912331278615

Desch, L. W., Gaebler-Spira, D., & The Council On Children With Disabilities. (2008). Prescribing assistive-technology systems: Focus on children with impaired communication. *Pediatrics, 121*(6), 1271–1280. doi:10.1542/peds.2008-0695

Garcia, A. (2012). *How we do it: Using AAC to repair communication breakdowns*. Retrieved from http://praacticalaac.org/praactical/how-we-do-it-using-aac-to-repair-communication-breakdowns/

Goossens, C., Elder, P., & Crain, S. (1992). *Engineering the preschool environment for interactive symbolic communication*. Birmingham, AL: Southeast Augmentative and Alternative Communication Conference Publications.

Gulens, M., & AAC Mentor Project Team (2000). *What is AAC?* University Park, PA: Penn State University. Retrieved from http://mcn.ed.psu.edu/~mentor/Public/aac.html

Hanson, E. K. (2014). My clients talk! Do I still need to consider AAC in my treatment planning? Speech supplementation strategies: AAC for clients who talk! *SIG 12 Perspectives on Augmentative and Alternative Communication, 23,* 124–131. doi:10.1044/aac23.3.124

Hanson, E. K., Yorkston, K. M., & Beukelman, D. R. (2004). Speech supplementation techniques for dysarthria: A systematic review. *Journal of Medical Speech-Language Pathology, 12*(2), ix–xxix.

Hunt Berg, M., & Loncke, F. (2000). Assessing gestures. *Augmentative Communication News, 13*(1&2).

Individuals with Disabilities Education Improvement Act of 2004, 20 U.S.C. §1400 et seq.

King, A. M., Hengst, J. A., & DeThrone, L. S. (2013). Severe speech sound disorders: An integrated multimodal intervention. *Language, Speech, and Hearing Services in the Schools, 44,* 195–210.

Light, J., & Drager, K. (2012). *Early intervention for young children with autism, cerebral palsy, Down syndrome, and other disabilities.* Retrieved from http://aackids.psu.edu/index.php/page/show/id/12/index.html

Mathis, H., Sutherland, D., & McAuliffe, M. (2011). The effect of pause time upon the communicative interactions of young people who use augmentative and alternative communication. *International Journal of Speech-Language Pathology, 13*(5), 411–421, doi:10.3109/17549507.2011.524709

Millar, D. C., Light, J. C., & Schlosser, R. W. (2006). The impact of augmentative and alternative communication intervention on the speech production of individuals with developmental disabilities: A research review. *Journal of Speech, Language, and Hearing Research, 49*(2), 248–264.

Oommen, E. R., & McCarthy, J. W. (2015). Simultaneous natural speech and AAC interventions for children with childhood apraxia speech: Lessons form a speech-language pathologist focus group. *Augmentative and Alternative Communication, 31*(1), 63–76. doi:10:3109/07434618.2014.1001520

Schlosser, R. W., & Wendt, O. (2008). Effects of augmentative and alternative communication intervention on speech production in children with autism: A systematic review. *American Journal of Speech-Language Pathology, 17,* 212–230. doi:1058-0360/08/1703-0212

Soto, G. (2009). Academic adaptations for students with AAC needs. In G. Soto & C. Zangari (Eds.), *Practically speaking language, literacy, and academic development for students with AAC needs.* Baltimore, MD: Brookes.

Romski, M., Sevcik, R. A., Adamson, L. B., Cheslock, M., Smith, A., Barker, R. M., & Bakeman, R. (2010). Randomized comparison of augmented and nonaugmented language interventions for toddlers with developmental delays and their parents. *Journal of Speech, Language, and Hearing Research, 53,* 350–365.

Romski, M., Sevick, R. A., Barton-Hulsey, A., & Whitmore, A. S. (2015). Early intervention and AAC: What a difference 30 years makes. *Augmentative and Alternative Communication, 31*(3), 181–202. doi:10.3109/07434618.2015.1064163

United States Society of Augmentative and Alternative Communication (USSAAC). (2018). *AAC devices.* Retrieved from http://www.ussaac.org/aac-devices

Zabala, J. (2005). *Using the SETT framework to level the learning field for students with disabilities.* Retrieved from http://www.joyzabala.com/

CHAPTER 21

THE DAILY RESEARCHER

A clinician is a daily researcher whose investigations answer such questions as: "What treatment approach should I take with this child?"; "How do I know what I am doing is helping?"; "How do I change what I'm doing if it is not working?" This chapter discusses three essential topics in everyday clinical research:

- Evaluating Treatment Approaches
- Assessing Treatment Progress
- Dynamic Assessment

Learning Objectives

I hope on completing the chapter you will

- Understand the purpose of evidence-based practice.
- Know the SIGN framework.
- Appreciate the difficulty of determining why a treatment approach succeeds.
- Understand the value of assessing treatment progress.
- Describe the importance of dynamic assessment.

Key Words

Key words you will encounter in this chapter

Evidence-based practice (EBP)
Scottish Intercollegiate Guidelines
    Network (SIGN)
Pre- and posttests
Ongoing information gathering
Consumer interview
Single-subject design experiment
Dynamic assessment

Evaluating Treatment Approaches

If your doctor recommends a procedure, you likely will ask what's involved—how it's performed, what is the recovery time, what are possible complications, and so forth. Your doctor expects those questions and they will likely give you answers even if you don't ask, because you have a right to know the research support for decisions that affect you.

Most clinicians recognize the importance of research support, both from their doctors and for themselves. As discussed in several places in this book, **evidence-based practice** (EBP) embodies the clinician's goal of providing expert care based on current research and in accordance with the wishes, values, and beliefs of those we serve. It is "the integration of best research evidence with clinical expertise and patient values" (Sackett, 2000), what Apel and Self (2003) call, "the marriage of research and clinical services."

Looking at Research

A useful way to look at research support is through a framework that organizes your thoughts. The **Scottish Intercollegiate Guidelines Network (SIGN)** is a well-respected system used to evaluate the clinical support of a treatment approach (Scottish Intercollegiate Guideline Network. ,2011; Harbour & Miller, 2001). The American Speech-Language-Hearing Association (ASHA) has adopted the framework, as have researchers in the field (Williams, McLeod, & McCauley, 2010).

The SIGN System

SIGN divides types of research support into levels, the strongest research support being Level Ia. Table 21–1 shows the levels. Level Ia is a well-designed meta-analysis of more than one randomized controlled trial. The next highest level, Level Ib, involves

TABLE 21–1. Levels of Research Support

Level	Description
Ia	Well-designed meta-analysis of >1 randomized controlled trial
Ib	Well-designed randomized controlled study
IIa	Well-designed controlled study without randomization
IIb	Well-designed quasiexperimental study
III	Well-designed nonexperimental studies, that is, correlational and case studies
IV	Expert committee report, consensus conference, and clinical experience of respected authorities

well-designed randomized controlled studies. Next, in Level IIa comes well-designed controlled studies without randomization, followed by well-designed quasiexperimental studies in Level IIb. Lower on the strength scale are well-designed nonexperimental studies, including correlational studies and case studies in Level III; followed by expert committee reports, consensus conference reports, and clinical experience of respected authorities in Level IV.

SIGN and Speech

Baker and McLeod (2011a) reviewed treatment research for speech sound disorders and placed each study in its appropriate SIGN level. Their review comes from 134 treatment studies on speech sound disorders published from 1979 to 2009. See Baker and McLeod (2011a, 2011b) for further discussion, including a list of the 134 treatment studies. They found

- The studies represent 46 distinct successful treatment approaches and seven successful approaches to selection of treatment sounds.
- Most studies (41.5%) were Level IIb (quasiexperimental studies), followed by Level III (nonexperimental case studies) (32.6%).
- The largest number of studies (27.2%) described one child, followed by 2 to 5 children (18.2%), and 6 to 10 children (18.2%).

Observations

Baker and McLeod (2011a) offer an excellent beginning place to discuss research support for treatment approaches for speech sound disorders. Let's consider what their findings mean. Here are three observations and an additional thought

1. Number of studies: 134

   The number of treatment studies (134) means research support exists on which to base clinical decisions. It also suggests that a considerable number of people in our profession dedicate their time and efforts on behalf of children with speech sound disorders. The human hours needed to carry out a research study can be staggering. We are fortunate, I believe, to have colleagues who devote their careers to developing and testing intervention approaches. That said, 134 studies averaged over 30 years is less than five studies per year. This suggests our clinical area needs to continue to draw, train, and support researchers, hopefully in greater number in the future.

2. Number of approaches: 46

   The number of approaches, 46, indicates that many ways exist to treat speech sound disorders successfully. The high number also suggests that at present, no speech treatment approach appears so superior that it has replaced all others. The Van Riper Approach (also called The Traditional Approach) perhaps is the closest the profession ever came to a single dominant method to treat speech sound disorders (Van Riper, 1978). That approach led the field in part because it was intuitive and practical. It also helped that Van Riper wrote extremely well. Additionally, it appeared early in the profession when obtaining a consensus among clinicians was easier since the children we served were less diverse and faculty and students were trained in fewer and more similar programs.

Importantly, the large number of successful approaches does not imply that "anything works." Due to the nature of academic publishing, editors do not typically accept studies for publication that fail to report success. Journals require time, effort, and expense, and, if a study either shows no successful results or simply replicates the results of a previous study, an editor is likely to ask why they should publish it. As a result, we seldom hear about treatment approaches that do not show success.

3. Level of research support: quasiexperimental and case studies
   Most of the reviewed studies fall into the lower levels of research support, nearly 75% being quasiexperimental studies (41.5%) or nonexperimental case studies (32.6%). These designs provide an excellent way to explore a clinical idea, a successful study suggests to investigators they are "on the right track" and serves as an impetus to perform additional investigations. Often, this level of research focuses on a small number of children, many times less than 10 and sometimes fewer than five.

   In research designs at these levels, the investigator knows the purpose of the project (in fact, in most cases, for practical reasons, the investigator and the approach developer are the same person). Because intervention research is difficult and time consuming, most investigators do not undertake it unless they are passionate about their treatment idea. This passion, commendable in its own way, can influence the study's results, which raises the question: If someone with less passion for the approach did the study, would they achieve the same results?

An Additional Thought

An additional thought: even when a treatment approach succeeds, it is notoriously difficult to determine *why* it succeeds. The temptation is to credit success to the theory or principle that underlies the treatment. To illustrate, if a phonological treatment succeeds, the temptation is to conclude that success was due to its good application of phonological principles. Though that may be true, it also could be that success resulted from factors unrelated to the theoretical framework of the study. This is because any treatment approach contains many components, which alone or in combination may contribute to treatment success. For example, treatment activities, characteristics of the children, socioeconomic scale, time of day of treatment, and so forth all may contribute to a successful approach. In a practical sense, this means you should accept that a treatment approach succeeded more quickly than you should accept the explanation for *why* it succeeded.

Assessing Treatment Progress

Another task of a daily researcher is to assess the success of treatment of an individual child. As well as being a legal requirement, self-assessment of treatment progress is essential to a clinician who wants to grow and improve (Baker & McLeod, 2011b; Smit, Brumbaugh, Weltsch, & Hilgers, 2018; Williams, McLeod, & McCauley, 2010).

Standardized Tests: A Risky Choice

To a new professional, a published standardized speech assessment instrument may seem an ideal choice to assess treatment progress, since all you need to do is give the test before treatment begins and after treatment is over. The difficulty with this is that standardized tests often fail to measure small incremental changes that typically occur in clinic work, because the test assesses many sounds in addition to the treatment sound (Eisenberg & Hitchcock, 2010; Gillam & Justice, 2010).

To illustrate the problem, suppose you are treating [s] at the beginning of words and wish to assess your progress. A standardized test containing 100 different words probably only contains three or four [s] words, and it might have only one word to assess [s] word initially. If your treatment is successful, a standardized test would show that the child's score improved by one point out of 100 total possible points. Even if your treatment was wildly successful and resulted in a correct [s] in all positions, a standardized test would only show that the child's score improved by 3 or 4 points out of 100 total points.

Reasonable Assessment Options

Fortunately, many good options exist to assess a child's treatment progress. Three of the most important options are pre- and posttests, ongoing information gathering, and consumer interviews. Each is a reasonable choice for use by itself or in conjunction with the other two. A fourth option exists called single-subject design experiments. It offers a careful, time-consuming approach to assessment of treatment.

Pre- and Posttests

As the names suggest, you administer pretests prior to the onset of treatment and posttests either at a major treatment juncture or at the end of treatment. **Pre- and posttests** usually are quick and easy to give and do not take your attention away from a child during a treatment session. You can assess any treatment goal using a pre- and posttest.

Examples

- Count infant vocalizations during mealtime, provide treatment to promote more vocalizations, and then recount vocalizations when you believe the child has reached the goal.
- Count the number of different words in a toddler's expressive vocabulary, provide treatment to increase expressive vocabulary, and then recount expressive vocabulary when you believe the child has reached the goal.
- Count the correct productions of [s] on a consonant assessment probe, provide treatment for [s], and then readminister the assessment probe when you believe student has reached the goal. To illustrate, the following might be part of a pre-

and posttest for [s], given before you begin treatment and after treatment is over (see Consonant Probes in Six Informal Assessments on the companion website):

#___		S___S		___#	
sun	___	icy	___	bus	___
soap	___	messy	___	kiss	___
sit	___	castle	___	face	___
say	___	bossy	___	hiss	___
see	___	Bessie	___	horse	___

- Count the number of words on an assessment probe showing a fronting process, provide treatment to reduce fronting, and then readminister the assessment probe when you believe preschooler has reached the goal. To illustrate, the following might be a probe list to assess elimination of fronting at the beginning of words before and after treatment (see Phonological Process Probes in Six Informal Assessments on the companion website):

Fronting

Definition: Substitution of an alveolar stop for a postalveolar or velar consonant.

Focus: Listen to the underlined postalveolar and velar consonants. If said as alveolar consonants, the child likely has a fronting process.

Word	Transcription	Yes/No
key	ki	___
cheap	tʃip	___
bug	bʌg	___
bush	bʊʃ	___
itch	ɪtʃ	___
pick	pɪk	___
sheep	ʃip	___
jump	dʒʌmp	___
go	goʊ	___
edge	ɛdʒ	___
Total:		___/___

Ongoing Information Gathering

For many clinicians, **ongoing information gathering** (collection of data during a treatment session) is the gold standard for assessing treatment progress. Like pre- and posttests, you can assess any treatment goal using this method. On the plus side for ongoing information gathering, it allows a clinician to monitor a child's treatment progress closely.

Its potential disadvantage is that it can be time consuming and some clinicians feel that keeping data during a treatment session interferes with their interactions with the child.

Example

You might tabulate a child's rate of success as a percentage value during each treatment session. To illustrate, perhaps the child is 50% accurate in producing a treatment sound during session one, 58% accurate in session two, 64% accurate in session three, and so on.

Consumer Interviews

One of the most straightforward ways to evaluate clinic progress is to ask the consumer —that is, obtain a **consumer interview**. For younger children, this usually means asking a parent or teacher (or preferably both) to speak on the child's behalf. Though a consumer interview can be as simple as a question ("Is ____ speaking more at home?"), rating scales offer the advantage of objectivity ("____ reported that ____'s intelligibility improved from 3 at the onset of treatment to 5 at the end of treatment as measured on a 7-point scale."). A 5-point or 7-point scale typically performs better than a 3-point scale because of the tendency to avoid giving extreme scores. To illustrate, on a 3-point scale people often give many scores of 2, making clinical progress difficult to measure. A 5-point scale offers a greater range of midpoint scores from which to select (2, 3, 4), and a 7-point scale offers an even greater range of midpoint choices.

Example

You may want to include a consumer interview along with other forms of assessment. For example, if treating a preschooler for an **[s]** problem, include a consumer interview at the end of treatment along with a pre and posttest or ongoing information gathering. The same is true if treatment focused on goals such as improvement in story retell, phonological awareness, treatment sound production at home, and so forth.

Single-Subject Design Experiments

Clinicians seldom assess treatment using a **single-subject design experiment** (a demonstration that improvement in the child results from the clinician's treatment rather than from extraneous factors such as time and maturation). I include it here because it offers a design option if you want a rigorous evaluation of your treatment approach, perhaps with the idea of publication in mind. As discussed earlier in the chapter, the largest percentage of speech treatment studies (41.5%) are single-subject design experiments.

Example

The description that follows illustrates the basic steps and logic behind one type of a single-subject design experiment, called a multiple baseline design.

Multiple Baseline Design Experiments. Multiple baseline design is a single-subject design experiment that applies well to treatment of speech sound disorders. A multiple baseline design can evaluate treatment if (1) the child has at least two potential treatment sounds and (2) the child's treatment sounds are distinct enough that the child does not improve on both sounds when you treat one of them. For example, [p] and [b] would probably not be suitable treatment sounds in a single-subject design experiment, because in many cases when you focus on [p] (or [b]), the cognate also improves. Better treatment sounds for a single-subject design experiment might be [p] and [s], because improving one would not likely improve the other.

Components of Multiple Baseline Design Experiments. Multiple baseline design experiments consist of two phases: A (baseline) and B (treatment). During the baseline, you do not provide treatment on the treatment sound. The baseline and treatment phases each must be at least three intervals (usually treatment sessions) in length. For example, collect data baseline for at least three treatment sessions, and then provide treatment for at least the same (and most likely more) number of sessions. Changes in percentage values between the baseline and treatment phases are typically the means to demonstrate treatment progress.

Steps: The following are steps in a multiple baseline experiment.

1. Selection
   Select at least two treatment sounds that are distinct enough that a child's progress in achieving one sound doesn't affect the other sound.

2. Baseline
   Begin collecting baseline data on both sounds during the first session. For example, ask the child to pronounce 20 words beginning with the first treatment sound and 20 different words beginning with the second treatment sound. Graph the data as percentage of correct productions. Continue to collect baseline data for both treatment sounds during at least three sessions. If the child begins to show improvement on the first treatment sound prior to the end of baseline, continue collection of baseline data until the percentage of correct productions is the same for two sessions in a row or until the last session of baseline shows fewer correct productions than the session that preceded it. The purpose of collecting the additional baseline data is to ensure that improvement is occurring without treatment. If this occurs, you should abandon the experiment because the child may not need treatment for that treatment sound.

3. Treatment (First Treatment Sound)
   Begin treatment for the first treatment sound while continuing to collect baseline data for the second treatment sound.

4. Treatment (Second Treatment Sound)
   After the child reaches criterion (typically 75% correct) for the first sound, begin treatment for the second treatment sound. Continue to provide treatment for the second treatment sound until the child reaches criterion for it as well.

Dynamic Assessment

Dynamic assessment is a third type of daily research.

Definition

Dynamic assessment identifies and, if need be, alters supports that facilitate a child's speech making abilities (Bain & Olswang, 1995; Glaspey & Stoel-Gammon, 2005, 2007; Hasson & Joffe, 2007; Strand, 2009). This discovery process begins in the speech evaluation and continues throughout treatment. Dynamic assessment is something that most clinicians do every day (probably without calling it dynamic assessment): they adjust a clinical plan to fit the needs of an individual child. And adjust it again. And again. And perhaps again, depending on the child's responses and the clinician's intuitions, knowledge, and experiences about what they need to alter to help the child learn.

Examples

Any aspect of treatment is subject to dynamic assessment. To illustrate, you may decide that a metaphor selected for [s] is not successful with a child and so change to another. A few more examples may help clarify the point without, I hope, belaboring the obvious:

- A student appears confused by a description of a treatment sound, so you switch to a different description and add a demonstration.
- A preschooler bursts into tears when he loses a game of speech sound bingo, so you shelf the game and change to speech sound drawing, which the child loves.
- A second grader is inattentive in therapy because she misses her friends, so you decide to include the student's friends in therapy activities.
- A child with elective mutism may appear uneasy in treatment, so you alter your typical therapy manner to be less animated.

The Importance of Dynamic Assessment

Why should it matter that a clinician makes small to large adjustments during treatment? I believe it relates to the findings of several large review studies (meta-analyses) in psychology that ask: "Why do clients improve in treatment?" and "Is it primarily the approach that the clinician uses or is it the clinician's treatment skills?" After reviewing the evidence, the investigators concluded that the preponderance of evidence illustrated that clients improved primarily because of clinician's treatment skills rather than because of the specific approach they used (Lambert, 2004; Staines, 2008). The following is two thoughts about those results:

1. The investigators did not suggest that treatment approaches are unimportant, or that "any old treatment approach will do." That is, a clinician's treatment skills are

not the *only* reason why a child improves, though it appears to be a *primary* one. Nor were the authors implying that other aspects of treatment are unimportant. I believe everyone recognizes a child's motivation, length of time in treatment, previous treatment experiences, family involvement, and so forth all may play a part in influencing treatment success. Instead, the study weighed the relative importance of two important treatment variables, clinical skills and treatment approach, rather than to say all other aspects of treatment lack importance.

2. We don't know with certainty why the clinician matters so much to a child's treatment success, nor do we know if the results for psychology apply to treatment of speech sound disorders. But here is a hypothesis: children with speech sound disorders improve in treatment *not* because a clinician has found and executes the best, most-perfect treatment approach, but because a clinician selects a treatment approach that appears a good match to a child's speech needs, and during treatment they adjust and modify their treatment based on the child's responses. That is, the primary reason a child succeeds in speech treatment is due to the experience, judgment, and intuition of a skillful clinician and his/her ability to undertake dynamic assessments from the beginning and throughout treatment.

Conclusions

These are the major ideas in this chapter

1. A clinician is an everyday researcher.
2. Evidence-based practice embodies the clinical goal of providing expert care based on current research in accordance with the wishes, values, and beliefs of those we serve.
3. Options to assess a child's treatment progress include pre- and posttests, ongoing information gathering, consumer interviews, and, much less frequently, single-subject design experiments.
4. Dynamic assessment identifies and, if need be, alters supports that facilitate a child's speech making abilities.

Review Questions

1. Explain in your own words the meaning of *everyday researcher.*
2. What is Scottish Intercollegiate Guideline Network (SIGN)?
3. What is the level of research support for the greatest number of treatment studies of speech sound disorders?
4. Why do you think so many successful approaches exist?
5. Why is it difficult to determine *why* a treatment approach succeeds?
6. Explain in your own words why a clinician typically does not use a standardized test to assess treatment progress.
7. Create an example of a pre- and posttest to assess treatment of prevocalic voicing.

8. What is the value and possible problems with ongoing information gathering?
9. Develop a consumer interview pre- and posttest to assess intelligibility in a story retelling activity.
10. Why are single-subject design experiments discussed in this chapter?
11. What is dynamic assessment?

References

Apel, K., & Self, T. (2003). Evidence-based practice: The marriage of research and clinical services. *The ASHA Leader, 8*(16), 6–7.

Bain, B. A., & Olswang, L. B. (1995). Examining readiness for learning two-word utterances by children with specific expressive language impairment: Dynamic assessment validation. *American Journal of Speech-Language Pathology, 4*(1), 81–91.

Baker, E., & McLeod, S. (2011a). Evidence-based practice for children with speech sound disorders: Part 1 narrative review. *Language, Speech, and Hearing Services in Schools, 42*, 102–139.

Baker, E., & McLeod, S. (2011b). Evidence-based practice for children with speech sound disorders: Part 2 application to clinical practice. *Language, Speech, and Hearing Services in Schools, 42*, 140–151.

Eisenberg, S. L., & Hitchcock, E. R. (2010). Using standardized tests to inventory consonant and vowel production: A comparison of 11 tests of articulation and phonology. *Language, Speech, and Hearing Services in Schools, 41*(4), 488–503.

Gillam, S., & Justice, L. (2010). RTI progress monitoring tools: Assessing primary-grade students in response-to-intervention programs. *The ASHA Leader, 15*(11), 12–15.

Glaspey, A., & Stoel-Gammon, C. (2007). A dynamic approach to phonological assessment. *Advances in Speech-Language Pathology, 9*(4), 286–296.

Glaspey, A. M., & Stoel-Gammon, C. (2005). Dynamic assessment in phonological disorders: The scaffolding scale of stimulability. *Topics in Language Disorders: Clinical Perspectives on Speech Sound Disorders, 25*(3), 220–230.

Harbour, R., & Miller, J. (2001). A new system for grading recommendations in evidence based guidelines. *British Medical Journal, 11*, 334–336.

Hasson, N., & Joffe, V. L. (2007). The case for dynamic assessment in speech and language therapy. *Child Language Teaching and Therapy, 23*(1), 9–25.

Lambert, M. (2004). *Bergin and Garfield's handbook of psychotherapy and behavior change.* New York, NY: John Wiley.

Sackett, D. (2000). *Evidence-based medicine: How to practice and teach EBM* (2nd ed.). Edinburgh, Scotland: Churchill Livingstone.

Scottish Intercollegiate Guideline Network. (2011). Retrieved from http://www.sign.ac.uk

Smit, A., Brumbaugh, K., Weltsch, B., & Hilgers, M. (2018). Treatment of phonological disorder: A feasibility study with focus on outcome measures. *American Journal of Speech Language Pathology, 27*, 536–552.

Staines, G. (2008). The relative efficacy of psychotherapy: Reassessing the methods-based paradigm. *Review of General Psychology, 12*(4), 330–343.

Strand, E. (2009). Dynamic assessment of motor speech disorders in children. In C. Bowen (Ed.), *Children's speech sound disorders* (pp. 265–269). Oxford, UK: Wiley-Blackwell.

Van Riper, C. (1978). *Speech correction: Principles and methods* (6th ed.). Englewood Cliffs, NJ: Prentice-Hall.

Williams, L. McLeod, S. & McCauley, R. (Eds.), *Interventions for speech sound disorders in children*. Baltimore, MD: Brookes,

CHAPTER 22

SOUND DECISIONS

The topic of the final "learn by doing" chapter is treatment. The exercises connect the dots between treatment sounds and other treatment areas, including developmental goals, talking with children, talking about speech, assistive technology, and the clinician as researcher. As elsewhere in this book, the purpose is less to present "the right way" and more to describe the logic and implication of the many decisions that arise in clinical work. Some speech samples in this chapter are from previous assessment exercises, while others are new. Topics in this chapter include:

- Definitions
- Exercises

Learning Objectives

I hope on completing the chapter you will

- Appreciate the role of speech acquisition in treatment sound decisions.
- Know how to carry out most and least knowledge methods to select treatment sounds.
- Recognize the difference between different ways to select treatment sounds.
- Understand the difference between discrimination training and promoting awareness.
- Know treatment sound options for students.

Key Words

Key words you will encounter in this chapter

Established
Emerging
Early 8
Key environment
Frequency of occurrence
Tilde
Highest 8
Discrimination training
Promoting speech awareness
Late 8

Definitions

Many treatment decisions prove useful with speech acquisition, and so, for convenience, information referred to frequently is included here.

Early, Mid, and Late 8

Early 8: m b j n w d p h

Mid 8:   t ŋ k g f v ʧ ʤ

Late 8: s ʃ θ ð z r l ʒ

Phonological Processes

Consonants

Place Changes

- **Fronting:** Substitution of an alveolar stop for a postalveolar or velar consonant.
- **Velar assimilation:** Consonants assimilate to the place of production of a velar consonant.
- **Labial assimilation:** Consonants assimilate to the place of production of a labial consonant.
- *Backing:* Alveolar (and sometimes postalveolar) consonants are pronounced as velar stops.
- *Glottal replacement:* Replacement of a consonant with a glottal stop.

Changes in Manner

- **Stopping:** Substitution of a stop for a fricative or affricate.
- **Gliding:** Substitution of a glide for a liquid.
- **Lateralization:** Sounds typically produced with central air emission (most commonly [s] and [z], but sometimes [ʃ], [ʒ], [ʧ], and [ʤ]) are pronounced with lateral air emission.
- *Affrication:* Stops or fricatives (both usually alveolars) are pronounced as affricates.
- *Nasalization:* Nasal stop replaces nonnasal consonants (usually oral stops).
- *Denasalization:* Oral consonants (usually oral stops) replace nasal consonants.

Sound Reversal

- **Metathesis (meTAthesis):** The reversal of two sounds in a word; for example, saying *pet* as **[tɛp]**.

Consonant Cluster Changes

- **Cluster reduction:** Deletion of a consonant in a consonant cluster.
- **Epenthesis (ePENthesis):** Insertion of a vowel between consonants in a consonant cluster.

Vowels

- **Vowel neutralization:** A neutral vowel (schwa, [ʊ], or [ɪ]) replaces another vowel.
- **Vocalization:** A neutral vowel (schwa, [ʊ], or [ɪ]) replaces a syllabic consonant.

Syllables

Entire Syllable

- **Reduplication:** Repetition of a syllable.
- **Syllable deletion:** Deletion of an unstressed syllable.

Beginning of Syllables

- **Prevocalic voicing:** Consonants before a vowel are voiced.
- ***Initial consonant deletion:*** The initial consonant in the word is deleted.

End of Syllables

- **Final consonant devoicing:** Obstruents are voiceless at the ends of words.
- **Final consonant deletion:** Deletion of a consonant at the end of a syllable or word.

Exercises

Exercise 1

This exercise explores the role of stimulability in selecting a treatment sound with a toddler or early preschooler. The child is E, who was born prematurely and who received a tracheostomy when she was approximately 3 months old due to bronchopulmonary dysplasia (BPD), a lung problem sometimes resulting from medical efforts to save children whose immature lungs are too weak to provide the breaths of life (Bleile, Stark, & Silverman McGowan, 1993). The following is E's entire expressive vocabulary at 2;8.

Speech Sample

Intended Words	E's Words*
1. daddy	dædə
2. hi	haɪ
3. down	da
4. mom	mam
5. hop	bap
6. water	wawa
7. book	bʊk
8. bow	boʊ
9. baby	bʌbʌ
10. up	ʌp
11. please	baɪ
12. bye	baɪ
13. bag	baɪ
14. bubble	bʌ
15. pop	bap
16. ball	bɔ
17. Pop Pop	pap pap

*If E seems familiar, she should: her speech development was the subject in exercises both in Chapter 10, "Speech Puzzles," and in Chapter 14, "Phonetic Inventories."

Questions

1. E's speech contains both **established** consonants (consonants that occur in two or more words) and **emerging** consonants (consonants that occur in one word). To begin, list E's established and emerging consonants in the beginning of words.

2. Many options for treatment sounds exist in E's few sounds, some likely and others less so. To narrow the list, first look at established sounds ([d] and [b]]. What would E learn about speech if you select these sounds? *This and the following are possible sound choices.*

3. Why might you select established sounds as treatment sounds?

4. Next, look at emerging sounds. If you select [m] as a treatment sound, what does E learn about speech?

5. If you select [h] or [p] as a treatment sound, what does E learn?

6. Comparing [h] and [p], which is the least knowledge choice for E? Why?

7. What does E learn about speech if you select [w]?

8. Next, list E's established and emerging consonants in the end of words.

9. Perform the same analysis for word final consonants as you did for word initial consonants.

10. Which consonant is the least knowledge choice in word final position?

Answer Sheet

1. **Established**   **Emerging**

   Beginning of Word   **Beginning of Word**

2. Established sounds:

3. Established sounds:

4. [m]:

5. [h] or [p]:

6. Least knowledge:

7. [w]:

8. **Established Emerging**

   End of Word   **End of Word**

9. [p]:

   [m]:

   [k]:

10. Least knowledge:

Exercise 2

This exercise focuses on selecting a nonstimulable treatment sound with a younger child. The child is Johnny, a boy with Down syndrome whose entire expressive vocabulary at 3 years, 11 months consists of eight words.

Speech Sample

Intended Words	Johnny's Words
1. bubble	bʌ
2. baby	bʌ
3. pig	pi
4. dog	gɔ
5. go	gɔ
6. pop	gɔ
7. in	gɔ
8. moo	gɔ

Questions

1. To begin, a somewhat unusual phonological process limits Johnny's range of word initial consonants. What is the name of the process?
2. What is the name of the phonological process that affects all consonants at the end of words?
3. Sometimes, with a small expressive vocabulary, you can identify established and emerging consonants at a glance. Try that. Look at the sample and find which consonants are established (two or more words) and which are emerging (one word).
4. Though the major focus is on nonstimulable sounds in this exercise, one option is to select [**p**], which is an emerging stimulable sound. If you select [**p**], what will Johnny learn about speech that he doesn't know already?
5. Next, suppose you decide to select a nonstimulable word final treatment sound. How might it benefit Johnny's speech development if you can help him learn to make words ending in consonants?
6. You have many choices for a treatment sound among word final consonants, including selecting all nonstimulable consonants to treat each session, as Miccio and Williams (2010) recommend. For this exercise, suppose you decide to teach a small number of word final nonstimulable consonants in high functional words using early acquired consonants as your treatment sounds (selecting later acquired consonants might prove challenging with Johnny, though you might do so with other children.) According to the discussion in Chapter 17, "Treatment Sounds," which consonants are the **early 8** (first consonants that children typically acquire)? (**Hint:** For convenience, this information appears at the beginning of the present chapter.)

7. Now, eliminate early 8 consonants that do not occur word finally in English. Which consonants remain?

8. We now are down to the early 5, which might be the number you want. For this exercise, reduce this list of potential treatment sounds further through the following **key environment** (**Hint:** A key environment is a phonetic environment that facilitates speech): *consider establishing voiceless consonants at the end of syllable.* If you follow this suggestion, which consonants do you eliminate?

9. The early 8 is now the early 1. What is this consonant and what does Johnny learn about speech if you teach it?

10. Alternately, suppose you decide to teach one of the Early 8 nasal consonants.

    a. What does Johnny learn about making speech sounds at the end of words if you select [m]?

    b. What does Johnny learn about making speech sounds at the end of words if you select [n]?

Answer Sheet

1. Process:

2. Process:

3. **Beginning of Word**

4. *Established*   *Emerging*

5. [p]:

6. Word final consonants:

7. Early 8:

8. Early 8 word finally:

9. Eliminated consonants:

10. Consonant:

11. a. [m]:

    b. [n]:

Exercise 3

Intelligibility, as estimated by **frequency of occurrence** (relative frequency with which a sound occurs in a language), offers another possible method to select treatment sounds. This exercise focuses on Mike, who was born in Korea and was adopted by an American couple when he was 2 years, 2 months. Mike is approximately 4 years, 8 months (Pollock, 1983). Cognitive and receptive language testing indicate he is functioning within age-normal limits. Mike's entire expressive vocabulary consists of 10 words. In common with many children with severe speech challenges, Mike's speech impairment would benefit from an approach that included both speech and assistive technology. The present exercise focuses on the speech aspect of treatment.

Speech Sample

Intended Words	Mike's Words
1. balls	da
2. dish	dɪ
3. hat	næ
4. fast	dæ
5. got	da
6. mask	næ
7. stand	dæ
8. sun	da~dan
9. right	na
10. tent	dɛ

Questions

1. To begin, what does the **tilde** (~) mean in word #8?

2. As with Johnny in Exercise 2, a quick glance is sufficient to identify Mike's established consonants (Mike has no emerging consonants word initially). Which established consonants appear word initially?

3. Which distinctive features do these two sounds share? How do the two sounds differ?

4. Which consonant occurs word finally as an alternate in one word?

5. Suppose you select intelligibility to guide selection of treatment sounds in the beginning of words. Go to Chapter 17, "Treatment Sounds," find the table on frequency of occurrence, and copy the **Highest 8** (8 highest frequency English consonants).

6. What sound class are the six English consonants with the highest frequency? What sound class are the remaining two?

7. I suggest removing the liquids from consideration for this child due to the severity of his speech involvement. Of the remaining six sounds, Mike already produces [d] and [n]. How might selecting [d] and [n] benefit Mike's communication development? (**Hint:** The same question arose in Exercise 2.)

8. If we eliminate [d] and [n], we are down to the Highest 4 [t s k m]. List what Mike learns about speech for each consonant.

9. As with Johnny in Exercise 2, a key environment gives you additional information to make the decision of which sound to select: *consider establishing voiced consonants before a vowel as in bee.* Based on this key environment, which of the highest 4 might be easiest for Mike to learn? Why?

10. Lastly, use your analysis to answer the following questions.

   a. Which of the highest 4 may be easiest for Mike to learn?

   b. Which two consonants are the least knowledge choices?

   c. Which consonant helps Mike learn one distinctive feature?

Answer Sheet

1. Tilde:

2.

3.

4. Word finally:

5. Highest 8:

6. Highest 6:

   Remaining 2:

7. Possible benefit:

8. a. [t]:

   b. [s]:

   c. [k]:

   d. [m]:

9. Easiest:

10. a.

   b.

   c.

   d.

Exercise 4

This exercise shifts from treatment sound selection to perceptual training and speech practice in younger children. The child is Dora (Wolfe, 1994). She's 2 years, 9 months, and her communication history is unremarkable except for having an older brother receiving services for speech problems. Dora's hearing and language abilities are within normal limits.

Speech Sample

Intended Words	Dora's Words
1. puppy	✓*
2. pillow	piwʊʊ
3. pretty	pʌti
4. telephone	bæbən
5. tricycle	taɪtɪtoʊ
6. car	tar
7. carrot	tɛrət
8. kitty cat	tɪʔi tæt
9. cup	tʌp
10. king	tɪn
11. cookie	tuti
12. bird	bʊd
13. bed	bɛ
14. bananas	nænəz
15. big	✓
16. bottle	baʔə
17. Barney	✓
18. bus	bʌs
19. ball	ba
20. bib	bɪ
21. blocks	bwaʃ
22. doggy	daʔi
23. give	dib
24. go	doʊ

*✓ = Word does not contain speech errors.

Questions

1. To begin, consider phonological processes in Dora's speech.

    a. What phonological process affects velar consonants in words #5 to #11, #23, #24?

    b. Are there any words in which Dora makes a velar consonant correctly?

    c. What phonological process affects intervocalic oral stop consonants in words #8, #16, and #22?

    d. Are there words in which Dora makes an intervocalic stop consonant correctly?

2. For this exercise, suppose you select reduction of fronting as your developmental goal and [k] and [g] as your treatment sounds. What metaphor would you use to refer to [k]? (***Hint:*** Feel free to either develop your own, use one you've heard, or use one listed in Chapter 19, "Talking About Speech.")

3. What is a possible touch cue for [k]? (***Hint:*** As with metaphors, feel free to either develop your own, use one you've heard, or use one listed in Chapter 19, "Talking About Speech.")

4. Dora probably is too young to benefit much from reflection on speech. How may metaphors and touch cues help her? (***Hint:*** You'll probably need to flip pages between this chapter and Chapter 17, "Treatment Sounds," for the remainder of this exercise.)

5. Speech practice for a child Dora's age may take a variety of forms. If you select imitation, what are its advantages and disadvantages?

6. What are the advantages and disadvantages of picture or object naming as a form of speech practice?

7. A child under 3 years sometimes benefits from a combination of facilitative talk and more direct instruction that includes metaphors, touch cues, imitation and naming, and so forth. List naturally occurring facilitative talk forms to try with Dora as part of a dynamic assessment (see Chapter 21, "A Daily Researcher").

8. List three modified facilitative talk forms that you might also try.

Answer Sheet

1. a.

    b.

    c.

    d.

2. Possible metaphors:

3. Possible touch cue:

4. Possible help:

5. Imitation:

6. Object of picture naming:

7. Facilitative talk forms:

8. Modified facilitative talk forms:

Exercise 5

This exercise looks at treatment sound decisions in a late preschooler (3;6 to 5;0). The child is Tess, who is 4 years, 4 months (Kim, 1995). Tess's mother reports a normal prenatal and birth history, but that Tess did not say her first words until 2 years. A hearing evaluation indicates hearing within normal limits.

Speech Sample

Intended Words	Tess' Words*
1. popcorn	patə
2. cannot	tænə
3. cat	tæ-tæt
4. coffee	tapi
5. cookie	tʊti
6. Cookie Monster	tuti montə
7. cow	taʊ
8. crab	dəwæb~tu.æ
9. clown	taʊn
10. because	bita
11. broken	bɔti.ɛn
12. doctor	dotə
13. grandma	dænəma~dæma
14. sticker	tɪtə
15. skate	peɪt
16. chicken	tɪtɛm
17. homework	hɔmwʊ
18. look	jut
19. okay	oʊteɪ

*I simplified details of the child's background for this exercise.

Questions

1. This small sample of Dora's speech contains many phonological processes.

   a. Which two phonological processes occur in Dora's pronunciation of "clown"? (word #9).

   b. Which phonological process affects the first consonant in "look"? (word #18)

2. Suppose you decide to make either (or both) [k] and [l] your treatment sounds. What does Dora learn about speech if [k] is the treatment sound?

3. What does Dora learn about speech if [l] is the treatment sound?

4. Between [k] and [l], which is the least knowledge choice?

5. To determine stimulability, develop a small five-word list of probe words for both [k] and [l] to test those consonants at the beginning of words. At least three words in each list should be in one of these key environments. Consider establishing alveolar consonants before a front vowel as in *tea*, and establishing velar consonants before or after a high back vowel as in *coo* and *duke*. *The first word in each list is an example.*

6. If you select a sound Dora is unable to produce on the probe, you have selected a nonstimulable treatment sound. What is the underlying logic of this selection?

7. If you select a sound Dora can produce on the probe, you have selected a stimulable sound. What is the underlying logic of this selection?

Answer Sheet

1. a.

   b.

2. [k]:

3. [l]:

4. Least knowledge choice:

5. a. [l]

      i. *leak*

     ii.

     iii.

     iv.

      v.

   b. [k]

      i. *Coo*

     ii.

     iii.

     iv.

      v.

6. Underlying logic:

7. Underlying logic:

Exercise 6

This exercise explores the clinical implications of two different concepts of perception training. The student is Bobby, who is 5 years, 7 months, attends a public elementary school, and wears bilateral PE tubes because of a history of chronic otitis media (Seo, 1995).

Speech Sample*

Intended Words	Bobby's Words
1. car	tar
2. carrots	tæwɛts
3. cornflake	toʊrnfweɪt
4. ran	wæn
5. country	tʌntʃwi
6. green	gwin
7. grow	gwoʊ
8. glue	gwu
9. secret	sikwɛt
10. ice cream	aɪs kwim

*I simplified the speech sample slightly for this exercise.

Questions

1. This small speech sample suggests that Bobby has difficulty pronouncing which class of consonants?

2. Which phonological process does Bobby use in place of this class of consonants?

3. Assume for this and questions 4 to 6 that you view perception training as correcting a problem in discrimination (see Chapter 17, "Treatment Sounds"). What is the goal of **discrimination training**?

4. How would you know that Bobby needs discrimination training?

5. Would you provide discrimination training before beginning speech practice, ongoing with speech practice, or after completing speech practice?

6. What type of activity would you likely use to develop Bobby's discrimination abilities?

7. Now, assume for this and the following questions that you view perception training as promoting Bobby's speech awareness (see Chapter 17, "Treatment Sounds"). What is the goal of **promoting speech awareness**?

8. How would you know that Bobby needs help promoting awareness?

9. Would you promote speech awareness before beginning speech practice, ongoing with speech practice, or after completing speech practice?

10. What activities might you select from to promote Bobby's speech awareness?

11. *For discussion:* Discrimination training and promoting awareness reflect two different concept of perception training. In your own words, describe the concepts underlying both perspectives.

Answer Sheet

1. Class of consonants:

2. Phonological process:

3. Goal of discrimination training:

4. Need:

5. Discrimination training:

6. Activity:

7. Goal of promoting speech awareness:

8. Need:

9. Promoting speech awareness:

10. Activities:

11. *For discussion:*

Exercise 7

This exercise focuses on speech decisions with students. The student is Dee, who is 7 years, 5 months (Lee, 1994), and was diagnosed with a communication disorder at 3 years. Dee does well in school and receives speech-language services twice a week through a speech and hearing clinic.

Speech Sample*

Intended Words	Dee's Words	Intended Words	Dee's Words
1. patch	✓	28. dinosaur	✓
2. pig	✓	29. dish	✓
3. potatoes	✓	30. dive	✓
4. teeth	tit	31. dog	✓
5. telescope	tɛləkoʊp	32. duck	✓
6. tub	✓	33. gate	deɪt
7. train	tʃɛn	34. goat	✓
8. cage	✓	35. gun	✓
9. cake	keɪt	36. meow	miwaʊ
10. candy	tændi	37. milk	✓
11. kangaroo	tændəwə	38. mother	mʌdʊ
12. carrots	kæwəts	39. mouth	maʊt
13. cat	✓	40. knife	naɪ
14. cup	✓	41. nose	✓
15. coat	✓	42. feather	fɛdʊ
16. cow	✓	43. fish	✓
17. crab	kæb	44. fire	faɪ.ə
18. crayon	kɛwən	45. flag	fæg
19. clown	kaʊn	46. thumb	tʌm
20. balloon	✓	47. Santa Claus	sæntə kɔz
21. bat	✓	48. seal	si.ə
22. bed	✓	49. sun	✓
23. boat	✓	50. star	ta.ə
24. book	✓	51. stove	toʊv
25. bus	✓	52. snake	neɪk
26. butterfly	bʌdəfaɪ	53. sled	sɛd
27. bridge	bɪdʒ	54. sheep	✓

Intended Words	Dee's Words	Intended Words	Dee's Words
55. shoe	✓	68. yard	jʌd
56. van	✓	69. yellow	lɛloʊ
57. vest	✓	70. wagon	✓
58. this	dɪs	71. watch	✓
59. the	də	72. rabbit	wæbɪt
60. zipper	zɪpə	73. radio	weɪdi.oʊ
61. zoo	✓	74. rain	weɪn
62. chair	tʃɛ.ə	75. rope	woʊp
63. church	tʃɜ	76. lamp	✓
64. jelly	✓	77. leaf	✓
65. judge	dʒʌd	78. lion	✓
66. hand	✓	79. elephant	✓
67. hat	✓	80. umbrella	əmbwɛji.ə

*✓ = Dee says the word correctly.

Questions

1. Dee's speech contains many phonological processes and individual sound errors. *Kangaroo* (word #11) and *gate* (word #33) are examples of a phonological process in its last stage. What is the name of the phonological process?

2. Dee's speech also contains several phonological processes affecting consonant clusters.

   a. What is the phonological process that affects words #7, #17, #19, #27, #45, #47, and #50 to #53?

   b. A different process affects the consonant cluster in *crayon* (word #18). What is its name?

3. Dee's speech also contains phonological processes affecting several nonstimulable late 8 consonants (last acquired English consonants).

   a. What phonological process affects interdental consonants in words #38, #39, #42, #46, #58, and #59?

   b. What is the name of the phonological process that affects [r] in words #72 to #75?

4. For this exercise, the first developmental speech goal is to complete the elimination of fronting. Our treatment sounds are [k] and [g]. Even though fronting is a phonological process associated with preschoolers, Dee brings the cognitive and attention abilities of a student to her speech work, which changes the clinical tool set. To illustrate, compare the perception enhancing tools typically available to an early preschooler working on [k] with those available to a student. (**Hint:** See Chapter 17, "Treatment Sounds.")

5. Go to the Treatment Resources on the companion website to find one description and one demonstration for velar consonants and explain them here.

6. Students (and selected late preschoolers) also have multipurpose higher technology options to establish speech, train perception, and practice speech. List three higher technology options appearing in Chapter 19, "Talking about Speech."

7. A student has many ways available to practice speech. List three ways to provide mass practice of [k] and other sounds (see Chapter 17, "Treatment Sounds").

8. List five ways a student can practice speech in a language context.

9. For this exercise, the second treatment sound is [r], one of Dee's nonstimulable late 8 consonants. Dee's treatment options for [r] are the same as for [k], with the addition of a technique (really, two closely related techniques) to transform a nonstimulable sound into a stimulable one. What are the names of these techniques?

10. What's the difference between phonetic placement and shaping?

11. The Treatment Resources on the companion website contains over 100 techniques for phonetic placement and shaping. Go to that resource and find one phonetic placement and one shaping technique for [r] and explain them here.

Answer Sheet

1. Phonological process:

2. a. Phonological process:

   b. Phonological process:

3. a. Phonological process:

   b. Phonological process:

4. a. Early preschooler:

   b. Student:

5. Description:

   Demonstration:

6. Higher technology options:

7. Mass practice:

8. Language:

9. Techniques:

10. Difference:

11. Phonetic placement:

    Shaping:

Conclusions

Major ideas in this "learn by doing" chapter include

1. Many reasonable clinical options exist to select, establish, train perception, and practice speech.
2. For younger children through students, selection of treatment sounds entails making clinical decisions about stimulability and speech knowledge.
3. Speech acquisition, intelligibility, and key environments all can help to select between choices of treatment sounds.
4. Several conceptions of perceptual training exist, each with different implications for treatment sound clinical decisions.
5. Students have a wide range of treatment sound choices, including ways to transform nonstimuable sounds into stimulable ones.

Review Questions

1. What are the definitions of stimuable and nonstimulable?
2. What is most knowledge and what is least knowledge?
3. How may speech acquisition and frequency of occurrence affect selection of treatment sounds?
4. What are key environments and how may they affect selection of treatment sounds?
5. What higher technology options exist to describe and demonstrate speech?
6. What clinical option for students convert a nonstimulable sound into a stimulable one?

References

Bleile, K., Stark R., & Silverman McGowan, J. (1993). Evidence for the relationship between babbling and later speech development. *Clinical Linguistics and Phonetics*, *7*, 319–337.

Kim, J. (1995). *Student research project*. Honolulu, HI: University of Hawaii.

Lee, S. (1994). *Student research project*. Honolulu, HI: University of Hawaii.

Pollock, K. (1983). Individual preferences: Case study of a phonologically delayed child. *Topics in Language Disorders*, *3*, 10–23.

Seo, R. (1995). *Student research project*. Honolulu, HI: University of Hawaii.

Wolfe, D. (1994). *Student research project*. Honolulu, HI: University of Hawaii.

APPENDIX A

SPECIAL SYMBOLS AND DIACRITICS

The special symbols (additional phonetic symbols) and diacritics (modifications of existing symbols) on the following page are for transcribing persons with speech disorders (International Phonetic Association, 2015).

extIPA SYMBOLS FOR DISORDERED SPEECH
(Revised to 2015)

CONSONANTS (other than those on the IPA Chart)

	Bilabial	Labio-dental	Labio-alveolar	Dento-labial	Bidental	Linguo-labial	Inter-dental	Alveolar	Retroflex	Palatal	Velar	Velo-pharyngeal	(Upper) pharyngeal
Plosive		p̪ b̪	p͆ b͆	p̺ b̺			t̼ d̼	t̪ d̪					ꞯ ʛ
Nasal		m̪ m̪	m̺ m̺			n̼ n̼	n̪ n̪						
Trill						r̼	r̪					ʩ ʩ	
Fricative, median		f̪ v̪	f̺ v̺	h̺ h̺	θ̼ ð̼	θ̪ ð̪	θ̠ ð̠					ʩ ʩ	
Fricative, lateral						ꞎ ꞎ	ꞎ ꞎ		ꞎ ꞎ	ʎ̝ ʎ̝	ʟ̝ ʟ̝		
Fricative, lat. + med.								ls lz					
Fricative, nasal	m̥ m̃	m̥ m̃					n̥ ñ	n̥ ñ	ɲ̥ ɲ̃	ŋ̥ ŋ̃			
Approxt., lateral						l̼	l̪						
Percussive	ʬ ʬ				ʭ								

DIACRITICS

◌̼	labial spreading	s̺	◌̃, ◌̃	denasal, partial denasal	m̃ h̃	◌̰	main gesture offset right	s̺
◌̺	strong articulation	f̺	◌̃	fricative nasal escape	v̂	◌̰	main gesture offset left	s̺
◌̥	weak articulation	v̥	◌̃	velopharyngeal friction	s̃ ʒ̃	◌̥	whistled articulation	s̃
\	reiteration	p\p\p	↓	ingressive airflow	p↓	◌◌	sliding articulation	θs

CONNECTED SPEECH, UNCERTAINTY ETC.

(.) (..) (...)	short, medium, long pause
f, ff	loud(er) speech: [{f laʊd f}]
p, pp	quiet(er) speech: [{p kwaɪət p}]
allegro	fast speech: [{allegro fast allegro}]
lento	slow speech: [{lento sloʊ lento}]
crescendo, ralentando etc. may also be used	
◯, Ⓒ, Ⓥ	indeterminate sound, consonant, vowel
Ⓕ, Ⓟ etc.	indeterminate fricative, probably [p] etc.
( )	silent articulation, e.g. (ʃ), (m)
(( ))	extraneous noise, e.g. ((2 sylls))

VOICING

◌̬	pre-voicing		z̬
◌̬	post-voicing		z̬
◌̥	partial devoicing		z̥ ʒ̥
◌̥	initial partial devoicing		z̥ ʒ̥
◌̥	final partial devoicing		z̥ ʒ̥
◌̬	partial voicing		s̬
◌̬	initial partial voicing		s̬
◌̬	final partial voicing		s̬
◌=	unaspirated		p=
ʰ◌	pre-aspiration		ʰp

OTHER SOUNDS

ɹ̺	apical-r
ɹ̈	bunched-r (molar-r)
s̻ z̻	laminal fricatives (incl. lowered tongue tip)
kꞎ etc.	[k] with lateral fricated release etc.
tˡˢ dˡᶻ	[t, d] with lateral and median release
tʰ̪	[t] with interdental aspiration etc.

t͡θ	linguolabial affricate etc.
ƛ ɡ̆ ȵ	velodorsal oral and nasal stops
ᵻ	sublaminal lower alveolar percussive
ǃᵻ	alveolar click with sublaminal percussive release
D͡r̼	buccal interdental trill (raspberry)
*	sound with no available symbol

© ICPLA 2015

Source: IPA Chart. (2015). Retrieved from http://www.internationalphoneticassociation.org/content/ipa-chart

APPENDIX B
DEFINITIONS

This resource contains definitions of speech terminology to describe speech sound disorders. Not all—or even a large portion—of these terms appear in this book, though you may encounter them in other books and articles, and so, I have included them here. You can access the information two ways. If you know the term, simply look it up in the alphabetical list. If you are unsure of the term, but know the topic, you can look up a topic and then look for the term there. Terminology appears first, then topics. The topics are

- Places of Production
- Manners of Production
- Vowels
- Names for Sounds
- Transcription
- Abbreviations
- Speech Characteristics
- Speech Environments
- Assimilations
- Common Names for Speech Disorders
- Names for Speech Errors
- Major Phonological Processes
- Prespeech and Early Speech
- [s], [l], and [r]

Definitions

Affricate. A consonant with a stop onset and fricative release. The English affricates are [ʧ] and [ʤ].

Affrication. A phonological process in which a person pronounces stops or fricatives as affricates; for example, *see* is [**tsi**].

Allophone. A variant of a phoneme that does not affect meaning; for example, unaspirated [**p°**] and aspirated [**pʰ**] are allophones of the phoneme /p/.

Alveolar. A class of consonants produced with constriction between articulators at the alveolar ridge, which lies immediately posterior to the upper front teeth. The English alveolar consonants are [**t**], [**d**], [**s**], [**z**], [**n**], [**1**], and [**r**].

Ambisyllabic. A consonant sometimes belongs to two syllables; for example, some investigators consider the second [**m**] in *mama* to be ambisyllabic.

Approximant. Liquids and glides. The English approximants are [**l**], [**r**], [**j**], and [**w**].

Arrestor. A consonant occurring after a vowel in the same syllable; for example, *t* is the arrestor consonant in *bit.*

Articulation error. A speech error resulting from problems in speech motor control.

Articulation disorder. As defined in this book, an articulation disorder results from problems in speech motor control. Some authors use the term articulation disorder to refer to problems in both phonology and speech motor control.

Aspiration. A burst of air arising after the release of a voiceless stop in positions such as the beginning of a word; for example, the English [**t**] in *tube* [**tʰub**].

Assimilation. The influence of speech elements on each another. See also **progressive assimilation** and **regressive assimilation**.

Babble. A prespeech vocalization in which repetitions of syllables predominate.

Back vowels and diphthongs. Vowels in which the back of the tongue is the major articulator; the English back vowels and diphthongs are [**u**], [**ʊ**], [**oʊ**], [**ɔ**], [**ɔɪ**], [**ʌ**], and [**ɑ**].

Backing. A phonological process in which velar consonants replace alveolar consonants; for example, *tee* is [**ki**].

Bilabial. Consonant made using the two lips. The English bilabial consonants are [**p**], [**b**], [**m**], and [**w**].

Bladed [s]. An [**s**] produced with the tongue blade raised rather than the tongue tip.

Blends. Consonant clusters.

Brackets. Transcriptions enclosed by square brackets indicate only that a person made the sounds, without claiming whether or not the sounds are phonemes of the language. For example, placing *b* within brackets (i.e., [**b**]) indicates a person made the sound, but does not indicate whether [**b**] is a phoneme. See **phoneme** and **square brackets**.

Broad transcription. Transcription of phonemes. Enclose broad transcriptions within slashes. See **phoneme** and **slashes**.

Buccal (pronounced "buckle") speech. Speech produced by trapping air between the cheeks; it is sometimes called "Donald Duck speech." Children with tracheostomies often discover they can make words and short phrases using buccal speech.

Bunched [r] and [ɚ]. Production of [r] and [ɚ] with the tongue tip lowered and the bulk of the tongue raised. See **retroflex [r] and [ɚ]**.

C. Consonant.

Canonical babbling. A no-speech vocalization in which syllables predominate. See **babble**.

Capital "E" (pronounced [i]). The name for the sound transcribed [i].

Caret. The name for the sound transcribed [ʌ].

Central. Sounds made with air flowing over the tongue midline. All the English consonants are central, except [l], which is lateral.

Central vowel. Vowel in which the tongue blade is the major articulator. The English central vowel is [ə].

Childhood apraxia of speech (CAS). A neurological speech disorder in which the precision and consistency of movements underlying speech are impaired in the absence of neuromuscular deficits.

Close. Vowels and diphthongs produced with the tongue raised toward the roof of the mouth. The category "close" replaces "high" in the revised International Phonetic Alphabet (International Clinical Phonetics and Linguistics Association, 1992). The English close vowels and diphthongs are [i], [ɪ], [u], and [ʊ].

Close-mid. Vowels and diphthongs produced with the tongue in a relatively neutral position. The category "close-mid" replaces "mid" in the revised International Phonetic Alphabet (International Clinical Phonetics and Linguistics Association, 1992). The English close-mid vowels and diphthongs are [eɪ], [oʊ], and [ə].

Cluster Reduction. A phonological process in which a consonant or consonants in a consonant cluster are deleted; for example, *speed* is pronounced as [pid] or [sid].

Coalescence. The merger of two or more sounds; for example, the pronunciation of [sp] in *spy* as [f], which appears be a coalescence of the place of production of [p] (labial) and the manner of production of [s] (fricative).

Coarticulation. The theory that sounds blend together during speech production.

Cognates. Two sounds that differ only in voicing; for example, [p] and [b] are cognates.

Complementary distribution. Sounds that never occur in the same phonetic environment; for example, English [h] and [ŋ] are in complementary distribution.

Consonant. A sound made with marked constriction somewhere along the vocal tract.

Consonant cluster. Two or more consonants occurring within the same syllable in which the sequence of consonants is uninterrupted by vowels.

Continuants. Sounds sustained for extended periods. The English continuant sound classes are fricatives, nasals, liquids, glides, vowels, and diphthongs.

Cooing. A prespeech vocalization containing consonants and vowels produced at the back of the mouth.

CV. Consonant-vowel.

CVC. Consonant-vowel-consonant.

Dark [l]. An [l] produced in the velar area. Also called velarized [l].

Deletion. Failure to produce a sound; for example, the pronunciation of *deep* as [di].

Denasalization. A phonological process in which oral stops replace nasal consonants; for example, *me* is *bi*.

Dental. Consonants produced with the tongue tip against the back of the upper front teeth. In English, alveolar consonants typically dentalize when they occur prior to an interdental consonant, as in *tenth*.

Dentalized. See **dental**.

Devoicing. Production with partial voicing or complete lack of voicing of sounds typically produced with voicing.

Diacritics. Modifications made to phonetic symbols to describe phonetic details; for example, a small raised [ʰ] is a diacritic used to indicate aspiration. The diacritic system is that of the International Clinical Phonetics and Linguistics Association (1992).

Dialect. A variation of speech caused by the influence of region, social class, or ethnic or racial identification.

Digraph. The name for the sound transcribed [æ].

Diphthong. A sequence of two vowels in which only one is syllabic. The English diphthongs are [eɪ], [aɪ], [aʊ], [ɔɪ], and [oʊ].

Discrimination training. See **perception training**.

Distinctive features. Attributes of sounds that distinguish one sound from another.

Distortion. A close approximation of a sound; a sound made slightly different than the intended sound.

Dynamic assessment. Assessment of a child's speech using various types of support.

Dysarthria. Motor speech disorders arising from impairments originating in the peripheral or central nervous system.

Eggressive. The outward flow of air from the mouth or nose.

Environments. See **phonetic environments**.

Epenthesis (ePENthesis). A phonological process in which a vowel inserts between consonants in a consonant cluster; for example, *treat* is [tərit].

Epsilon. The name for the sound transcribed [ɛ].

Excessive stress or equal stress (EES). Excessive or equal stress on syllables.

Final consonant deletion. A phonological process in which a consonant occurring at the end of a syllable or word deletes; for example, *beet* is [**bi**].

Final consonant devoicing. A phonological process in which voiced obstruents devoice at the end of a syllable or word; for example, *mead* is [**mit**].

Fricative. A consonant produced with a sufficiently small distance between the articulators to cause a "hissing sound." The English fricatives are [**f**], [**v**], [**θ**], [**ð**], [**s**], [**z**], [**ʃ**], and [**ʒ**].

Front vowels and diphthongs. Vowels in which the tongue tip is the major articulator; the English front vowels and diphthongs are [i], [ɪ], [eɪ], [ɛ], [æ], [a], [aɪ], and [aʊ].

Frontal lisp. See **lisping**.

Fronting. A phonological process in which alveolar consonants replace velar consonants (and sometimes postalveolar affricates); for example, *key* is [**ti**].

Glide. Consonants produced with relatively little constriction between articulators. The English glides are [**j**] and [**w**].

Gliding. A phonological process in which a fluid consonant is pronounced as a glide; for example, *Lee* is pronounced [**wi**] or (less typically) [**ji**].

Glottal. Sounds produced at the vocal folds; for example, [**h**] is a glottal glide.

Glottal replacement. A phonological process in which a glottal stop replaces other consonants; for example, *boot* is [buʔ].

High vowels. Vowels produced with the tongue raised toward the roof of the mouth. The English high vowels are [i], [ɪ], [u], and [ʊ].

Homonyms. Words that sound alike but have different meanings; for example, *reed* and the present tense of *read* are homonyms.

Homorganic. Sounds produced at the same place of production; for example, in English [b], [p], [m], and [w] are homorganic.

Horseshoe. The name for the sound transcribed [ʊ].

Independent analysis. A type of analysis in which a child's speech abilities are described without reference to the language of the child's community; for example, an independent analysis might describe a child's speech as containing [p b t d], but would not indicate if these consonants are produced correctly relative to the adult language (Stoel-Gammon & Dunn, 1985). See also **relational analysis**.

Ingressive. Sounds made with the inward movement of air.

Initial consonant deletion. A phonological process in which the consonant beginning a word deletes; for example, *bee* is [i].

Initial sound. A sound beginning a word or syllable.

Interdental. Consonants produced with the tongue tip protruding between the upper and lower front teeth. The English interdental consonants are [θ] and [ð].

Intervocalic. Consonants occurring between vowels; for example, the second [b] in *baby* is intervocalic. Also see **syllable position**.

Interword variability. Variation in the pronunciation of speech elements in different words.

Intonation. Pitch changes that occur when speaking as part of prosody. See **prosody**.

Intraword variability. Variation in the pronunciation of speech in the same word; for example, the initial sound in *bee* pronounced as [b], [p], or [mb].

Jargon. Canonical babbling under an adultlike intonation contour.

Labial. Bilabial and labiodental consonants. The English labial consonants are [p], [b], [m], [w], [f], and [v].

Labial assimilation. A phonological process in which consonants assimilate to the place of production of a labial consonant; for example, *bead* is [bib].

Labialization. Pronunciation of consonants with greater-than-expected lip rounding.

Labiodental. Consonants produced with the upper lip and lower teeth. The English labiodental consonants are [f] and [v].

Late 8. The last eight consonants typically acquired by students. The late 8 are [s], [ʃ], [θ], [ð], [z], [tʃ], [r], and [l].

Late 8 + One. In this book, the late 8 + [ɚ], which sometimes is remediated in conjunction with [r].

Lateral. Sounds produced with air flowing over the sides of the tongue. The English lateral is [l].

Lateral lisp. See **lisping**.

Lateral [s]. An [s] produced with air flowing over the sides of the tongue. The symbol for lateral [s] is [ls].

Lateralization. A phonological process in which sounds typically produced with central air emission (most commonly [s] and [z]) are pronounced with lateral air emission; for example, *see* is pronounced [**lsi**] (see **diacritics**).

Light [l]. An [l] made at the alveolar place of production. Light [l] typically occurs in syllable-initial position in English.

Lip rounding. See **rounding**.

Lips spread. See **spreading**.

Liquid. A class of sounds made with a relatively large aperture between the tongue and the roof of the mouth. The English liquids are [l] and [r].

Lisping. An error in which alveolar consonants (typically fricatives) occur with the tongue either on or between the front teeth. Also called a frontal lisp. Lateral lisps are the same as lisping except the airflow comes over the sides of the tongue.

Long "s" (pronounced [ɛs]). The name for the sound transcribed [ʃ].

Manner of production. The degree of narrowing in the vocal tract and direction of airflow that occurs during the production of sounds. The English manner of production classes are stops (oral and nasal), affricates, fricatives, liquids, glides, vowels, and diphthongs.

Mature jargon. Sentencelike units in which the sounds occur with little phonetic accuracy. Children who produce jargon "know the tune before the words."

Maximal pair. See **word pair**.

Medial sound. See **word-medial position**.

Metalinguistics. The ability to reflect on language.

Metathesis (MeTAthesis). A phonological process in which the order of sounds in a word reverse; for example, *peek* is [**kip**].

Minimal pair. See **word pairs**.

Multisyllabic. More than one syllable.

Narrow transcription. Transcription containing diacritics to indicate the actual speech sounds produced by a speaker. Brackets enclose narrow transcriptions. See also **brackets**.

Nasal stop. A consonant made with the velum lowered and complete closure somewhere in the oral tract.

Nasality. Production of a sound with the velum lowered.

Nasalization. Nasal stops replace nonnasal consonants (usually oral stops).

Nasals. A class of consonants made with a lowered velum. The English nasal stops are [**m**], [**n**], and [**ŋ**]. See also **nasal stop**.

Neutral vowels. Vowels that "stand-in" for many other vowels and diphthongs in unstressed syllables; for example, [ə], [ɪ], and [ʊ] are neutral vowels for many English speakers.

Noncontrastive. See **complementary distribution**.

Nonreduplicated babbling. Babbling in which consonants and vowels vary within syllables; for example, *ba-di-du* or *mu-mi*. See also **reduplicated babbling**.

Obstruent. Oral stops, affricates, and fricatives.

Omission. See **deletion**.

Onset. A linguistic unit theorized by some researchers to occur at the beginning of syllables; for example, [**sp**] in *spy* and [**t**] in *toe* are considered onsets in some linguistic theories of syllable structure.

Open. Vowels and diphthongs produced with the tongue lying relatively flat on the floor of the mouth. "Open" replaces "low" in the revised International Phonetic Alphabet (International Clinical Phonetics and Linguistics Association, 1992). The English open vowels and diphthongs are [a], [ɑ], [aɪ], and [aʊ].

Open "o" (pronounced [oʊ]). The name for the sound transcribed [ɔ].

Open syllable. Syllable ending with a vowel or diphthong; for example, *bay* and *toe* have open syllables.

Open-mid. Vowels and diphthongs produced with the tongue raised slightly from the floor of the mouth. The category of "open-mid" replaces "mid" in the revised International Phonetic Alphabet (International Clinical Phonetics and Linguistics Association, 1992). The English open-mid vowels and diphthongs are [ɛ], [ʌ], [ɔɪ], and [ɔ].

Oral stop. Stop consonants made with a raised velum. The English oral stops are [p], [b], [t], [d], [k], and [g].

Palatal. Place of production at which the tongue approximates the hard palate. The English palatal consonant is [j].

Perception training. Clinical philosophy that training helps to improve a child's ability to distinguish between different sounds, syllables, and words.

Pharyngeal fricative. A fricative produced in the pharyngeal region. Pharyngeal fricatives sometimes occur in the speech of children with repaired cleft palates.

Phone. A sound of a language. Every consonant, vowel, and diphthong is a phone.

Phoneme. A sound that is capable of distinguishing between words; for example, [p] and [b] are English phonemes as illustrated by the words *bee* and *pea*.

Phonemic transcription. Transcription of the phonemes of a language.

Phonetic environments. Syllable positions in which sounds occur; for example, [t] in *beet* occurs in the syllable-final position and [d] in *buddy* occurs in the intervocalic position.

Phonetic transcription. Transcription of the sounds of a language.

Phonetically consistent form (PCF). A word made up by a child (typically, an infant) that does not appear to be based on an adult model. Also called a proto word.

Phonetics. The study of the acoustic, psychoacoustic, and production aspects of speech.

Phonological awareness. Conscious knowledge of the sound structure of a language.

Phonological disorder. In this book, a phonological disorder results from problems in language knowledge. Some authors use the term phonological disorder to refer to problems in both phonology and speech motor control.

Phonological error. A speech error resulting from absent or limited knowledge of the phonological system of the language.

Phonological knowledge. A person's knowledge of the phonological organization of his or her language.

Phonological processes. Descriptions of systematic differences between the child's speech and the speech of adults in the child's community.

Phonological rule. A description of the systematic relationship between units in a phonological system.

Phonology. The study of the linguistic organization of sound.

Phonotactics. The rules for the sequential arrangement of speech sounds; for example, an English phonotactic rule is that [sp] is an acceptable word-initial consonant cluster but [ps] is not.

Place of production. The point in the vocal tract at which maximum constriction occurs during production of a sound. Place of production is sometimes called place of articulation.

Postalveolar. A place of production immediately posterior to the alveolar ridge. "Postalveolar" replaces "alveopalatal" in the revised edition of the International Phonetic Alphabet (International Clinical Phonetics and Linguistics Association, 1992). The English postalveolar consonants are [tʃ], [dʒ], [ʃ], and [ʒ].

Postvocalic. Consonants occurring after a vowel in the same syllable; for example, [t] in *eat* [it].

Prevocalic voicing. A phonological process in which voiced consonants replace voiceless consonants before a vowel; for example, *pea* is [bi].

Primary stress. The major stress in a word; for example, the syllable *tween* carries the primary stress in *between.*

Print "a" (pronounced [eɪ]). The name for the sound transcribed [a].

Progressive assimilation. Assimilation due to the influence of an earlier occurring sound on a later occurring sound; for example, [r] is often pronounced with rounded lips in *shriek* because of the lip rounding that occurs in [ʃ]. See also **regressive assimilation**.

Prosody. Modifications in intonation, rate, and stress of sounds as they occur in phrases and sentences.

Pure vowel. A vowel that remains relatively unchanged throughout its production; the English pure vowels are [i], [ɪ], [æ], [a], [ɑ], [ə], [ʌ], [ɔ], [ʊ], and [u].

R-colored vowel. See **rhotic vowel**.

Reduplicated babbling. Babbling in which syllables are repeated; for example, *ba-ba-ba* or *da-da*. See also **nonreduplicated babbling**.

Reduplication. A phonological process in which a syllable repeats; for example, *water* is [wɑwɑ].

Regressive assimilation. Assimilation resulting from the effect of a later occurring sound on an earlier occurring sound; for example, [n] in *tenth* is often produced as a dental consonant because of the influence of interdental [θ]. See also **progressive assimilation**.

Relational analysis. Analysis that compares the child's speech to the speech of the child's community (Stoel-Gammon & Dunn, 1985). An example of a relational analysis is the statement, "The child produced [k] as [t]." See also **independent analysis**.

Residual error. A speech error that persists beyond age 9 and into adulthood.

Resyllabification. Movement of a sound from its original syllable; for example, [t] in the phrase *It is* often is resyllabified to *I tis* in casual speech.

Retroflex [r] and [ɚ]. [r] and [ɚ] are produced in one of two ways: bunched or retroflexed. Retroflex [r] and [ɚ] occur with the tongue body slightly retracted, the tongue tip raised, and the sides of the back of the tongue against the inside of the teeth. See also **bunched [r] and [ɚ]**.

Rhotic vowel. Production of a schwa with an [r]-coloring; for example, the vowel in *merge* and the vowels in *murder.* Non-rhotic vowels are vowels and diphthongs made without [r] coloring. See also **[r] colored vowel, schwa [r]**, and **schwar**.

Rime (also called Rhyme). A linguistic unit within a syllable theorized to include the vowel and any final consonants; for example, the vowel + [nt] in *bent* is a rime in some linguistic theories of syllable structure.

Rounding. Lip puckering that accompanies [w] and some back vowels and diphthongs. For many speakers, some lip rounding also accompanies [ʃ]. The English back unrounded vowels are [ʊ], [ʌ], and [ɑ] and the English back rounded vowels are [u], [oʊ], [ɔ] and [ɔɪ].

S. Syllable.

Schwa. The name for the sound transcribed as [ə].

Schwa [r]. A vowel made with [r] coloring; for example, the vowel in *merge* and the vowels in *murder*. See also **rhotic vowel**.

Schwar. A name sometimes given for schwa [r].

Semivowels. A consonant that can "stand-in" for a vowel. The English semivowels are [j] and [w].

SFWF. Syllable final word final; for example, the position of [t] in *beat* is SFWF. In the word *rub* /b/ is SFWF.

SFWW. Syllable final within word; for example, [m] in steamboat is SFWW.

Sibilant. Alveolar and postalveolar fricatives and the fricative portion of alveolar and postalveolar affricates.

Singleton. A consonant produced adjacent to a vowel. For example, [t] in *too* is a singleton.

SIWI. Syllable initial word initial; for example, the position of [s] in *see* is SIWI.

SIWW. Syllable initial within word; for example, the position of [t] in *between* is SIWW.

Slashes (virgules). Transcriptions enclosed by slashes indicate that the sounds are phonemes of the language; for example, /p/ is a phoneme of English. See **phoneme**.

SODA. A system for describing speech errors (substitution, omission, deletion, addition).

Sonorants. Sounds produced with relatively unobstructed airflow. The English sonorant sound classes are nasals, liquids, glides, and vowels.

Special symbols. Within this book, additional transcription symbols used to describe a child's speech errors in addition to those listed in Table 2–1. The symbol system is that of the International Clinical Phonetics and Linguistics Association (1992).

Speech sound disorders. A neutral term to describe speech errors without commitment to the cause of the disorder. Within this book, a speech sound disorder (1) arose during childhood and is not directly attributable to damage to the speech mechanism, sensory systems, peripheral nervous system, or central nervous system; (2) is not the result of dialect or non-English language influences; and (3) is considered a disorder either by the child or members of the child's community. See also **articulation disorder** and **phonological disorder**.

Spreading. A smilelike stretch of the lips that accompanies [s] and [z] and English front vowels and diphthongs.

Square brackets. See **brackets**.

Stimulability. Capacity to pronounce a speech element. To illustrate, if a person can pronounce [t] in imitation or another means, the person is stimulable for [t].

Stop. A class of consonants made with complete closure at some point in the vocal tract. The English oral stops are [p], [b], [t], [d], [k], and [g] and the English nasal stops are [m], [n], and [ŋ].

Stopping. A phonological process in which an oral stop replaces a continuant (typically a fricative); for example, *see* is [ti].

Stridency deletion. Deletion of strident consonants. See **strident**.

Strident. Sounds characterized by noisiness resulting from a fast rate of airflow. The English strident consonants are fricatives and affricates in labiodental [f v], alveolar [s z], and postalveolar [tʃ dʒ ʃ ʒ] places of production.

Substitution. Replacement of one sound with another; for example, a substitution of [s] for [t] results in *see* being said as *tee*.

Suprasegmental. In English, major suprasegmental components include intonation, rate, and stress. See **prosody**. In some linguistic theories, suprasegmentals are features that spread over more than one segment. For example, velar assimilation entails spreading the velar feature over a word, as in the pronunciation of *peak* as [kik].

Syllable deletion. A phonological process in which an unstressed syllable deletes; for example, *banana* is [næ nə].

Syllable final position. The end of a syllable; for example, [t] in *pit*, [nt] in *mint*, and [p] in *captain* occur in syllable final position.

Syllable initial position. The beginning of a syllable; for example, [b] in *bug*, [sp] in *spy*, and [t] in *captain* occur in syllable initial position.

Theta. The name for the sound transcribed [θ].

Thorn. The name for the sound transcribed [ð].

Unaspirated. Production of a typically aspirated oral stop without aspiration; for example, the pronunciation of *pea* [pʰi] as [pᵒi].

V. Vowel.

Variegated babbling. Canonical babbling produced under an adultlike intonation contour. See **jargon**.

Velar. Place of production made by raising the back of the tongue toward the soft palate. The English velar consonants are [k], [g], and [ŋ]. Vowels and diphthongs also occur in the velar position, but people call them back vowels and back diphthongs rather than velar vowels and velar diphthongs.

Velar assimilation. A phonological process in which consonants assimilate to the place of production of a velar consonant; for example, *teak* is [kik].

Velarized [l]. See **dark [l]**.

Vocalization. A phonological process in which a neutral vowel replaces a syllabic consonant; for example, *beetle* is [biʔu].

Voiced. Sound made with vocal fold vibration.

Voiceless. Sound made without vocal fold vibration.

Voicing. Vibration of the vocal folds.

Vowel. A sound made without marked constriction in the vocal tract.

Vowel neutralization. A phonological process in which a neutral vowel replaces another vowel; for example, *bat* is [bət].

Word pairs. Words that differ by a single sound; for example, *pea* and *bee* are word pairs. Word pairs that differ by one distinctive feature in one sound are called minimal pairs (e.g., [p] and [b] in *pea* and *bee*). Word pairs that differ by more than one distinctive feature in one sound are called maximal pairs (e.g., [p] and [m] in *pea* and *me*).

Word-final position. Sounds ending a word (word finally); for example, [t] in *boat* is in word-final position.

Word-initial position. Sounds beginning a word (word initially); for example, [p] in *pit* is in word-initial position.

Word-medial position. Sounds in the middle of a word (word medially); for example, [n] in *final* and [d] in *window* are in word-medial position.

References

International Clinical Phonetics and Linguistics Association. (1992). *Clinical Linguistics and Phonetics, 6,* 259–262.

Stoel-Gammon, C., & Dunn, C. (1985). *Normal and disordered phonology in children.* Austin, TX: Pro-Ed.

Topics

Places of Production

Alveolar

Bilabial

Dental

Glottal

Interdental

Labial

Labiodental

Palatal

Place of production

Postalveolar

Velar

Manners of Production

Affricate

Approximant

Central

Continuants

Fricative

Glide

Lateral

Liquid

Manner of production

Nasal stop

Nasals

Obstruent

Oral stop

Semivowels

Sibilant

Sonorants

Stop

Strident

Vowels

Close

Diphthong

Neutral vowels

Open

Open-mid

Pure vowel

R-colored vowel

Rhotic vowel

Schwa

Schwa [r]

Vowel

Names for Sounds

Capital "E"

Caret

Digraph

Epsilon

Horseshoe

Long "s"

Open "o"

Print "a"

Schwa

Schwar

Theta

Thorn

Transcription

Brackets (square brackets)

Broad transcription

Diacritics

Narrow transcription

Phone

Phoneme

Phonemic transcription

Phonetic transcription

Phonetics

Slashes

Special symbols

Abbreviations

C

CV

CVC

S

SFWF

SFWW

SIWI

SIWW

SODA

V

Speech Characteristics

Aspiration

Blends

Cognates

Consonant

Consonant cluster

Dialect

Distinctive features

Eggressive

Homonyms

Homorganic

Ingressive

Intonation

Lip rounding

Lips spread

Multisyllabic

Nasality

Primary stress

Prosody

Rounding

Singleton

Spreading

Suprasegmental

Unaspirated

Voiced

Voiceless

Voicing

Speech Environments

Ambisyllabic

Arrestor

Environments

Initial sound

Intervocalic

Medial sound

Onset

Open syllable

Phonetic environments

Postvocalic

Resyllabification

SFWF

SFWW

SIWI

SIWW

Syllable initial position

Syllable final position

Word-final position

Word-initial position

Word-medial position

Assimilations

Assimilation

Coalescence

Progressive assimilation

Regressive assimilation

Common Names for Speech Disorders

Articulation disorder

Phonological disorder

Speech sound disorder

Names for Speech Errors

Articulation error

Deletion

Distortion

Omission

Phonological error

Phonological processes

Phonological rule

Residual error

Substitution

Major Phonological Processes

Affrication

Backing

Cluster reduction

Denasalization

Epenthesis (ePENthesis)

Final consonant deletion

Final consonant devoicing

Fronting

Gliding

Glottal replacement

Initial consonant deletion

Labial assimilation

Lateralization

Metathesis (MeTAthesis)

Prevocalic voicing

Reduplication

Stopping

Syllable deletion

Velar assimilation

Vocalization

Vowel neutralization

Prespeech and Early Speech

Babble

Canonical babbling

Cooing

Intraword variability

Interword variability

Jargon

Nonreduplicated babbling

Phonetically consistent form (PCF)

Reduplicated babbling

Variegated babbling

[s], [l], and [r]

Bladed [s]

Bunched [r]

Dark [l]

Dentalized

Fricative

Frontal lisp

Gliding

Lateral

Lateral lisp

Lateral [s]

Late 8

Lateralization

Light [l]

Lip rounding

Lisping

Pharyngeal fricative

Residual error

Retroflex [r]

Velarized [l]

DIALECT AND ACCENT

This appendix lists major speech characteristics of nine of the many different varieties of English, including

- African American English (AAE)
- Spanish-influenced English
- Asian-influenced English
- Bosnian-influenced English
- Hawaiian Creole
- Russian-influenced English
- Hindi-influenced English
- Singapore Colloquial English (SCE)
- Turkish-influenced English

None of these speech variations is a speech sound disorder. However, the speech variations contain patterns that may contain speech characteristics similar to those in the speech of children with speech disorders, and so, may be confused with them. Three varieties are dialects (African American English, Hawaiian Creole, Singapore Colloquial English) and the six others are accents. When sufficient information exists, the descriptions include consonants and consonant classes, vowels, and prosody. When information is less complete, the descriptions are more abridged.

African American English (AAE)

African American English (AAE) is a variety of English spoken by many African Americans. AAE varies by region, social class, and formality of setting.

Pattern	Word	Pronunciation	AAE
Consonants			
Stops			
Coarticulated glottal stop with devoiced final stop	bad	bæd	bæt?
Devoicing of final consonants	tube	tub	tup
Deletion of final alveolar stops	pad	pæd	pæ
Nasals			
Absence of final nasal consonants	pan	pæn	pæ
Fricatives			
Word initial [d] for [ð]	they	ðe	de
Intervocalic and word final [f] for [θ] and [v] for [ð]	brother	brʌðɚ	brʌdɚ
Liquids			
Deletion of postvocalic [r] and [l]	more	mor	mo
Consonant clusters			
[k] for [t] in [str] clusters	street	strit	skrit
Final consonant simplification, especially when both members of the consonant cluster are voiced or voiceless	desk	dɛsk	dɛs
Metathesis of consonants in a cluster	ask	æsk	æks
Vowels			
The diphthongs [aɪ], [aʊ], and [ɔɪ] often neutralize to [a], [a], and [ə], respectively			
Prosody			
Absence of initial unstressed syllables	about	əbaʊt	baʊt
Stress on the first rather than the second syllable	Detroit	Detróit	Détroit
Use of wide-range of intonation contours and vowel elongations			

Pattern	Word	Pronunciation	AAE
Use of more level and falling final contours and rising contours			
Replacement of absent final consonants with nasalization or lengthening of preceding vowel	cone	kon	ko: or kõ

Spanish-Influenced English

Spanish contains 18 consonants and five vowels. Consonant clusters occur in syllable initial position and contain a stop consonant followed by either a flap or [l]. Five consonants can appear in word-final position: [l r d n s]. The following consonants exist in English, but not Spanish: [v θ ʔ h].

Pattern	Word	Pronunciation	Spanish-Influenced English
Addition	stamp	stæmp	estæmp
Affrication	she	i	ʧi
Consonant devoicing	he's	hiz	his
Nasal velarization	fan	fæn	fæŋ
Stopping	vase	ves	bes
	thought	θat	tat
	though	ðo	do

Asian-Influenced English

Asian-influenced English is an "umbrella term" for a wide variety of languages including Chinese, Japanese, and other variations from locations such as the Philippines, Korea, and southern and southeast Asia.

Pattern	Word	Pronunciation	Asian-Influenced English
Epenthesis	blue	blu	bəlu
	beak	bik	bik
Final consonant deletion	gate	get	ge
Syllable deletion	potato	potato	teto
[l] for [r]	ray	re	le
Stopping	vase	ves	bes
[ʃ] for [ʧ]	cheap	ʧip	ip

Bosnian-Influenced English

For many years, the people of Bosnia and Herzegovina have spoken the same language, Serbo-Croatian. However, after the war, each ethnic group claims to have a separate language. There are five vowels and 25 consonant phonemes in Bosnian, as well as several differences between the two languages that contribute to the "Bosnian accent."

Pattern	Word	Pronunciation	Bosnian-Influenced English
Consonants			
[v] for [w]	we	wi	vi
Stopping	these	ðiz	diz
	thought	θat	tat
Production of [ʧ], [ʤ], [ʒ] in overly hard manner	church	ʧɝʧ	ʧɝʧ
	judge	dʒʌdʒ	dʒʌdʒ
	beige	beɪʒ	beɪʒ
[r] for [ɹ]	room	ɹum	rum
Vowels			
[e] for [æ]	bag	bæg	beg
[a] for [ɑ]	arm	ɑrm	arm
[a] for [ə]	afresh	əfreʃ	afreʃ
[a] for [ʌ]	but	bʌt	bat
[o] for [ɔ]	long	lɔŋ	loŋ

Hawaiian Creole

Major characteristics of Hawaiian Creole include the following.

Pattern	Word	Pronunciation	Hawaiian Creole
Stopping of [θ] and [ð]	thought	θat	tɑt
Deletion of [r] after a vowel	more	mor	moə
Deletion of final consonants	beak	bik	bi
Backing and affrication of alveolar consonants in [r] clusters	tree	tri	ʧri

Russian-Influenced English

There are six vowels and 36 consonant phonemes in Russian. The most common vowel is /a/. The most common consonants are /t n s/; the least common consonants are /g f/. Phonemes that appear in English and do not exist in Russian are /θ ð ŋ w r/. Phonemes that appear in Russian but do not exist in English are central close unrounded /i/, trilled /r/, velar fricative /x/, and retroflex fricative /s/. In Russian, phonology, stops /t d/ as well as nasals /l n/ are pronounced as either dental or postalveolar /t' d' n' l'/.

Stress and intonation in Russian language depends on the number of words in a sentence. Typically, stress falls on every word in a sentence, except for particles and conjunctions, producing an impression of "flat" intonation as compared to American English.

Pattern	Word	Pronunciation	Russian-Influenced English
Consonants			
Fricatives			
Alveolar for dental before high and mid front vowels	this	ðɪs	zɪs or dɪs
[w] for [v]	votka	vɑtkə	wɑtkə
[v] for [w]	we	wi	vi
Velar for glottal	hello	helo	xɛlo
Stops			
Postalveolar for alveolar	trendy	trɛndi	t'rɛnd'i
Devoicing of final consonants	tube	tub	tup
Nasals			
[n] for [ŋ]	pink	pɪŋk	pink
Vowels			
[i] for [ɪ]	big	bɪg	big
Prosody			
Impression of "flat" intonation			

Hindi-Influenced English

The Indian subcontinent is home to approximately 225 languages and 845 dialects. Hindi is the national language and is spoken by the majority of people. Hindi contains 11 different vowels and 40 different consonants.

Pattern	Word	Pronunciation	Hindi-Influenced English
Consonants			
[v] pronounced as [ß]	very	vɛri	ßɛri
Stopping of interdental fricatives	thank	qæŋk	tæŋk
Retroflex production of [d]	deep	dip	dip
Deaspiration of initial stops	pen	pɛn	poɛn
Affrication	she	ʃi	ʧi
Depalatalization	show	ʃo	so
Addition	station	steʃən	isteʃən
Epenthesis	blade	bled	bəled
Metathesis	ask	æsk	æks
Vowels			
Lowering of tongue	roll	rol	rɔl
Tensing of [ɪ] and [ʊ]	rim	rɪm	rim
Use of lax vowel	gate	get	gɛt
[ɛ] for [æ]	at	æt	ɛt
Prosody			
Substitution of one vowel for another due to change in stress placement			
Intonation contours of Hindi differ from English, decreasing intelligibility			

Singapore Colloquial English (SCE)

Singapore Colloquial English (SCE) shares many similarities with Chinese in terms of its syntax and semantic and pragmatic features, which give the impression of English words embedded in Chinese sentence structures. Code switching is common in Singapore, where people frequently switch from SCE to standard English and back to SCE depending on the communication context and the parties involved in the communication. Code switching often occurs when the formality of the conversation or the communicative partner is changed, standard English being used in formal settings and SCE being used during informal, day-to-day interactions. Interlanguage switches between English, Malay, Mandarin, or other dialects also are common, usually in informal settings. These switches can occur at phrase level, where the speaker changes languages from one phrase to the next; or they can occur within the phrase, where words of another language are embedded into the phrase structure of the original language.

Pattern	Word	Pronunciation	Singapore Colloquial English
Consonants			
Initial interdental fricatives are stopped and dentalized	the	də	də
Initial voiceless consonants partially voiced and unaspirated	pan	pæn	poæn
Deletion of initial /w/ preceding /u/	woo	wu	u
/dz/ for /z/	zoo	zu	dzu
Final consonants unaspirated	fat	fæt	fæt
	bad	bæd	bæd
Final interdental fricatives are labiodentals	tooth	tuq	tuf
Final cluster reduction	don't	dont	don
Devoicing of final fricatives	ooze	uz	us
Vowels			
Vowels may be shortened	bee	bi	bɪ
Vowels may be more closed	bag	bæg	bɛg

Turkish-Influenced English

Turkish is an Indo-European language, belonging to the Altaic branch of the Ural-Altay linguistic family. The language now spoken in Turkey is accepted as standard Turkish and is the descendant of Ottoman Turkish and its predecessor, the so-called Old Anatolian Turkish. Turkish contains eight vowels and 21 consonant phonemes. Vowels are short. Turkish does not permit initial consonant clusters. Obstruents are voiceless in syllable-final position, and syllable final consonant clusters typically are sonorants + voiceless stops (examples: [rk rt nk]). The syllable final consonant clusters [nç st] may occur in borrowed words. Vowel and consonant harmony (assimilation) is a unique characteristic of Turkish and results in vowels and consonants within words sharing distinctive features. Turkish is a syllable-timed language in which syllables recur at regular intervals in words, phrases, and sentences.

Pattern	Word	Pronunciation	Turkish-Influenced English
Consonants			
Labiodentals as bilabials	vote	vot	ßot
Stopping of interdentals	this	ðɪs	dɪs
Final consonant devoicing	tube	tub	tup
Cluster reduction	steep	stip	sip or tip
	beast	bist	bis or bit
Epenthesis	blade	bled	bəled
Palatalization of [ŋ]	king	kiŋ	kiɲ
Final devoicing of syllable-final nasals	mean	min	min̥
Vowels			
Vowel shortening	bee	bi	bɪ
Prosody			
Vowel and consonant assimilations may occur			
Errors in placement of stress may result from stress-timed alternations in words, phrases, and sentences			

Index

Note: Page numbers in **bold** reference non-text material.